Bandolier's
Little Book
of Pain

Bandolier's Little Book of Pain

Andrew Moore
Jayne Edwards
Jodie Barden
Henry McQuay
Pain Research
Churchill Hospital, Oxford

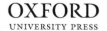

Great Clarendon Street, Oxford OX2 6DP
United Kingdom

Oxford University Press is a department of the University of Oxford.
It furthers the University's objective of excellence in research, scholarship,
and education by publishing worldwide. Oxford is a registered trade mark of
Oxford University Press in the UK and in certain other countries

Published in the United States of America by Oxford University Press
198 Madison Avenue, New York, NY 10016, United States of America

British Library Cataloguing in Publication Data
Data available

Library of Congress Cataloging in Publication Data
Data available

ISBN 978-0-19-870519-2

Contents

Section 3
Migraine and headache

Section 4
Chronic pain

Section 5
Arthritis

Section 6
Complementary and alternative therapies

Section 7
Cancer and palliative care

Introduction

Background

Holywell Manor is the graduate student part of Balliol College in Oxford. All four authors have Balliol links, and three have lived in the Manor at some time over the last 35 years. The Manor was the place this book was conceived in a series of discussions about the future of evidence-based medicine between two of us (RAM and HJM) and David Sackett and Muir Gray in the late 1990s.

There were three themes. The first was that good evidence was likely to come from good systematic reviews of good clinical trials. For all sorts of reasons, many of which are discussed in later pages, too much of the medical literature can be misleading, or is just plain wrong. The second theme was that of knowing good from bad, and having the good and useful knowledge in one place so that one could refer to it when needed. The third theme was that of the individual versus the population as a whole – because unique biology, choice and circumstance often dictate what happens, and evidence is but one part of a complex equation. Evidence-based medicine is about tools, not about rules.

Clearly what was needed was an evidence toolbox. This toolbox was more than just a filing cabinet full of papers. David Sackett's work showed that few professionals had much time for all the reading they would need to do just to keep up. We already had the proven success of Bandolier, by that time with about 25,000 paper copies a month, and a success as much because it demystified evidence and the way that results were collected. Bandolier even had a small if used Internet site.

The solution was obvious: find all the good evidence about a topic, write a short and simple abstract with some quality filters, and make sure that it can demonstrate quality in its assessments. Since pain was at the leading edge of systematic reviews and methodological development, it seemed a good idea, so we started to do it, and launched the Oxford Pain Internet Site in 1998.

The book of the Internet site

People seemed to like the Pain Internet Site, and the Bandolier Internet site has replicated it in other areas. One of the interesting things was that people started asking for all those Internet pages to be collected into a book, partly because people find it hard to read for long periods on-screen. Enough did so to make us (and Oxford

University Press) believe them, and so Bandolier's Little Book of Pain has collected much of the information on the Internet and set it to paper, with a bit of organisation.

This book is therefore a snapshot of evidence available as of mid-2002. It is supported by the Internet site (www.ebandolier.com or www.jr2.ox.ac.uk/bandolier). New material will be added to the site as new reviews are done and more good evidence becomes available. Books are hopeless places to store some forms of information. For instance, there is a list of several hundred systematic reviews with pain as an outcome on the Internet site (www.jr2.ox.ac.uk/bandolier/painres/MApain.html). These would be hopeless in a book. The two are therefore self-supporting, and it will be interesting to us to find out what readers and users think of this arrangement.

Who is the book for? An interesting question, this. The simple answer is that it is for any professional with an interest in pain, and who wants to use the best evidence available for the good of their service and their patients.

About Bandolier and pain research at Oxford

Bandolier and Pain Research live with the Oxford Pain Relief Unit based at the Churchill Hospital in Oxford. As part of the NHS the Pain Relief Unit treats over 100 patients with chronic pain a week, who come mainly from the centre of England, but also from elsewhere in the UK, and from abroad. Academically Pain Research is part of the Nuffield Department of Anaesthetics at the University of Oxford. There are some complicated relationships, though, with many of us wearing more than one hat.

The Oxford Pain Relief Trust

The Trustees of the Pain Research Trust are Dr Chris Glynn, Dr Tim Jack, Professor Henry McQuay and Dr Andrew Moore. Among them they have published around 1000 scientific articles.

This charity was established initially to raise money for the current Pain Unit building, used for both treating patients and for research. Over £850,000 was raised and the building opened in 1998. The Trust is now planning further developments, including specialist training provision for UK and overseas doctors, and support for pain-related research locally and elsewhere. A long-term goal is the creation of a permanent pain research team within the University of Oxford.

Pain research

Research is conducted under the auspices of the University of Oxford and headed by Henry McQuay, Professor of Pain Relief. Henry McQuay and Andrew Moore have been working together on pain and related topics for over 25 years. Pioneering work has taken place over the last 8 years into the development and application of evidence-based methods for research and practice. The team is internationally recognised for innovative thinking in many different areas.

PaPaS

International collaboration is an important part of our work. Housed within Pain Research is the Cochrane collaborative research group on Pain, Palliative and Supportive Care, and an International Association for the Study of Pain Special Interest Group on systematic reviews in pain. These groups are crucial to the development of global improvement in pain therapy, and in supportive and palliative care.

Bandolier

Bandolier is a bulletin about evidence-based healthcare. The first issue of Bandolier was published in February 1994. It has been produced monthly ever since. It has become the premier source of evidence-based healthcare information in the UK and worldwide. The electronic version of Bandolier was voted best NHS Internet site for 1999, and has over 500,000 visitors every month from all over the world. While many are health professionals, this is also a source of high quality information for many patients and their carers, as well as for organisations who commission and pay for healthcare.

People we want to thank

In the book are lots of systematic reviews, and in the reviews lots of trials. All of us are indebted to the hundreds of thousands of patients who agreed to participate in randomised trials. We should also be grateful to the thousands of researchers who undertook those trials, and the hundreds of reviewers for pulling them all together.

The BUPA Foundation, The Gwen Bush Foundation, and Merck, Sharp and Dohme Ltd have all supported the creation of Internet pain material that finds its way into this book. They have all been very brave, because we only accept sponsorship if there is absolutely no control from the sponsoring body over what we write.

There are also many people to thank. Martin Baum at OUP has been incredibly patient with us as we have amended our thinking. That we eventually got fingers to keyboard was due to the organisational ability and project management skills of Maureen McQuay. The development of the Internet site owes much to the way that Anna Oldman originally set it up, with considerable help from Lesley Smith and Jayne Edwards. Between them, they brought the pain, migraine and complementary therapy pages to life.

Many people have worked with us over the years and helped shape our thoughts, or just helped shape our thoughts, including Dawn Carroll, Ed Charlton, Sally Collins, David Gavaghan, Geoff Gourlay, Alex Jadad, Eija Kalso, John Reynolds, Kate Seers, Martin Tramèr, Phil Wiffen, and all the people who contributed to the ICECAP meeting in

Alicante in September 2001.

Chris Glynn and Tim Jack, our clinical colleagues, are always useful sounding boards, and the nurses on the Pain Relief Unit helped us broaden our thinking. Maura Moore and Carole Newton provided much organisational support. Our old mentor, John Lloyd, helped set us on the quest for greater understanding and better treatments.

Andrew Moore   Jayne Edwards
Jodie Barden   Henry McQuay
Pain Research
The Churchill Hospital, Oxford
January 2003

Section 1
Understanding EBM

1.1 **Pain – there's a lot of it about**

Pain relief has been a major medical interest since Sumerian times 6000 years ago, when poppy juice was first used. Yet there is still a lot of pain about, it is a source of great disability, it detracts from the quality of life, and is often poorly treated. What is needed is more (and perhaps different) research, a concentration on evidence of what works and what does not, and education and dissemination of knowledge to make better use of what we have now.

What is not likely is a magic bullet of a treatment that cures all pain without doing any harm. What we have is actually quite effective. The problem is that while the best pain relief can be very good indeed, all too often the best is not attained. Reasons are often simple, and have nothing to do with complicated science.

To get the best we need an overview of everything from the best bench science to how best to give the tablets. That is the goal of the Oxford Pain Relief Trust. The following paragraphs illustrate some of the problems, and suggest some solutions.

Chronic non-malignant pain

A study carried out in Scotland examined chronic pain in the community [1]. About 5000 questionnaires were sent to people and four out of five replied. The definition of chronic pain used was 'pain or discomfort, that persisted continuously or intermittently for longer than three months'.

Half of the respondents reported having chronic pain. This increased with age in women and men from about one-third of those aged 25–34 to almost two-thirds in those older than 65 years (Figure 1.1.1).

What pains and when?

The two most common reasons for chronic pain were back pain, which varied little with age, and arthritis, which rose dramatically with age to afflict a quarter of people in their 60s or older. Angina was also more common in older age groups. A brief summary of a review of chronic pain prevalence [2] gives more detail on how common different non-malignant pains are (Table 1.1.1). Studies included were full journal publications, studied adult community or clinic-based populations in Europe or North America, used clear and established diagnostic criteria for disease/pain conditions of interest, presented prevalence and/or incidence data for the disease/pain condition of interest and reported survey/study response rates.

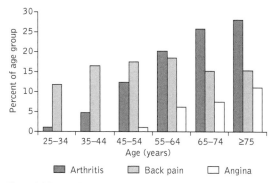

Figure 1.1.1 Pain is more common in older people.

While not all of the persons affected will necessarily seek help from their GP, or be referred on to secondary or even tertiary care, it is clear that even within this limited selection that primary care organisations will have large numbers of patients with chronic pain. In general, as the population ages, the problem will increase in magnitude, or will already be a bigger problem where there are large retirement populations.

And its not just chronic pain. Large surveys in hospitals show us that about a third of surgical or medical inpatients have pain present all or most of the time, the pain is often severe, and many have to ask for treatments which often take time to arrive [3].

Chronic pain causes real problems

In Scotland the severity of chronic pain was measured and the disability it caused. A quarter of people with chronic pain had pain that was highly disabling and at least moderately limiting. A further quarter had pain that was of high intensity, and all of this despite treatment (Table 1.1.2).

Many pain days

Even simple back of envelope calculations demonstrate that the number of days someone has pain is large. If even 10% of the population had pain every day (likely from the Scottish survey and others), then there would be over 2 billion days of pain in the UK. That is 30–40 days of pain for every one of us!

Impact of pain on quality of life

In Holland research has shed light on how chronic diseases affect quality of life [4]. Eight large data sets were found and analysed by quality of life factors. Ranking different conditions showed that

Table 1.1.1 Common non-malignant chronic pain conditions

Condition	Comments	Prevalence per 100,000	Incidence per 100,000
Musculoskeletal pain			
Back pain	For self-reported low back pain in the community 6% of the population reported pain persisting for at least a year and 3% were still unable to work a year later. In a UK primary care organisation population of 100,000 people there might be as many as several thousand with back pain that is disabling and limiting	Several thousand	
Neck pain	Significantly disabling chronic neck pain	About 5000	
Fibromyalgia	Severe chronic widespread pain defined as fibromyalgia by current criteria	200–1000	
Polymyalgia rheumatica		500	50
Face or head pain			
Migraine	Using International Headache Society criteria. Only about one patient in six seeks help from a doctor.	10,000 women	
Chronic tension headache	Using International Headache Society criteria 1000–3000	2000 men	10
Trigeminal neuralgia	First episode for incidence	100	2–5
Neuropathic pain			
Diabetic neuropathy	Sensory neuropathy occurs in about 15% of diabetics, and painful neuropathy in about 10%–25%	200–500	
Postherpetic neuralgia	Postherpetic neuralgia occurs in 13–26% of patients with zoster (340/100,000 per year with zoster infection), and is more common in over 60s	50–150	34
Multiple sclerosis	MS has crude prevalence of 100/100,000 in England, and about twice that in Scotland. Pain occurs in about half of patients	50	
Vascular pain			
Intermittent claudication	Higher rates in older people	400–800	200
Angina	About a third of prevalent cases severe	4000	500
Chronic postoperative pain			
Phantom limb pain	Post amputation, phantom and/or stump pain		
Pain after operation	After breast surgery, or thoracotomy, or cholecystecomy chronic pain at or near wound site is relatively common, affecting up to 25% of patients	25	

Table 1.1.2 Pain, its intensity and how it affects daily living

Description of pain and its effects	Percent of people with chronic pain
Low disability/low intensity	49
Low disability/high intensity	24
High disability/moderately limiting	11
High disability/severely limiting	16

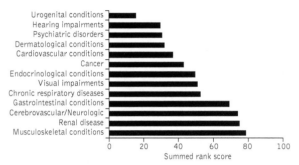

Figure 1.1.2 High scores show greater negative effects on the quality of life.

musculoskeletal conditions (including arthritis and back pain), renal disease, cerebrovascular/neurological conditions and gastrointestinal conditions impacted most severely on quality of life. This impact of everyday pain on quality of life is something that has yet to be fully appreciated perhaps by those who organise our health services and allocate resources (Figure 1.1.2).

Acute pain

An audit of patients in hospital [5] has shown that as many as 87% of patients (medical and surgical) said that they experienced pain of moderate or severe intensity at some time (Table 1.1.3). One of the problems was that for many, even though they asked for treatment for their pain, it did not arrive immediately. Acute pain, where there is a large number of possible treatments of known efficacy, effectiveness may be hampered by the inability of a service to deliver efficacious interventions.

How to make things better

No one thing will accomplish this. We need more and better basic research, the most tangible products of which are likely to come from

Table 1.1.3 Audit of acute pain in hospital

Pain description	Number/total	Percent
Pain was present all or most of the time	1042/3162	33
Pain was severe or moderate	2755/3157	87
Pain was worse than expected	182/1051	17
Had to ask for drugs	1085/2589	42
Drugs did not arrive immediately	455/1085	41

the major pharmaceutical companies. But experience is that wonderful new and effective treatments are rare beasts.

Clinical research and practice are much more likely to make a difference now, helping to make existing evidence sensible and understandable so that people can use it. Examples are the league tables of relative effectiveness of treatments for acute pain and migraine. These do not dictate what analgesic to use for a particular patient, but they can help in making choices about treatments based on their effectiveness, their propensity for harm, and their cost.

Then there's education and dissemination. This is the process of getting the information out to the real world – Grimsby on a wet Tuesday afternoon, rather than the dreaming spires of Oxford on a sunny summer day. We hope and expect that some of the things we do in research and dissemination will help make that come about.

References

1. Elliott, A. M. *et al.* (1999). The epidemiology of chronic pain in the community, *Lancet* 354: 1248–52.
2. McQuay, H. J. *et al.* (in press). Chronic non-malignant pain, *Health Care Needs Assessment*.
3. Bruster, S. *et al.* (1994). National survey of hospital patients, *BMJ* 309: 1542–6.
4. Sprangers, M. A. G. *et al.* (2000). Which chronic conditions are associated with a better or poorer quality of life? *Journal of Clinical Epidemiology* 53: 895–907.
5. Bruster, S. *et al.* (1994). National survey of hospital patients, *BMJ* 309: 1542–1546.

1.2 **Measuring pain**

Pain is a personal experience which makes it difficult to define and measure. It includes both the sensory input and any modulation by physiological, psychological and environmental factors. Not surprisingly there are no objective measures – there is no way to measure pain directly by sampling blood or urine or by performing neurophysiological tests. Measurement of pain must therefore rely on recording the patient's report. The assumption is often made that because the measurement is subjective it must be of little value. The reality is that if the measurements are done properly, remarkably sensitive and consistent results can be obtained. There are contexts, however, when it is not possible to measure pain at all, or when reports are likely to be unreliable. These include impaired consciousness, young children, psychiatric pathology, severe anxiety, unwillingness to co-operate, and inability to understand the measurements. Such problems are deliberately avoided in trials.

Measurement scales

Anyone who spends a few hours reading research papers on pain will soon be mystified by the incredible number of measurement scales that have been used. It is probable that at least several hundred measurement methods have been used (Alex Jadad, personal communication). Only for very few will there have been any attempt to discuss systematically with patients what constitutes a worthwhile change. Despite this there are some commonly used measurement methods, some available for decades, that have proved to be reliable.

Acute pain

Most acute pain analgesic studies include measurements of pain intensity and/or pain relief, and the commonest tools used are categorical and visual analogue scales.

Categorical and visual analogue scales. Categorical scales use words to describe the magnitude of the pain (Figure 1.2.1). They were the earliest pain measure [1]. The patient picks the most appropriate word. Most research groups use four words (none, mild, moderate and severe). Scales to measure pain relief were developed later. The commonest is the five category scale (none, slight, moderate, good or lots, and complete).

For analysis numbers are given to the verbal categories (for pain intensity, none = 0, mild = 1, moderate = 2 and severe = 3, and for relief none = 0, slight = 1, moderate = 2, good or lots = 3 and

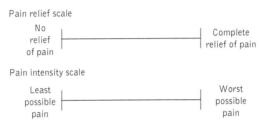

Figure 1.2.1 Categorical pain scale.

Pain relief scale

No relief of pain ├─────────────────┤ Complete relief of pain

Pain intensity scale

Least possible pain ├─────────────────┤ Worst possible pain

Figure 1.2.2 Visual analogue scales.

complete = 4). Data from different subjects is then combined to produce means (rarely medians) and measures of dispersion (usually standard errors of means). The validity of converting categories into numerical scores was checked by comparison with concurrent visual analogue scale measurements. Good correlation was found, especially between pain relief scales using cross-modality matching techniques [2,3]. Results are usually reported as continuous data, mean or median pain relief or intensity. Few studies present results as discrete data, giving the number of participants who report a certain level of pain intensity or relief at any given assessment point. The main advantages of the categorical scales are that they are quick and simple. The small number of descriptors may force the scorer to choose a particular category when none describes the pain satisfactorily.

Visual analogue scales (VAS), lines with left end labelled 'no relief of pain' and right end labelled 'complete relief of pain', seem to overcome this limitation (Figure 1.2.2). Patients mark the line at the point corresponding to their pain. The scores are obtained by measuring the distance between the no relief end and the patient's mark, usually in millimetres. The main advantages of VAS are that they are simple and quick to score, avoid imprecise descriptive terms, and provide many points from which to choose. More concentration and coordination are needed, which can be difficult postoperatively or with neurological disorders.

Pain relief scales are perceived as more convenient than pain intensity scales, probably because patients have the same baseline relief (zero) whereas they could start with different baseline intensity (usually moderate or severe). Relief scale results are then easier to compare. They may also be more sensitive than intensity scales. A theoretical drawback of relief scales is that the patient has to remember what the pain was like to begin with.

Other tools. Verbal numerical scales and global subjective efficacy ratings are also used. Verbal numerical scales are regarded as an alternative or complementary to the categorical and VAS scales. Patients give a number to the pain intensity or relief (for pain intensity 0 usually represents no pain and 10 the maximum possible, and for pain relief 0 represents none and 10 complete relief). They are very easy and quick to use, and correlate well with conventional VAS [4].

Global subjective efficacy ratings, or simply global scales, are designed to measure overall treatment performance. Patients are asked questions like 'How effective do you think the treatment was?' and answer using a labelled numerical or a categorical scale. Although these judgements probably include adverse effects they can be the most sensitive discriminant between treatments. One of the oldest scales was the binary question 'Is your pain half gone?' Its advantage is that it has a clearer clinical meaning than a 10 mm shift on a VAS. The disadvantage, for the small trial intensive measure pundits at least, is that all the potential intermediate information (1–49% or how much greater than 50%) is discarded.

Analgesic requirements (including patient-controlled analgesia, PCA), special paediatric scales, and questionnaires like the McGill are also used. The limitation to guard against is that they usually reflect other experiences as well as or instead of pain [5].

Judgement of the patient rather than by the carer is the ideal. Carers overestimate the pain relief compared with the patient's version.

Analysis of scale results – summary measures

In the research context pain is usually assessed before the intervention is made and then on multiple occasions. Ideally the area under the time-analgesic effect curve for the intensity (sum of pain intensity differences; SPID) or relief (total pain relief; TOTPAR) measures is derived (Figure 1.2.3). TOTPAR, for example, is measured by calculating the area under the curve for pain relief against time. If a patient had complete pain relief immediately, and sustained it for the full 6 h of measurement, then the maximum TOTPAR would be attained (in this case a score of 4 points times 6 h, giving a TOTPAR of 24, the maximum achievable). Another patient who had a score of 12 would have 50% of the maximum, or 50%maxTOTPAR (Figure 1.2.3).

These summary measures reflect the cumulative response to the intervention. Their disadvantage is that they do not provide information about the onset and peak of the analgesic effect. If onset or peak are important then time to maximum pain relief (or reduction in pain intensity) or time for pain to return to baseline are necessary.

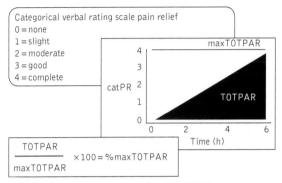

Figure 1.2.3 Calculating TOTPAR and %maxTOTPAR.

Migraine

People with migraines have a whole range of symptoms. Pain is perhaps the most obvious, but many are nauseated and may have other associated symptoms like photophobia or phonophobia. This page describes some of the outcomes measured in clinical trials, and that might be expected to be reported in trials and collected in systematic reviews.

Pain. Pain is usually measured using a simple scale, in which sufferers describe it as no pain, mild pain, moderate pain, or severe pain. Pain has to be moderate or severe before a treatment is taken in clinical trials, and the reason is that if there is no pain, or the pain is only mild, the effectiveness of treatments in taking away the pain cannot be measured.

These scales have proved highly robust in clinical trials in acute and chronic pain over decades. Pain is measured before a treatment is taken, and then at 0.5, 1, 1.5, 2 h, and possibly longer, though after 2 h the relevance declines because headaches get better by themselves.

The two outcomes most often reported and used are described below.

Headache response. This is when pain which is initially moderate or severe becomes mild, or where there is no pain. This can be measured at any time, but usually the 2-h response is taken (Figure 1.2.4).

Pain free. This is when pain which is initially moderate or severe becomes no pain. This can be measured at any time, but usually the 2-h response is taken (Figure 1.2.4).

Sustained response. Patients who have a headache response at 2 h have headache that becomes no worse, and take no other headache medicine over the period of 2–24 h (Figure 1.2.5).

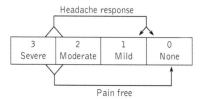

Pain free at 2h is now the preferred IHS
primary endpoint for clinical trials

Figure 1.2.4 Headache response and pain free at 2 h. IHS is an abbreviation for International Headache Society.

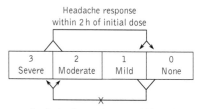

Figure 1.2.5 Sustained headache response and pain free.

Sustained pain free. Patients who are pain free at 2 h, have no recurrence of headache, and take no other headache medicine over the period of 2–24 h (Figure 1.2.5).

Other outcomes. Symptoms associated with migraine are nausea, photophobia or phonophobia. Not every patient with migraine has some, or all, of these associated symptoms. The number or proportion of patients who have these symptoms initially, but where the symptoms are completely relieved by (say) 2 h, are important outcomes.

Functional disability is measured on a 4 point scale, from grade 0 where there is no functional disability to grade 3 where patients are restricted to bed. The number or proportion of patients who have some functional disability initially, but where there is no disability at (say) 2 h, is an important outcome.

Clearly other outcomes could be measured, and sometimes are, but these are the main ones used in clinical trials.

Chronic pain

This is a much more difficult area because, unlike acute pain and migraine trials, pain measurement has not been subject to standardisation. Indeed, standardisation may not even be possible across all chronic pain conditions. What patients might want is to be pain free without any adverse effects, but this is rarely achievable. More often it is a balance of pain relief against the bearability of adverse effects that is sought, often by a process of titration.

What we often get in clinical trials reporting on chronic pain is some form of outcome that approximates to patients achieving some level of pain relief, or some degree of global improvement.

One of the most commonly used chronic pain measurement tools is the McGill Pain Questionnaire, either in its long or short form [6]. In this the patient is asked to describe their pain using a number of criteria, using words that describe the sensory and affective qualities, and using evaluative words that describe the overall intensity of the total pain experience.

In arthritic pain a series of different measures of pain have been used. Most recent studies use the Western Ontario and McMaster Universities Osteoarthritis Index visual analogue scales (WOMAC), which have a number of patient and physician scoring elements [7]. Most commonly reported is a visual analogue scale for pain walking on a flat surface, but other domains include pain at rest, for instance. In rheumatoid arthritis pain scales can be used with other measures, like the number of painful or swollen joints, or surrogate measures like grip strength.

In all chronic and acute pain there will be psychological and functional overtones. Though not strictly pain measurements, these are incredibly important if hard for ordinary folk. Fortunately they are now being examined systematically and explained well [8].

Comment

There will always be circumstances where pain measurement is difficult. Examples are where communication is difficult in adults through language or illness, and particularly in children, though measures are being improved [9].

The bewildering array of pain measures should not obscure some very obvious things.

First, in most circumstances patients know best. Ask the patient about their pain and do not jump to conclusions. Someone who can stand having teeth drilled without local anaesthetic can be an agonised wretch with a hand in ice-cold water for just a few seconds. Some people just do not need analgesics after surgery. Every study of postoperative opioid consumption using PCA demonstrates wild inter-patient differences.

Second, measuring pain is a key to treating it. Pain measurement is not just for clinical research, nor even for audit. It should be something done regularly, like taking a temperature, or measuring blood pressure.

References

1. Keele, K. D. (1948). The pain chart, *Lancet* 2: 6–8.
2. Scott, J. and Huskisson, E. C. (1976). Graphic representation of pain, *Pain* 2: 175–84.
3. Wallenstein, S. L. *et al.* (1980). Clinical evaluation of mild analgesics: The measurement of clinical pain, *British Journal of Clinical Pharmacology* 10: 319S–327S.
4. Murphy, D. F. *et al.* (1988). Measurement of pain: a comparison of the visual analogue with a nonvisual analogue scale, *Clinical Journal of Pain* 3: 197–9.
5. Jadad, A. R. and McQuay, H. J. (1993). The measurement of pain. In: Pynsent, P., Fairbank, J., Carr, A. (eds), *Outcome Measures in Orthopaedics*, Butterworth Heinemann, Oxford, pp. 16–29.
6. Melzack, R. and Katz, K. (1999). Pain measurement in persons in pain. In: Wall, E. D. and Melzack, R. (eds), *Textbook of pain*, (4th edn.) Churchill Livingstone, Edinburgh, pp. 409–26.
7. Bellamy, N. *et al.* (1988). Validation and study of WOMAC, *Journal of Rheumatology* 15: 1833–40.
8. de C Williams, A. C. (1999). Measures of function and psychology. In: Wall, E. D. and Melzack, R. (eds), *Textbook of pain* (4th edn.) Churchill Livingstone, Edinburgh, pp. 427–44.
9. McGrath, P. J. and Unruh, A. M. (1999). Measurement and assessment of paediatric pain. In: Wall, E. D. and Melzack, R. (eds), *Textbook of pain* (4th edn.) Churchill Livingstone, Edinburgh, pp. 371–84.

1.3 **Outcomes**

Outcomes and measurement are closely related one to another, so closely related in fact that taking them as separate sections requires some explanation. There are several dictionary definitions for outcome: 'the issue; consequence; result'. The result of a trial or review is not necessarily the issue that interests us.

Robert Macnamara once said, in another context, that we must stop making what is measurable important, and find ways to make the important measurable. Gertrude Stein is supposed to have said in the 1920 that for a difference to *be* a difference it has to *make* a difference. Once we take messages like this on board, then what we might regard as an outcome may be completely different from the result of a trial, or what the researchers have actually measured. We need to think differently.

Who is involved?

For a start there are a number of different people or organisations who can have different ideas about the relative value of different outcomes.

1. The patient probably just wants the pain to go away, or not come back, at minimal cost in adverse effects or inconvenience.

2. Professionals probably want the same, but in addition will have in mind how difficult it may be to achieve this goal. There will be issues of training and expertise, or number of available clinic visits, or known or suspected dangers from treatments for other co-morbid conditions, or age or ethnicity.

3. Providers will have the same concerns as professionals, but overlain by concerns about costs, or resources or other services needed like diagnostic tests or imaging, or staff and beds.

However it is looked at, the issue of outcomes is more than just some bald result of a clinical trial. But the results of clinical trials have to be examined to see what outcomes might usefully be obtained, especially when systematic reviews or meta-analyses are being performed. Reviewers have particular responsibility for extracting useful outcomes.

Acute pain outcomes

In acute pain trials, analgesic information is most often reported using some form of pain intensity or pain relief scale. These scales may be used to produce several forms of outcome, some of which include:

1. Peak pain relief: Usually a time curve of pain relief (or pain intensity difference) is plotted, and the time of the peak mean relief reported. This should not be confused with the mean time to peak relief calculated from all the individual times of peak relief.

2. Number of patients with pain half gone (at least 50% pain relief).

3. Summed pain intensity difference (SPID): This is the summed differences between initial pain intensity and pain intensity at time points after the intervention (area under the pain intensity difference-time curve). SPID is complicated by the fact that numerical scores are higher for severe pain (3) than moderate pain (2). Differences between groups might in some circumstances be explained by different proportions of patients with baseline moderate or severe pain.

4. VASSPID: This is the visual analogue equivalent of SPID.

5. Total pain relief (TOTPAR): the area under the curve for pain relief against time. Since all patients have an initial pain relief of zero, the problems found with SPID are not encountered.

6. VASTOTPAR: The visual analogue equivalent of TOTPAR. [Note that SPID and TOTPAR are usually measured over 4 or 6 h, but 2 h or 8 h equivalents are not uncommon.]

7. The number or proportion of patients with at least half pain relief (at least 50% maxTOTPAR). This is commonly used in meta-analysis of 4 and 6 h acute pain studies using standard methods and used to calculate a number needed to treat. This outcome dichotomises continuous information, and useful information (like 49% of maximum pain relief) can be lost. There are reasons (section 1.7) why this is a very useful outcome, however.

8. Number or proportion of patients with good or excellent results using patient (or sometimes physician) global estimate.

9. Time to first (or next) analgesia. Sometimes given as a mean or median, sometimes as a survival curve, and sometimes as the number of patients remedicating at particular times.

10. Analgesic consumption, either by tablets or PCA.

There are probably many more outcomes. The quality of each can vary. For instance, when calculating SPID, patients requesting additional analgesia usually have their pain intensity taken as the original pain intensity, and their pain relief as zero. Some researchers use the 'last observation carried forward' method. Few researchers tell us which method they have actually used. The result can be a degree of uncertainty about whether like is always being compared with like.

The utility of each is interesting to contemplate, and much depends on the questions being asked in an individual trial or in a review.

Perhaps one of the more useful, if less often reported, outcomes, is time to remedication, as in the context of clinical trials this is driven by the patient not the system. An example of how this outcome can be used can be seen in Figure 1.3.1, where available information for placebo and some common analgesics is shown. By about 2 h half the patients given placebo need another analgesic, and over 90% do so by

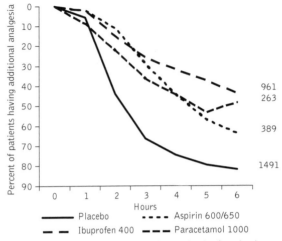

Figure 1.3.1 Proportion of patients needing analgesic after placebo, aspirin 600/650 mg, ibuprofen 400 mg and paracetamol 1000 mg (from an unpublished systematic review of randomised double-blind trials). Numbers at right indicate number of patients given each treatment.

6 h. Paracetamol, aspirin and ibuprofen all generate less need for additional analgesia, so that with ibuprofen 400 mg only about 40% of the patients need additional analgesia by 6 h.

When we have seen (section 1.1) that delivery of analgesic is a major problem for treating acute pain in hospital, this sort of information might prove particularly useful for nurses and doctors organising acute pain services. This sort of information is actually quite useful for patients as well, and particularly useful for professionals in training.

The point here is not to sell this outcome over any other, but to indicate that different outcomes are reported, and that different outcomes can be used in different ways.

Migraine

For migraine we have at least some idea of what it is that patients want from therapy. Representative American households were identified by random digit survey in 1998. About 5100 were contacted by telephone using a computer-assisted interview to identify people with migraine according to IHS criteria [1]. There were 688 individuals identified as having migraine in the past year, a prevalence of 18% in women and 6% in men. About a third had never consulted a doctor.

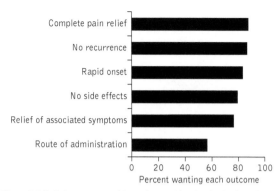

Figure 1.3.2 Outcomes wanted by patients with migraine in the USA.

Patients with migraine want the headache to go away now, completely, and not come back (Figure 1.3.2). They also want any associated symptoms, like nausea, to be relieved also. The bulk of them want a tablet or rapidly dissolving tablet, and are not impressed by subcutaneous or intranasal delivery systems. Fortunately the measurements in clinical trials of migraine (section 1.2), especially those over 24 h, go a long way to providing answers for these outcomes.

Chronic pain

In chronic pain a number of different outcomes are used. Often this will be the number or proportion of patients having what is deemed a useful reduction in their pain, or degree of pain relief. In trials and systematic reviews figures like 25%, 50% and even 75% pain relief have been used.

In 144 arthritis trials of non-steroidal anti-inflammatory drugs (NSAIDs) the number of outcomes commonly used in arthritis research that are measured on ordinal or interval scales, and therefore potentially useful for meta-analysis (global evaluation, pain, number of tender joints and grip strength) was examined [2]. Optimal outcomes were reported on the original ordered categories (number in each category), and usable required information on patients in two or more ordered categories. The main results are shown in Table 1.3.1. Global evaluation, pain, joint count and grip strength were used in most of the trials, but reported in a useful way in few.

In rheumatoid arthritis a primary or major outcome is often the percentage of patients responding to American College of Rheumatology 20 criteria. These are a 20% improvement in tender and swollen joint counts and 20% improvement in three of five remaining core measures. Not an easy outcome to understand or explain, this.

Table 1.3.1 Reporting outcomes in arthritis trials

	Global evaluation	Pain	Joint count	Grip strength
Number of trials	127	98	123	124
Percent optimal	41	28	33	27
Percent usable	69	48	40	33

Comment

When it comes to outcomes reported by individual trials and by systematic reviews, we need to be sure that the outcomes being reported are important for us, and that we can understand and use them. Often this is difficult. One of the big holes in pain research, and in clinical research in general, is work with patients, carers (professional and lay) and providers, about what constitutes a useful outcome and why. We can put all the effort we like into clinical trials and systematic reviews, but if we have no idea of the *human* importance of the result, we might begin to ask why we bother.

References

1. Headache Classification Committee of the International Headache Society (1988). Classification and diagnostic criteria for headache disorders, cranial neuralgias and facial pain, *Cephalalgia* 8 (Suppl 7): 19–28.
2. Gøtzsche, P. C. (2001). Reporting of outcomes in arthritis trials measured on ordinal and interval scales is inadequate in relation to meta-analysis, *Annals of Rheumatic Disease* 60: 349–52.

1.4 **Clinical trial methods**

If trials are not done properly, any results they produce will be worthless. We call this validity. What constitutes a valid trial depends on many factors, and so there are no absolute hard and fast rules that can cover every clinical eventuality. But for pain, we can make some important observations about what to look for in a valid clinical trial.

Randomisation

We randomise trials to exclude selection bias. Trials are usually performed where there is uncertainty as to whether a treatment works (is better than no treatment or placebo), or whether one treatment is better than another. We start from a position of intellectual equipoise. But trials are often done by believers, and belief, even subconscious belief, might influence our choice of patients to have one treatment or another if we could choose. To avoid this, and to ensure that the two groups of patients are identical, we make the choice randomly. This might be by tossing a coin, or more often by computer-generated randomisation. If we do not randomise we can end up with groups that are not the same, thus invalidating the trial, or with a trial that no one will believe because trials that are not randomised are often shown to be wrong (see later). Randomisation is essential in almost all cases.

Blinding

We conduct trials blind to minimise observer bias. It's belief again. Because, even if randomised, if we know that Mrs Jones has treatment A and Mr Smith treatment B, our observations may be biased by our belief that Mr Smith overstates his complaint and Mrs Jones understates hers. Only if we have no idea which treatment they received will we be free from a bias that is known to deliver incorrect results (again, see later). Blinding is essential in almost all cases.

Initial pain intensity

In the absence of pain, how do you measure the effect of an analgesic? With difficulty, of course. So, especially in acute pain, patients have to have pain of at least moderate intensity before they can be given a test intervention. Figure 1.4.1 shows what happened to 410 patients having minor orthopaedic surgery that lasted about 20 min [1].

A trained nursing sister was with them so that when pain was of at least moderate intensity they could enter a clinical trial. Most of them needed an analgesic by about 3 h, but some did not need analgesia until 12 h or more had elapsed, and 23 (6%) did not need any analgesia at all.

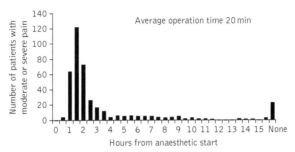

Figure 1.4.1 Requirement for analgesia after minor orthopaedic surgery.

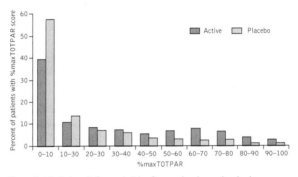

Figure 1.4.2 Pain relief over 4–6 h after analgesic or placebo in over 4000 patients.

Placebo

People in pain respond to placebo treatment. Some patients given placebo obtain 100% pain relief (Figure 1.4.2), and others get none [2]. Some people having treatment get 100% pain relief, and others get none. We cannot predict who will get what degree of analgesia, so in many cases to show that an intervention is effective we have to use patients given placebo.

There is no ethical problem, or at least should not be. In acute pain studies patients are allowed to use additional analgesia after some period, usually 60–90 min, after which time their pain scores revert to the initial value and their pain relief scores revert to zero. In chronic pain studies additional analgesic use is also permitted, and additional analgesic use is often a secondary outcome in trials.

One important point about Figure 1.4.2 is that the distribution is not normal. This is no bell-shaped curve, but is highly skewed. Despite this, many outcomes like SPID and TOTPAR are reported as means with standard deviations or standard errors. Unless we know that the distribution of data is normal, and especially where we know, like here, that there the distribution is well away from normal, we should treat outcomes reported as means with some caution.

Sensitivity

Particularly for a new analgesic, a trial should prove its internal sensitivity – that is that the study was an adequate analgesic assay. This can be done in several ways. For instance, if a known analgesic (paracetamol) can be shown to have statistical difference from placebo, then the analgesic assay should be able to distinguish another analgesic of similar effectiveness. Alternatively, two different doses of a standard analgesic (e.g. morphine) could be used – showing the higher dose to be statistically superior to the lower dose again provides confidence that the assay is sensitive. Failure to demonstrate sensitivity in one assay invalidates the results from that particular assay. The results could still be included in meta-analysis, however.

Equivalence

Studies of analgesics of an A versus B design are notoriously difficult to interpret, but we have guidance of what to expect from equivalence trials, and have useful guides about what features of equivalence trials are important in determining their validity [3]. The intellectual problem with equivalence (A versus B) trials is that the same result is consistent with three conclusions:

- both A and B are equally effective;
- both A and B are equally ineffective;
- trials inadequate to detect differences between A and B.

To combat the problems posed by the latter two conclusions, McAlister and Sackett [3] suggest several criteria in addition to those used for superiority trials (A and/or B versus placebo). These are shown in Table 1.4.1.

Control shown previously to be effective?

Ideally documented in a systematic review of placebo-controlled trials with benefits exceeding a clinically important effect. Without this information both may be equally ineffective.

Patients and outcomes similar to original trials?

Obvious, this one. If they are not, then any conclusion about equivalence is doomed. Beware, though, trials designed to show equivalent efficacy being used to demonstrate differences in harm or toxicity, for which they were not powered.

Table 1.4.1 Criteria for validity in superiority and active-control equivalence trials

Superiority trials	Active-control equivalence trials
Randomised allocation	Randomised allocation
Randomisation concealed	Randomisation concealed
All patients randomised accounted for	All patients randomised accounted for
Intention to treat analysis	Intention to treat analysis *on-treatment analysis*
Clinicians and patients blinded to treatment received	Clinicians and patients blinded to treatment received
Groups treated equally	Groups treated equally
Groups identical at baseline	Groups identical at baseline
Clinically important outcomes	Clinically important outcomes Active control previously shown to be effective Patients and outcomes similar to trials previously showing efficacy Both regimens applied in an optimal fashion Appropriate null hypothesis tested Equivalence margin pre-specified
Trial of sufficient size	Trial of sufficient size

Regimens applied in identical fashion?

The most common example is that of choosing the best dose of A versus an ineffective dose of B (no names, no pack drill, but no prizes for picking out numerous examples especially from pharmaceutical company sponsored trials showing 'our drug is better than yours'). Should be OK if licensed doses are chosen.

Other pitfalls to look out for are low compliance or frequent treatment changes, incomplete follow up, disproportionate use of cointerventions and lack of blinding.

Appropriate statistical analysis?

Equivalence trials are designed to rule out meaningful differences between two treatments. Often one-sided tests of difference are used. Lack of significant superiority is not necessarily the same as defining an appropriate level of equivalence and testing for it.

Intention to treat analysis confers the risk of making a false-negative conclusion that treatments have the same efficacy when they do not. In equivalence trials the conservative approach may be to compare patients actually on treatment. Both analyses should probably be used.

Prespecified equivalence margin?

How different is different? Equivalence trials should have a prior definition of how big a difference is a difference, and justify it. Even more than that, they have to convince you that the lack of that difference means that treatments would, in fact, be equivalent.

Size?

Most equivalence trials do not have enough power to detect even a 50% difference between treatments, and a 1994 review [4] found that 84% were too small to detect a 25% difference. Size is everything when we want to show no difference, and the smaller the difference that is important, the larger the trial has to be.

When can we say that drugs have a 'class effect'?

Class (noun): '*any set of people or things grouped together or differentiated from others*'. An increasingly asked question is that whether a set of drugs forms a class, and whether there is a 'class effect'. Class effect is usually taken to mean similar therapeutic effects and similar adverse effects, both in nature and extent. If such a 'class effect' exists, then it makes decision-making easy: you choose the cheapest.

Criteria for drugs to be grouped together as a class involve some or all of the following:

- drugs with similar chemical structure;
- drugs with similar mechanism of action;
- drugs with similar pharmacological effects.

Declaring a class effect requires a bit of thought, though. How much thought, and of what type, has been considered in one of that brilliant JAMA series on users guides to the medical literature [5]. No one should declare a class effect and choose the cheapest without reference to the rules of evidence set out in this section.

Levels of evidence for efficacy

These are shown in Table 1.4.2, though if it comes down to levels 3 and 4 evidence for efficacy, the ground is pretty shaky. Level 1 evidence is what we always want and almost always never get, the large randomised head to head comparison. By the time there are enough compounds around to form a class, there is almost no organisation interested in funding expensive, new, trials to test whether A is truly better than B.

Most of the time we will be dealing with randomised trials of A versus placebo or standard treatment and B versus placebo or standard treatment. This will be level 2 evidence based on clinically important outcomes (a healing event) or validated surrogate outcomes (reduction of cholesterol with a statin). So establishing a class effect will likely involve quality systematic review or meta-analysis of quality randomised trials.

What constitutes quality in general is captured in Table 1.4.2, though there will be some situation dependent factors. The one thing missing from consideration in Table 1.4.2 is size. There probably needs to be some prior estimate of how many patients or events constitutes a reasonable number for analysis.

Table 1.4.2 Levels of evidence for efficacy for class effect

Level	Comparison	Patients	Outcomes	Criteria for validity
1	RCT direct comparison	Identical	Clinically important	Randomisation concealment Complete follow up Double-blinding Outcome assessment must be sound
2	RCT direct comparison	Identical	Valid surrogate	Level 1 plus Validity of surrogate outcome
2	Indirect comparison with placebo from RCTs	Similar or different in disease severity or risk	Clinically important or valid surrogate	Level 1 plus Differences in methodological quality End points Compliance Baseline risk
3	Subgroup analyses from indirect comparisons of RCTs with placebo	Similar or different in disease severity or risk	Clinically important or valid surrogate	Level 1 plus Multiple comparisons, post hoc data dredging Underpowered subgroups Misclassification into subgroups
3	Indirect comparison with placebo from RCTs	Similar or different in disease severity or risk	Unvalidated surrogate	Surrogate outcomes may not capture all good or bad effects of treatment
4	Indirect comparison of nonrandomised studies	Similar or different in disease severity or risk	Clinically important	Confounding by indication, compliance, or time Unknown or unmeasured confounders Measurement error Limited database, or coding systems not suitable for research

Levels of evidence for safety

These are shown in Table 1.4.3. There are always going to be problems concerning rare, but serious, adverse events. The inverse rule of three tells us that if we have seen no serious adverse events in 1500 exposed patients, then we can be 95% sure that they do not occur more frequently than 1 in 500 patients.

Randomised trials of efficacy will usually be underpowered to detect rate, serious adverse events, and we will usually have to use other study designs. In practice the difficulty will be that soon after new treatments are introduced there will be a paucity of data for these other types of study. Only rarely will randomised trials powered to detect rare adverse events be conducted.

Most new treatments are introduced after being tested on perhaps a few thousand patients in controlled trials. Caution in treatments for chronic conditions is especially necessary if trials are only short-term, and where other diseases and treatments are likely.

Compliance

A difficult issue this, with a fragmented literature. But we do know that while compliance is usually high in clinical trials it may be lower

Table 1.4.3 Levels of evidence for safety in class effect

Level	Type of study	Advantages	Criteria for validity
1	RCT	Only design that permits detection of adverse effects when the adverse effect is similar to the event the treatment is trying to prevent	Underpowered for detecting adverse events unless specifically designed to do so
2	Cohort	Prospective data collection, defined cohort	Critically depends on follow up, classification and measurement accuracy
3	Case-control	Cheap and usually fast to perform	Selection and recall bias may provide problems, and temporal relationships may not be clear.
4	Phase 4 studies	Can detect rare but serious adverse events if large enough	No control or unmatched control Critically depends on follow up, classification and measurement accuracy
5	Case series	Cheap and usually fast	Often small sample size, selection bias may be a problem, no control group
6	Case report(s)	Cheap and usually fast	Often small sample size, selection bias may be a problem, no control group

in practice. Treatment schedules that are likely to improve compliance (once a day, for instance) might be important.

Cost

Economic studies are complicated beasts, and we need to treat this evidence with caution. Assumption of a class effect is usually done to justify choosing the cheapest drug in terms of acquisition (prescribing) costs. Terrific if this means that the costs of achieving the same ends are minimised. It may not be like that, and health economics in class effects need to be carefully thought through.

Problems

The correct design of an analgesic trial is situation dependent. In some circumstances very complicated designs have to be used to ensure sensitivity and validity.

No gold standard

There may be circumstances in which there is no established analgesic treatment of sufficient effectiveness to act as a gold standard against which to measure a new treatment, often the case in chronic pain. Clearly, the use of placebo or non-treatment controls is of great importance, especially when effects are to be examined over prolonged periods of weeks or months.

But it is paradoxically these very circumstances in which ethical constraints act against using placebo or non-treatment controls because of the need to do *something*. In acute pain studies, conversely, there is little problem with using placebos, since the failure of placebo (or any treatment) can be dealt with by prescribing additional analgesics that should work.

When there is no pain to begin with

Clearly, where there is no pain it is difficult to measure an analgesic response. Yet a number of studies seek to do this by pre-empting pain, or using an intervention where there is no pain (intraoperatively, for instance) to produce analgesia when pain is to be expected.

These are difficult, but not impossible, circumstances in which to conduct research. Meticulous attention to trial design is necessary to be able to show differences.

Comment

What makes a trial valid is governed by many factors. For the most part, when we consider a trial designed to show efficacy, it has to live up to rigorous standards. If not, then it could give the wrong answer. There is simply no escape from recognising that we need to understand the basics of good trial design if we are not to be misled. That is especially the case when we try to look at papers that try to demonstrate equivalence between two treatments, or where folks make hurried assumptions about class effects to justify choosing interventions with lower acquisition costs, and ignore differences in efficacy, effectiveness, or safety.

References

1. McQuay, H. J. *et al.* (1982). Some patients don't need analgesics after surgery, *Journal of the Royal Society of Medicine* 75: 705–8.
2. Moore, A. *et al.* (1996). Deriving dichotomous outcome measures from continuous data in randomised controlled trials of analgesics, *Pain* 66: 229–37.
3. McAlister, F. A. and Sackett, D. L. (2001). Active-control equivalence trials and antihypertensive agents, *American Journal of Medicine* 111: 553–8.
4. Moher, D. *et al.* (1994). Statistical power, sample size, and their reporting in randomized controlled trials, *JAMA* 272: 122–4.
5. McAlister, F. A. *et al.* (1999). Users' guides to the medical literature XIX Applying clinical trial results B. Guidelines for determining whether a drug is exerting (more than) a class effect, *JAMA* 282: 1371–7.

1.5 **Systematic review and meta-analysis**

Systematic reviews identify and review all the relevant studies, and are more likely to give a reliable answer. They use explicit methods and quality standards to reduce bias. Their results are the closest we are likely to get to the truth in the current state of knowledge. We will see (section 1.6) that even the best trials designed to tell us that an analgesic is better than placebo can give the wrong result just by the random play of chance. Systematic reviews (and meta-analysis, the statistical combining of information from many trials) are our best defence against making incorrect decisions based on inadequate data.

The questions a systematic review should answer for us are:

- how well does an intervention work (compared with placebo, no treatment or other interventions in current use) – or can I forget about it?
- is it safe?
- will it work and be safe for the patients in my practice?

Clinicians live in the real world and are busy people, and need to synthesise their knowledge of a particular patient in their practice, their experience and expertise, and the best external evidence from systematic review. They can then be pretty sure that they are doing their best. But the product of systematic review and particularly meta-analysis – often some sort of statistical output – is not usually readily interpretable or usable in day-to-day clinical practice.

Outputs, the way in which results of meta-analyses are expressed, are dealt with in section 1.7. This section is all about quality control, and about the problem of bias. Bias – *a one-sided inclination of the mind* – is a real problem, not least because researchers have found many examples where there is a propensity to get an incorrect answer in individual trials or reviews of trials. The job of a systematic review is to pull all the nuggets from piles of dross, not to give us one big pile of dross that may or may not have some nuggets in it. What we seek, but unfortunately do not always get, is a good review of good trials. Too often we get bad reviews, even bad reviews of good trials (Figure 1.5.1).

Searching for relevant trials

To produce valid reviews of evidence, the reviews need to be systematic. To be systematic they need to include all relevant randomised controlled trials (RCTs), or whatever other reports available. Identifying all the relevant trials is a 'fundamental challenge' [1] which is easily

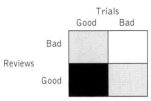

Figure 1.5.1 Trials and reviews – hopes and expectations.

underestimated, though the advent of the Cochrane Library with its CDROM or Internet database of about 300,000 controlled trials has made this much easier in recent years. We now have many more and easier electronic ways of searching, including PubMed (www4.ncbi. nlm.nih.gov/entrez), with searching freely and easily available over the Internet.

The first obstacle faced by any reviewer is finding out how many eligible RCTs exist. Commonly the total is unknown, unless it is a new intervention, when all the trials will have been done with industrial sponsorship. Thus only for newer interventions are reviewers likely to be sure that they have found all the RCTs available. Otherwise the only way to find how many RCTs there are would be to scan every record in every language, in every available bibliographic database, to search by hand all non-indexed journals, theses, proceedings and textbooks, to search the reference lists of all the reports found, and to ask investigators of previous RCTs for other published or unpublished information [2]. In practice, constrained by time and cost, reviewers have to compromise, and then hope that what they have found is a representative sample of the unknown total population of trials. The more comprehensive the searching the more trials will be found, and any conclusions will then be stronger. Comprehensive searches can be very time consuming and costly, so again this emphasises the necessary compromise, where the target is the highest possible yield for given resources.

Retrieval bias is the failure to identify reports that could have affected the results of a systematic review or meta-analysis [3]. This failure may be because trials are still ongoing, or completed but unpublished (publication bias) or because although published the search did not find them. Trying to identify unpublished trials by asking researchers had a very low yield [4], and was not cheap. Registers of ongoing and completed trials are another way to find unpublished data, but such registers are rare though increasingly becoming available.

For pain, extensive electronic and hand searching found 14,000 trials with pain as an outcome published between 1950 and 1994. How these were distributed by clinical setting and intervention is shown in Table 1.5.1. All of this work was made available to the Cochrane Collaboration, and has been included in the Cochrane Library. Other parts of the Cochrane collaboration continue to hand

Table 1.5.1 Pain trials 1950–94

	Acute	Chronic	Cancer	Total	Percent
Complementary	112	223	10	345	2
Invasive	1697	336	34	2067	14
Pharmacological	5390	4978	337	10,705	75
Physical	402	501	36	939	7
Psychological	100	191	10	301	2
Total	7701	6229	427	14,357	
Percent	54	43	3		

search journals, and the Cochrane Library should be the first port of call for anyone undertaking a systematic review, because it gives not only controlled trials, but also any reviews in the Cochrane Library and elsewhere.

Quality control

Systematic reviews of inadequate quality may be worse than none, because faulty decisions may be made with unjustified confidence. Quality control in the systematic review process, from literature searching onwards, is vital. How to judge the quality of a systematic review is encapsulated in the questions [5]:

1. Were the question(s) and methods stated clearly?
2. Were the search methods used to locate relevant studies comprehensive?
3. Were explicit methods used to determine which articles to include in the review?
4. Was the methodological quality of the primary studies assessed?
5. Were the selection and assessment of the primary studies reproducible and free from bias?
6. Were differences in individual study results explained adequately?
7. Were the results of the primary studies combined appropriately?
8. Were the reviewers' conclusions supported by the data cited?

This is all very methodological, and important, stuff. But the key to systematic review is to avoid allowing bias to creep in and colour the results.

Garbage in, garbage out

For the avoidance of doubt, the clinical bottom line is that wherever bias is found it almost always results in a large over-estimation of the effect of treatments. Poor trial design makes treatments look better than they really are. It can even make them look as if they work when actually they do not work. This is why good guides to systematic review suggest strategies for bias minimisation by avoiding including trials with known sources of bias. They further suggest performing sensitivity analysis to see whether different trial designs are affecting results in a systematic review.

But this advice is ignored more often than not. It is ignored in reviews, and it is ignored in decision-making. The result is that decisions are being made on incorrect information, and they will be wrong. There is no alternative to having some rudimentary knowledge of potential sources of bias and how badly it can hurt.

Bandolier bias guide

This guide can be used when examining a systematic review, or a single clinical trial. The guide is not to be used for observational studies, or for studies of diagnostic tests.

Randomisation. The process of randomisation is important in eliminating selection bias in trials. If the selection is done by a computer, or even the toss of a coin, then any conscious or subconscious attitude of the researcher is avoided.

Some of the most influential people in evidence-based thinking showed how inadequate design exaggerated the effect measured in a trial (Table 1.5.2). They compared trials in which the authors reported adequately concealed treatment allocations with those in which treatment was either inadequately or unclearly described, as well as examining the effects of exclusions and double binding.

The results were striking and sobering, as Table 1.5.2 shows. Odds ratios were exaggerated by 41% in trials in which there was an inadequate concealment of treatment allocation, and by 30% when the process of concealing allocation was unclearly stated.

The amount of bias arising from failure to randomise is one reason why many systematic reviews exclude non-randomised trials and why restricting systematic reviews to include only randomised studies makes sense for reviews of effectiveness. The reason is the many, many examples where non-randomised studies have led reviews to come to the wrong conclusion.

Examples abound. A classic example [6] is a review of transcutaneous nerve stimulation (TENS) for postoperative pain relief (Figure 1.5.2). Randomised studies overwhelmingly showed no benefit over placebo, while non-randomised studies did show benefit. Put another way, almost all the positive trials were not randomised, while almost all the negative ones were randomised.

The randomisation effect is particularly strong where a review counts votes (a study is positive or negative) rather than combines data in a meta-analysis. It applies especially to studies in alternative therapies.

Blinding. The importance of blinding is that it avoids observer bias. If no one knows which treatment a patient has received, then no systematic over-estimation of the effect of any particular treatment is possible.

Table 1.5.2 Sources of bias

Source of bias	Effect on treatment efficacy	Size of the effect	References
Randomisation	Increase	Non-randomised studies overestimate treatment effect by 41% with inadequate method, 30% with unclear method	Schultz, K. F., Chalmers, I., Hayes, R. J. and Altman, D. G. (1995). Empirical evidence of bias: Dimensions of methodological quality associated with estimates of treatment effects in controlled trials, *Journal of the American Medical Association* 273: 408–12.
Randomisation	Increase	Completely different result between randomised and non-randomised studies	Carroll, D., Tramèr, M., McQuay, H., Nye, B. and Moore, A. (1996). Randomization is important in studies with pain outcomes: systematic review of transcutaneous electrical nerve stimulation in acute postoperative pain, *British Journal of Anaesthesia* 77: 798–803.
Blinding	Increase	17%	Schultz, K. F., Chalmers, I., Hayes, R. J. and Altman, D. G. (1995). Empirical evidence of bias: Dimensions of methodological quality associated with estimates of treatment effects in controlled trials, *Journal of the American Medical Association* 273: 408–12.
Blinding	Increase	Completely different result between blind and non-blind studies	Ernst, E. and White, A. R. (1998). Acupuncture for back pain: A meta-analysis of randomised controlled trials, *Arch Int Med* 158: 2235–41.
Reporting quality	Increase	About 25%	Khan, K. S., Daya, S. and Jadad, A. R. (1996). The importance of quality of primary studies in producing unbiased systematic reviews, *Arch Intern Med* 156: 661–6. Moher, D. *et al.* (1988). Does quality of reports of randomised trials affect estimates of intervention efficacy reported in meta-analyses? *Lancet* 352: 609–13.
Duplication	Increase	About 20%	Tramèr, M., Reynolds, D. J. M., Moore, R. A. and McQuay, H .J. (1997). Effect of covert duplicate publication on meta-analysis; a case study, *BMJ* 315: 635–40.

Geography	Increase	May be large for some alternative therapies	Vickers, A., Goyal, N., Harland, R. and Rees, R. (1998). Do certain countries produce only positive results? A systematic review of controlled trials, *Control Clin Trial* 19: 159–66.
Size	Increase	Small trials may overestimate treatment effects by about 30%	Moore, R. A., Carroll, D., Wiffen, P. J., Tramèr, M. and McQuay, H. J. (1998). Quantitative systematic review of topically-applied non-steroidal anti-inflammatory drugs, *BMJ* 316: 333–8. Moore, R. A., Gavaghan, D., Tramèr, M. R., Collins, S. L. and McQuay, H. J. (1998). Size is everything – large amounts of information are needed to overcome random effects in estimating direction and magnitude of treatment effects, *Pain* 78: 217–20.
Statistical	Increase	Not known to any extent, probably modest, but important especially where vote-counting occurs	Smith, L. A., Oldman, A. D., McQuay, H. J. and Moore, R. A. (2000). Teasing apart quality and validity in systematic reviews: an example from acupuncture trials in chronic neck and back pain, *Pain* 86: 119–32.
Validity	Increase	Not known to any extent, probably modest, but important especially where vote-counting occurs	Smith, L. A., Oldman, A. D., McQuay, H. J. and Moore, R. A. (2000). Teasing apart quality and validity in systematic reviews: an example from acupuncture trials in chronic neck and back pain, *Pain* 86: 119–32.
Language	Increase	Not known to any extent, but may be modest	Egger, M., Zellweger-Zähner, T., Schneider, M., Junker, C., Lengeler, C. and Antes, G. (1997). Language bias in randomised controlled trials published in English and German, *Lancet* 350: 326–9.
Publication	Increase	Not known to any extent, probably modest, but important especially where there is little evidence	Egger, M. and Davey Smith, G. (2000). Under the meta-scope: potentials and limitations of meta-analysis. In Tramèr, M. (ed.), Evidence Based Resource in Anaesthesia and Analgesia. BMJ Publications.

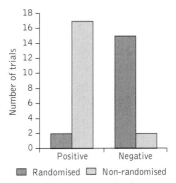

Figure 1.5.2 TENS for postoperative pain relief, randomised and non-randomised studies.

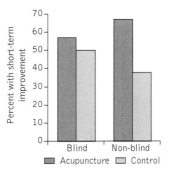

Figure 1.5.3 Effect of blinding on short-term outcomes after acupuncture for back pain.

Non-blinded studies over-estimate treatment effects by about 17% (Table 1.5.2). In a review of acupuncture for back pain (Figure 1.5.3), including both blinded and non-blinded studies changed the overall conclusion [7]. The blinded studies showed 57% of patients improved with acupuncture and 50% with control, a relative benefit of 1.2 (95% confidence interval 0.9–1.5). Five non-blinded studies showed a difference from control, with 67% improved with acupuncture and 38% with control. Here the relative benefit was significant at 1.8 (1.3–2.4).

Reporting quality. Because of the large bias expected from studies that are not randomised or not blind, a scoring system [8] that is highly dependent on randomisation and blinding will also correlate with bias. Trials of poor reporting quality consistently over estimate the effect of treatment [9,10]. This particular scoring system (Table 1.5.3)

Table 1.5.3 Oxford quality scoring system for controlled trials [8]

This is not the same as being asked to review a paper. It should not take more than 10 min to score a report and there are no right or wrong answers.

Please read the article and try to answer the following questions (see attached instructions):

1. Was the study described as randomised (this includes the use of words such as randomly, random and randomisation)?
2. Was the study described as double-blind?
3. Was there a description of withdrawals and drop outs?

Scoring the items:

Give a score of 1 point for each 'yes' and 0 points for each 'no'. There are no in-between marks.

Give 1 additional point if:

On question 1, the method of randomisation was described and it was appropriate (table of random numbers, computer generated, coin tossing, etc.)

and/or:

If on question 2 the method of double-blinding was described and it was appropriate (identical placebo, active placebo, dummy, etc.)

Deduct 1 point if:

On question 1, the method of randomisation was described and it was inappropriate (patients were allocated alternatively, or according to date of birth, hospital number, etc.)

and/or:

On question 2 the study was described as double-blind but the method of blinding was inappropriate (e.g. comparison of tablet vs. injection with no double dummy)

Advice on using the scale

1. *Randomisation*: If the word randomised or any other related words such as random, randomly, or randomisation are used in the report, but the method of randomisation is not described, give a positive score to this item. A randomisation method will be regarded as appropriate if it allowed each patient to have the same chance of receiving each treatment and the investigators could not predict which treatment was next. Therefore methods of allocation using date of birth, date of admission, hospital numbers or alternation should not be regarded as appropriate.

2. *Double-blinding*: A study must be regarded as double-blind if the word double-blind is used (even without description of the method) or if it is implied that neither the caregiver nor the patient could identify the treatment being assessed.

3. *Withdrawals and drop outs*: Patients who were included in the study but did not complete the observation period or who were not included in the analysis must be described. The number and the reasons for withdrawal must be stated. If there are no withdrawals, it should be stated in the article. If there is no statement on withdrawals, this item must be given a negative score (0 points).

has a range of 0–5 based on randomisation, blinding and withdrawals and dropouts. Studies scoring 2 or less consistently show greater effects of treatment than those scoring 3 or more.

Duplication. Results from some trials are reported more than once. This may be entirely justified for a whole range of reasons. Examples might be a later follow up of the trial, or a re-analysis. Sometimes, though, information about patients in trials is reported more than once without that being obvious, or overt, or referenced. Only the more impressive information seems to be duplicated, sometimes in papers with completely different authors. A consequence of covert duplication would be to overestimate the effect of treatment [11].

Intention to treat. Suppose 100 patients are randomised and enter a trial, but results are only reported on 50 of them because the other 50 dropped out or withdrew from treatment (a per-protocol analysis). What happened to the other 50 patients? Did they withdraw because of lack of efficacy, or because of adverse effects? Were there different reasons for withdrawal for treatment and control? If results are not reported and analysed according to all patients who entered the study, called intention to treat analysis, then bias may occur because we only see results in patients in whom the treatment worked.

Geography. Vickers and colleagues [12] showed that trials of acupuncture conducted in east Asia were universally positive, while those conducted in Australia/New Zealand, north America or western Europe were positive only about half the time. Randomised trials of therapies other than acupuncture conducted in China, Taiwan, Japan or Russia/USSR were also overwhelmingly positive, and much more so than in other parts of the world (Table 1.5.4).

This may be a result of an historical cultural difference, but it does mean that care should be exercised where there is a preponderance of studies from these cultures. Again, this is particularly important for alternative therapies, and it is probably one of the best arguments for the existence of publication bias. Do we really believe that every single

Table 1.5.4 Proportion of randomised trials, and acupuncture trials from different parts of the world

Country	Randomised or controlled trials		Acupuncture trials	
	Number	Positive (%)	Number	Positive (%)
England	107	75	20	60
China	109	99	36	100
Japan	120	89	5	100
Russia/USSR	29	97	11	91
Taiwan	40	95	6	100

acupuncture trial in China comes up with a positive result, or is it unacceptable for negative results that are contrary to accepted belief to be published?

Size. Clinical trials should have a power calculation performed at the design stage. This will estimate how many patients are needed so that, say, 90% of studies with X number of patients would show a difference of Y% between two treatments. When the value of Y is very large, the value of X can be small. More often the value of Y is modest, or small. In those circumstances, X is going to be larger, and more patients will be needed in trials for them to have a hope of showing a difference.

Yet clinical trials are often ridiculously small. The record is a ran-domised study on 3 patients in a parallel group design. But when are trials so tiny that they can be ignored? Many folk take a pragmatic view that trials with fewer than 10 patients per treatment arm should be ignored, though others may disagree.

There are examples where sensitivity in meta-analysis has shown small trials to have a larger effect of treatment than smaller trials (Table 1.5.2). The degree of variability between trials of adequate power is still large, because trials are powered to detect that there is a *difference* between treatments, rather than *how big* that difference is. The random play of chance can remain a significant factor despite adequate power to detect a difference, and this will be dealt with in section 1.6.

Statistics and data manipulation. Despite the best efforts of editors and peer reviewers, some papers are published that are just plain wrong. Wrong covers a multitude of sins, but two are particularly important.

Statistical incorrectness can take a variety of guises. It may be as simple as the data presented in a paper as statistically significant not being sig-nificant. It can often take the form of inappropriate statistical tests [13]. It can be data trawling, where a single statistical significance is obtained and a paper written round it. Reams could be written about this, but the simple warning is that readers or reviewers of papers have to be cautious of results of trials, especially where vote-counting is being done.

But also beware the power of words. Even when statistical testing shows no difference, it is common to see the results hailed as a success. While that may sound silly when written down, even the most cynical of readers can be fooled into drawing the wrong conclusion. Abstracts are notorious for misleading in this way.

Data manipulation is a bit more complicated to detect. An example would be an intervention where we are not told what the start condi-tion of patients is, nor the end, but that at some time in between the rate of change was statistically significant by some test with which we are unfamiliar. This is done only to make positive that which is not positive, and the direction of the bias is obvious (Table 1.5.2). Again, crucially important where vote-counting is being done to determine whether the intervention works or not.

Validity. Do individual trials have a design (apart from issues like randomisation and blinding) that allows them to adequately measure an effect? What constitutes validity depends on the circumstances of a trial, but studies often lack validity. A validity scoring system applied to acupuncture for head and neck pain demonstrated that trials with lower validity were more likely to say that the treatment worked than those that were valid [13]. This validity scoring system is described in detail in section 6.1, because it is particularly relevant to trials and reviews of complementary therapy where pooling data is less likely, and vote counting positive and negative trials more likely.

Language. Too often the search strategy for a systematic review or meta-analysis restricts itself to the English language only. Authors whose language is not English may be more likely to publish positive findings in an English language journal, because these would have a greater international impact. Negative findings would be more likely to be published in non-English language journals [14].

Publication. Finally there is the old chestnut of publication bias. This is usually thought to be the propensity for positive trials to be published and for negative trials not to be published. It must exist, and there is a huge literature about publication bias [15].

It is worth having some reservations about the fuss that is made, though. Partly this stems from the failure to include assessments of trial validity and quality. Most peer reviewers would reject non-randomised studies, or those where there are major failings in methodology. These trials will be hard to publish. Much the same can be said for dissertations or theses. One attempt to include theses [16] found 17 dissertations for one treatment. Thirteen were excluded because of methodological problems, mainly lack of randomisation, three had been published and were already included in the relevant review, and one could be added. It made no difference.

Funnel plots are not likely to be helpful. One often quoted, of magnesium in acute myocardial infarction [17], can more easily be explained by the fact that trials in a meta-analysis were trivially small to detect any effect and should never have been included in a meta-analysis in the first place (Figure 1.5.4).

But these are quibbles. If there is sufficient evidence available, large numbers of large, well conducted trials, then publication bias is not likely to be a problem. Where there is little information, small numbers of low quality trials, then it becomes more problematical.

Sensitivity analysis

Systematic reviewers should take these, and perhaps other, sources of bias into account when performing their reviews. One simple way of

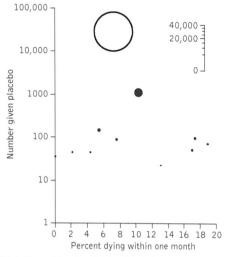

Figure 1.5.4 Size and baseline risk in trials included in a meta-analysis of magnesium in acute myocardial infarction (dark symbols) and a large randomised trial (white symbol).

checking for unknown (or unknowable) bias is to perform a sensitivity analysis. For example, our review might have properly conducted trials, but where some use one outcome and others use another. It is fairly simple not just to look at the results of all the trials, but also those with one or other outcome. If the results are the same, then fine. If they are not, we have something to explain. We can also do sensitivity analysis by trial quality, or by size, or by date of publication, or by any other criterion that seems to make sense. Reviewers who use sensitivity analysis are doing a good job. Reviews that do not mention sensitivity analysis are to be looked at closely to see whether it should have been done.

The one thing to be borne in mind is that sensitivity analysis can only be performed where there is sufficient information. If we have too few studies, then we end up salami-slicing small numbers of trials, and run the distinct risk of coming up with incorrect conclusions based on too little data.

Comment

This section is a brief review of some sources of bias in trials of treatment efficacy rather than a comprehensive discourse on the subject. Different sources of potential bias than those recounted here probably exist. Because bias is present, and exists in so many different forms, we have to be vigilant when reading about a clinical trial, and especially when taking the results of a single trial into clinical practice.

But systematic reviews and meta-analyses also suffer from quality problems. They should be considering potential sources of bias when they are being written. Many do not, and will therefore mislead. If systematic reviews or meta-analyses include poor trials or have poor reporting quality, then, just like individual trials, they too have a propensity for a greater likelihood of a positive result.

There is no doubt that meta-analyses can mislead. If they do, then it is because they have been incorrectly assembled or incorrectly used. The defence, indeed the only defence, is for readers to have sufficient knowledge themselves to know when the review or paper they are reading should be confined to the bin.

References

1. Chalmers, I. *et al*. (1992). Getting to grips with Archie Cochrane's agenda, *BMJ* 305: 786–7.
2. Jadad, A. R. and McQuay, H. J. (1993). A high-yield strategy to identify randomized controlled trials for systematic reviews, *Online Journal of Current Clinical Trials* [Serial Online] Doc No 33:3973
3. Simes, R. J. (1987). Confronting publication bias: a cohort design for meta-analysis, *Statistics in Medicine* 6: 11–29.
4. Hetherington, J. *et al*. (1989). Retrospective and prospective identification of unpublished controlled trials: lessons from a survey of obstetricians and pediatricians, *Pediatrics* 84: 374–80.
5. Oxman, A. D. and Guyatt, G. H. (1988). Guidelines for reading literature reviews, *Canadian Medical Association Journal* 138: 697–703.
6. Carroll, D. *et al*. (1996). Randomization is important in studies with pain outcomes: systematic review of transcutaneous electrical nerve stimulation in acute postoperative pain, *British Journal of Anaesthesia* 77: 798–803.
7. Ernst, E. and White, A. R. (1998). Acupuncture for back pain, *Archives of Internal Medicine* 158: 2235–41.
8. Jadad, A. R. *et al*. (1996). Assessing the quality of reports of randomized clinical trials: is blinding necessary? *Controlled Clinical Trials* 17: 1–12.
9. Khan, K. S. *et al*. (1996). The importance of quality of primary studies in producing unbiased systematic reviews, *Archives of Internal Medicine* 156: 661–6.
10. Moher, D. *et al*. (1998). Does quality of reports of randomised trials affect estimates of intervention efficacy reported in meta-analyses? *Lancet* 352: 609–13.
11. Tramèr, M. R. *et al*. (1997). Impact of covert duplicate publication on meta-analysis: a case study, *BMJ* 315: 635–9.
12. Vickers, A. *et al*. (1998). Do certain countries produce only positive results? A systematic review of controlled trials, *Controlled Clinical Trials* 19: 159–66.

13. Smith, L. A. *et al.* (2000). Teasing apart quality and validity in systematic reviews: an example from acupuncture trials in chronic neck and back pain, *Pain* 86: 119–32.

14. Egger, M. *et al.* (1997). Language bias in randomised controlled trials published in English and German, *Lancet* 350: 326–9.

15. Egger, M. and Davey Smith, G. (2000). Under the meta-scope: potentials and limitations of meta-analysis. In: Tramèr, M. (ed.), *Evidence based resource in anaesthesia and analgesia*, BMJ Publications.

16. Vickers, A. J. and Smith, C. (2000). Incorporating data from dissertations in systematic reviews, *International Journal of Technology Assessment in Health Care* 16: 711–3.

17. Egger, M. and Smith, G. D. (1995). Misleading meta-analysis. Lessons from 'an effective, safe, simple' intervention that wasn't, *BMJ* 310: 752–4.

1.6 **Size**

One of the single most important factors we have to get to grips with when evaluating evidence is size. We all occasionally meet people who will maintain that a clinical trial in which a new treatment used in 10 patients is statistically better than placebo in 10 other patients is sufficient evidence to take that new treatment into clinical practice, but that is wrong. Even conventional statistical significance is not very convincing. We conventionally use a 5% significance level, meaning that only one time in 20 should a particular result occur by chance. Yet when we play monopoly we are hardly surprised if we throw a double-six, one chance in 36.

Random play of chance

As well as all the other factors that can influence the result of a clinical trial or even meta-analysis, one we often forget is the random play of chance. If we have huge amounts of data, we can forget it. If we have moderate amounts of data, we must think about it, and if we have little data, then we are in trouble. Even if everything else is perfect, random chance can be a problem.

Let us consider ibuprofen for acute postoperative pain, where we have lots of trials in thousands of patients. All these trials are randomised, all are double blind, all had adult patients with initial pain of moderate or severe initial intensity, all were of high reporting quality, all measured pain relief in the same way over the same period of time, and results are expressed using the same outcome measure. Given such clear clinical homogeneity, our expectation would be that the results of these trials might be rather similar. If we represent the results as a L'Abbé plot where each symbol represents a trial (larger symbols larger trials), the similarity of the results is not obvious (Figure 1.6.1).

Some trials produced results in which all patients treated with ibuprofen had at least 50% pain relief while in others it was less than 20%. In some trials not one patient given placebo had at least 50% pain relief, while in others it was nearly 60%.

This huge variability should make us stop and think about the possible reasons for it. A number of explanations have been put forward, usually based on either different patient populations or different pain models, or both. The argument would be that women having an episiotomy in Venezuela would handle pain differently from men having a knee arthroscopy in Norway. This is a 'Welsh wimp versus Scottish stoic' argument. There is even a famous example of two trials of tramadol in acute pain, one of which said that it worked very well [1], and the other that it was no different from placebo [2]. The problem

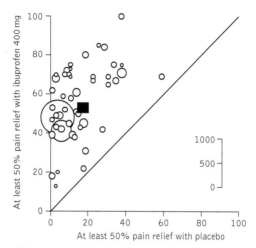

Figure 1.6.1 L'Abbe plot of randomised trials of ibuprofen 400 mg. Black square represents overall average.

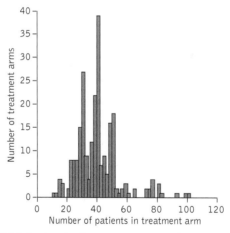

Figure 1.6.2 Number of patients per treatment arm in 244 treatment arms from 95 randomised trials in acute pain.

with both these trials, as with most done in acute and chronic pain, is that they are just too small.

Figure 1.6.2 shows the number of patients in each of 244 treatment arms from 95 randomised trials in acute pain, trials chosen from a systematic review in which fewer than 10 patients per trial arm was an exclusion criterion. It shows that the size was small, never more than 101 patients, and most usually 30, 40 or 50.

Before seeking any sophisticated explanation for the ibuprofen results, why not think first about what the effects of random chance would be when we have only 40 patients given ibuprofen and 40 patients given placebo. Fortunately the random effects can be calculated, and have been for exactly this eventuality, but taking individual patient data, examining the distribution of results, and simulating 10,000 trials. These trials have overall exactly the same success rate (experimental event rate) for ibuprofen and the same success rate (control event rate) for placebo as the actual trials. Size of trial also varied to mimic the size range found.

The results are shown in Figure 1.6.3, where the grey areas represent where any single trial could occur just by the random play of chance. Denser areas represent areas of greater probability. There is no other effect than random chance, not different patients, or pain models, or nice nurses or horrid doctors.

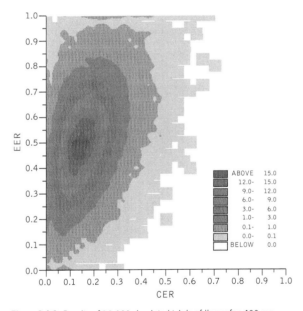

Figure 1.6.3 Results of 10,000 simulated trials of ibuprofen 400 mg versus placebo. Grey areas show where a trial can occur by chance when the mean size is 40 patients per treatment arm. EER is the experimental event rate (with ibuprofen) and CER the control event rate (with placebo).

Minimum number of events

If random chance is so important, then, how can we know when there is sufficient information for us not to be misled? Two simple things to bear in mind. First is that we have to recognise the difference between number of events and number of people. A sample of 10,000 people where there are only two events is not more impressive than a group of 40 patients in whom 20 events occur. We have to be mindful of the number of events as well as the number of patients in a sample.

If no events occur in, say, 5000 patients, then the best we can say is that we can be 95% confident that the event does not occur more frequently than once every 5000/3, or 16,667, patients [3]. This inverse rule of 3 is useful when we think that new treatments are often launched with experience in only a few thousand patients.

We can investigate the effect of numbers on our confidence by the simple expedient of feeding different numbers with the same percentage into a standard method of calculating confidence intervals of proportions. Let us use 30%. So we feed in 3 and 10, 30 and 100, 300 and 1000 and so on. The results of this can be seen graphically in Figure 1.6.4. Quite clearly our estimate of the proportion is quite tight when we have a total number of 1000 and 300 events. But when the

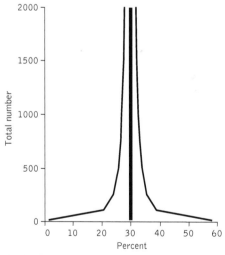

Figure 1.6.4 Confidence intervals around the proportion of 30% as number of observations increase. The vertical line represents the overall proportion and the other lines the upper and lower of the 95% confidence interval.

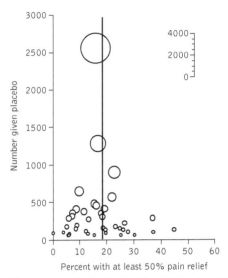

Figure 1.6.5 Percentage of patients with at least 50% pain relief with placebo in 56 meta-analyses in acute pain. Size of symbol is proportional to number of patients given placebo.

total is below 500, and especially below 100 when there are fewer than 30 events, we can have virtually no confidence in the result.

Let us now look at some real-life examples to see how they compare with the theoretical picture generated in Figure 1.6.4. There are three of them. The first (Figure 1.6.5) shows the percentage of patients with at least 50% pain relief with placebo in 56 meta-analyses in acute pain, with about 12,000 patients given placebo, and in which the overall mean was about 18%. All the trials were randomised, all double blind, and all used the same outcome, measured in the same way, over the same period of time, in similar pain models and patients. Only those meta-analyses with at least 1000 patients given placebo correctly measured the event rate with placebo. Where the number given placebo was small, the estimate varied widely from 0 to 60%.

Our next example is sperm counts. A review a decade ago [4] started us worrying about falling sperm counts, probably wrongly. If we take the data on sperm counts from that paper and calculate a weighted mean value in thousands of men, the mean is about 77 million sperm per mL. Large studies with many men confirm this, but small studies produce results that are all over the place (Figure 1.6.6). Small samples (some as few as seven men, which do not even show on the graph) produced widely differing results. For sperm counts, size really is everything.

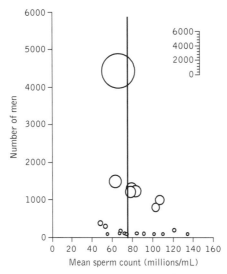

Figure 1.6.6 Sperm counts and size of study. Size of symbol is proportional to number of men.

The final example is the relative risk of perforation, ulcer, or bleed (PUB) in people taking NSAID compared with people not taking NSAID (Figure 1.6.7). The overall relative risk was 4. Studies with 1000 PUBs or more accurately measured this. Those with fewer did not. Below 200 PUBs the relative risks varied from no increased risk to an eightfold increased risk.

The lesson from these examples (and there are many others that could be used) is that we need reasonably large data sets to be confident of a result, and that conclusions drawn from limited amounts of information might mislead.

How much data do we need?

'How much data do we need for what?' would be the better question. Clinical trials are done to show, for example, that an analgesic in acute pain is better than placebo. Another question would be to ask how much data do we need to be confident of the size of an effect. The variables here are what happens with placebo, what happens with the treatment, and how confident we want to be. What we will do, therefore, is to calculate this for trials in acute pain.

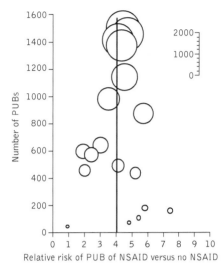

Figure 1.6.7 Relative risk of PUB in people taking NSAID compared with people not taking NSAID. Size of symbol is proportional to number of PUBs. Relative risks have been plotted from zero for convenience.

Statistical significance

Let us use a response rate of at least half pain relief with placebo of 16%, and vary the rate of what happens with treatment between 30% and 80%. Put in another way, our control event rate (CER) is 0.16 (a proportion) and the experimental event rate (EER) varies between 0.3 and 0.8. Table 1.6.1 gives us the number of patients in each treatment arm in each case [5].

For ibuprofen 400 mg, where the expected EER is 0.5, and when we want to be 95% confident that ibuprofen is better than placebo, we need 41 patients in each treatment arm (41 for ibuprofen, 41 for placebo) making a total of about 80 patients. This is the median number found in actual clinical trials (Figure 1.6.2). If we can afford to be less confident, we can make do with fewer patients. If we have an analgesic expected to be much better than ibuprofen, we can do with fewer patients. But if our analgesic is less efficacious than ibuprofen, we need many more patients.

Suppose, though, we want to be clinically confident of the result. First we need a definition of clinical confidence. For the sake of argument, let us say that we want to be 95% sure that the true number needed to treat (NNT, see section 1.7) is within ±0.5 of the observed NNT. So if the NNT is 3, we want to know that the true NNT is within 2.5–3.5.

Table 1.6.1 Number of patients required in each group for a statistically significant result that experimental is better than control

Probability	EER					
	0.30	0.40	0.50	0.60	0.70	0.80
0.50	83	26	17	13	10	7
0.75	137	40	27	21	14	10
0.90	200	57	34	29	20	13
0.95	244	68	41	33	23	16

Group sizes required to obtain a probability of 0.5, 0.75, 0.9 and 0.95 of obtaining a statistically significant result from the Chi-square test with a CER of 0.16 and EERs from 0.3 to 0.8

Table 1.6.2 Number of patients required in each group for a clinically relevant NNT ± 0.5

Probability	EER					
	0.30	0.40	0.50	0.60	0.70	0.80
0.50	>500	200	50	20	10	<10
0.75	>500	>500	150	60	25	10
0.90	>500	>500	320	110	50	20
0.95	>500	>500	470	180	80	40

Group sizes required to obtain a probability of 0.5, 0.75, 0.9 and 0.95 of obtaining a clinically relevant NNT (NNT within ± 0.5 of true value) with a CER of 0.16 and EERs from 0.3 to 0.8

In that case we need many more patients (Table 1.6.2). Now we need not 41 patients per group, but rather 470 per group or nearly 1000 in all. This is equivalent to more than 10 average sized RCTs designed for a statistical result only. Again if we can afford to be less confident, or have a better effect, we can do with fewer patients. But if we have a treatment that is less effective than ibuprofen, suddenly we need many, many patients.

We can carry this argument further, because computer simulations have been done that allow us to examine how likely clinical trials or meta-analyses are to accurately measure the clinical effect of a treatment, using the NNT as a measure of the clinical effect [5]. Table 1.6.3 shows that for ibuprofen 400 mg, 500 patients per group (1000 in all) will give us 95% confidence in the result. If we have only 200 patients per group (400 in total, five average trials) we can only be 81% confident. If the treatment is better than ibuprofen with a higher EER, then we can be very confident with small numbers of patients, but if we have small numbers with a treatment even marginally less effective, then the level of confidence drops off dramatically.

The lesson from all this is that we should beware small data sets with small numbers of events.

Table 1.6.3 Percentage of 100,000 simulated NNTs measured within ±0.5 of the true NNT with different event rates and group sizes

Group size	EER		
	0.40	0.50	0.60
25	26	37	57
50	28	51	73
100	38	61	88
200	55	81	96
300	63	89	99
400	71	93	99
500	74	95	100

Percent of trials in which the simulated NNT was within ±0.5 of the true NNT value, with increasing group size, and with a CER of 0.16 and EERs between 0.4 and 0.6

Does this thinking work in practice?

We can test whether this works in practice by looking at four large data sets with meta-analyses in acute pain. For four drugs and doses, ibuprofen 400 mg, aspirin 600/650 mg, paracetamol 975/1000 mg and ibuprofen 200 mg we have a sufficient number of trials to perform cumulative meta-analyses. In these we take the first trial to be published and calculate the NNT, then the first plus second, then the first, second and third, and so on. Over time, more and more information becomes available, and we can compare results at any one time with those with all the information available to us. And, remember, that these trials are all randomised and double blind, measuring the same outcome over the same period in the same way and with similar patients in similar clinical situations.

Figure 1.6.8 shows the data for ibuprofen 400 mg. The overall NNT was about 2.5 and the horizontal lines show ±0.5 NNT from this. The confidence interval was wide initially, but as the numbers of patients increased the confidence interval narrowed rapidly, and by the time about 1000 patients' worth of information was available, the confidence interval was within the boundary of ±0.5 of an NNT. This is just what we expected where the EER was about 0.55.

We have a similar pattern for aspirin 600/650 mg (Figure 1.6.9). Here, though, the NNT was 4.5 and the EER about 0.4. Again the confidence interval narrowed as more information became available, but only with almost 5000 patients was the interval within ±0.5 of an NNT unit. Again, this is about what we would have expected with a lower event rate.

For paracetamol 1000 mg the picture is somewhat different (Figure 1.6.10). The overall NNT is about 3.7, but early trials were wildly inaccurate, and overestimated the treatment efficacy (a lower

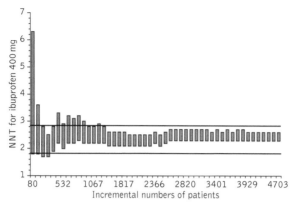

Figure 1.6.8 Cumulative meta-analysis for ibuprofen 400 mg.

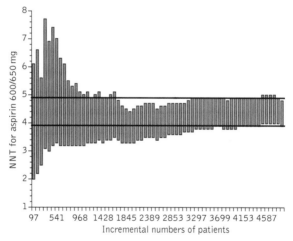

Figure 1.6.9 Cumulative meta-analysis for aspirin 600/650 mg.

NNT). Only as more information became available did the confidence interval come into line with that obtained from all the clinical trial information eventually available.

For ibuprofen 200 mg, we see a similar picture as for paracetamol, but in the opposite direction (Figure 1.6.11). Early trials wildly underestimated drug efficacy, and only as more information accumulated

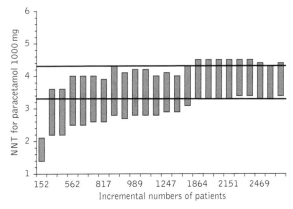

Figure 1.6.10 Cumulative meta-analysis for paracetamol 1000 mg.

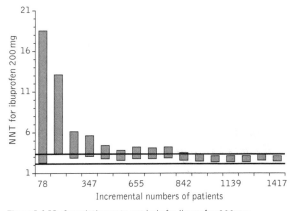

Figure 1.6.11 Cumulative meta-analysis for ibuprofen 200 mg.

did the result begin to give the same picture as for all clinical trial information.

Using cumulative meta-analysis

Cumulative meta-analysis, as used in Figures 1.6.8–1.6.11, is a useful technique for visually examining the results of all the trials as they are published, as well as having use as a quality control check for those doing systematic reviews. It has been used to examine the effects of size as well [6].

It is obvious that if we have a very small amount of information, from few patients, that the effects of random chance can be significant. As the amount of information or number of patients increases, then the effects of chance will diminish. In some circumstances, like acute pain trials, we can define how much information is needed for us to be confident not just that a treatment works, but how big is the effect of that treatment [5].

Confirmation that our estimate of the effect of treatment can be heavily dependent on size comes from a study from the USA and Greece [6]. Researchers looked at 60 meta-analyses of randomised trials where there were at least five trials published in more than three different calendar years. They were in either pregnancy and perinatal medicine or myocardial infarction.

For each meta-analysis trials were chronologically ordered by publication year and cumulative meta-analysis performed to arrive at a pooled odds ratio at the end of each calendar year. The relative change in treatment effect was calculated for each successive additional calendar year by dividing the odds ratio of the new assessment with more patients by the odds ratio of the previous assessment with fewer patients. This gives a 'relative odds ratio', in which a number greater than 1 indicated more treatment effect, and one less than 1 indicates less treatment effect. The relative odds ratio can be plotted against the number of patients included. The expected result is a horizontal funnel, with less change with more patients, and the relative odds ratio settling down to 1.

The two graphs they produced for pregnancy/perinatal medicine and myocardial infarction show exactly this expected pattern. Below 100 patients and the relative odds ratios vary between 0.2 and 6. By the time 1000 patients are included they are between 0.5 and 2. By the time we have about 5000 patients they settle down close to 1. The 95% prediction interval for the relative change in the odds ratio for different numbers for both examples is shown in Table 1.6.4.

Table 1.6.4 Effect of size on prediction of relative change in odds ratios with additional patients randomised [6]

Number of patients	Fixed effect prediction interval for relative change in odds ratio	
	Pregnancy/perinatal	Myocardial infarction
100	0.32–2.78	0.18–5.51
500	0.59–1.71	0.60–1.67
1000	0.67–1.49	0.74–1.35
2000	0.74–1.35	0.83–1.21
15,000	0.85–1.14	0.96–1.05

When evidence was based on only a few patients there was substantial uncertainty about how much the pooled treatment effect would change in the future. With only 100 patients randomised, additional information from more trials could multiply or divide by three the odds ratios we had at that point.

Comment

The lesson is simple. We need large amounts of information to get the true clinical efficacy of a treatment. Single small trials, even if performed impeccably, can give the wrong result because of the random play of chance. They can mislead. Together quality and size represent the keys to understanding clinical, as opposed to statistical, results. If we base practice on statistical results alone, we head for trouble. The need for size is the single biggest justification for using information from systematic reviews.

References

1. Sunshine, A. *et al.* (1992). Analgesic oral efficacy of tramadol hydrochloride in postoperative pain, *Clinical Pharmacology & Therapeutics* 51: 740–6.
2. Stubhaug, A. *et al.* (1995). Lack of analgesic effect of 50 and 100 mg oral tramadol after orthopaedic surgery: a randomized, double-blind, placebo and standard active drug comparison, *Pain* 62: 111–8.
3. Hanley, J. A. and Lippman-Hand, A. (1983). If nothing goes wrong, is everything alright? *JAMA* 249: 1743–5.
4. Carlsen, E. *et al.* (1992). Evidence for decreasing quality of semen during past 50 years, *BMJ* 305: 609–13
5. Moore, R. A. *et al.* (1998). Size is everything – large amounts of information are needed to overcome random effects in estimating direction and magnitude of treatment effects, *Pain* 78: 209–16.
6. Ioannidis, J. P. A. and Lau, J. (2001). Evolution of treatment effects over time: Empirical insight from recursive cumulative metaanalyses, *Proceedings of the National Academy of Sciences* 98: 831–6.

1.7 **Outputs and utility**

Output – 'quantity produced or turned out; data after processing by a computer'. This dictionary definition is the first clue to what this section is all about. If our best evidence comes from systematic reviews, then one of the most important things is how that systematic review gives us the result. From a clinical point of view we want to know how much benefit (or harm) a treatment will produce, and results of data processing might not be much help.

Utility – 'usefulness: the power to satisfy the wants of people in general'. This is the other part of the clue. If systematic reviews are to be useful, and therefore used, they have to present results in ways that are immediately accessible to ordinary professionals. When the average UK GP has just eight minutes to see a patient, working out what a hazard ratio or an effect size means will have little utility.

Definitions

Table 1.7.1 had a hypothetical trial of ibuprofen in acute pain. Not worrying too much at this stage about any other features or even the result itself, we will use this trial to present some of the more common

Table 1.7.1 Hypothetical acute pain trial

Treatment	Results of hypothetical randomised trial		
	Total number of patients treated	Number who achieved at least 50% pain relief	Number who did not achieve at least 50% pain relief
Ibuprofen 400 mg	40	22	18
Placebo	40	7	33
Calculations made from these results			
Experimental event rate (EER, event rate with ibuprofen)	22/40 = 0.55 or 55%		
Control event rate (CER, event rate with placebo)	7/40 = 0.18 or 18%		
Experimental event odds	22/18 = 1.2		
Control event odds	7/33 = 0.21		
Odds ratio	1.2/0.21 = 5.7		
Relative risk (EER/CER)	0.55/0.18 = 3.1		
NNT (1/(EER–CER))	1/(0.55–0.18) = 2.7		

definitions for presentation of results where information is available in dichotomous form. Dichotomous means the patient had the outcome or did not, and we have the numbers for each. In this trial, for instance, 22 of 40 patients given ibuprofen had adequate pain relief compared with only 7 of 40 given placebo. The term experimental event rate (EER) is used to describe the rate that good events occur with ibuprofen (22/40, or 55%) and control event rate (CER) to describe the rate that good events occur with placebo (7/40 or 18%).

Odds ratios. Table 1.7.1 shows first how to compute odds. Odds refers to the ratio of the number of people having the good event to the number not having the good event, so the experimental event odds are 22/18 or 1.2. The odds ratio is the ratio of the odds with experimental treatment and that of control, or here 1.2/0.21, 5.7. There are lots of different ways of computing odds ratios that give slightly different answers in different circumstances. Values greater than 1 show that experimental is better than control, and if a 95% confidence interval is calculated, statistical significance is assumed if the interval does not include 1.

For ibuprofen versus placebo the odds ratio is 5.7. Pick the bones out of that. How would you use that, other than knowing that an odds ratio that was far from 1 meant that ibuprofen was better than placebo.

Relative risk. Relative risk is a bit easier on the brain. It is simply the ratio of EER to CER, here 0.55/0.18 (or 55/18 for percentages), and is 3.1. Again values greater than 1 show that experimental is better than control, and if a 95% confidence interval is calculated, statistical significance is assumed if the interval does not include 1. Odds ratios and relative risk often give the same numerical value when they are low, but not when high. There is disagreement between eminent statisticians about which of these is 'best'. We use relative risk.

Again, knowing that the relative risk is 3.1 is not intuitively useful. Both relative risk and odds ratio are important ways of ensuring that there is statistical significance in our result. Unless there is statistical significance, we should not be using a treatment except in exceptional circumstances. So whatever else we do in the way of data manipulation, one or other of these tests has primacy for giving us the right to move on.

Number needed to treat. If we subtract the CER from the EER (EER–CER) then we have the absolute risk reduction (ARR), the effect due solely to ibuprofen, and nothing else. For every 100 patients with acute pain treated with ibuprofen, 37 (55–18) will have adequate pain relief because of the ibuprofen we have given them. Clearly then, we have to treat 100/37, or 2.7 patients with ibuprofen for one to benefit because of the ibuprofen they have been given. That is what numbers needed to treat (NNT) is (Table 1.7.1). This has immediate clinical relevance because we immediately know what clinical and other effort is being made to produce one result with a particular intervention.

The best NNT would be 1, where everyone got better with treatment and nobody got better with control, and NNTs close to 1 can be found with antibiotic treatments for susceptible organisms, for instance. Higher NNTs represent less good treatment, and the NNT is a useful tool for comparing two similar treatments. When doing so the NNT must always specify the comparator (e.g. placebo, no treatment, or some other treatment), the therapeutic outcome, and the duration of treatment necessary to achieve that outcome. If these are different, you probably should not be comparing NNTs. It is also worth mentioning that prophylactic interventions that produce small effects in large numbers of patients will have high NNTs, perhaps 20–100. Just because an NNT is large does not mean it will not be a useful treatment.

We can use the same methods for adverse events, when NNT become numbers needed to harm (NNH). Here small numbers are bad (more frequent harm) and larger numbers good. When making comparisons between treatments, the same provisos apply as for NNT, especially that for definition.

For both NNT and NNH we should recognise that we are working with an unusual scale which runs from 1 (everyone has outcome with treatment and none with control) to −1 (no-one has outcome with treatment and everyone has it with control), with infinity as the mid point where we divide by zero when EER equals CER. Once NNTs or NNHs are much above 10 the upper confidence interval gets closer to infinity and the upper and lower intervals look unbalanced.

Other outputs. There are masses of other outputs that people use for trials and epidemiological studies. These include effect size, relative risk reductions and so on. We do not find these useful, but their definitions are in Section 9.1.

Understanding different outputs

In order to see how the different outputs look, we can return again to a hypothetical trial of analgesic and placebo, though for convenience we use 1000 patients per group because we want to explore a range of possible results. In Table 1.7.2 we show six possible results in which the absolute proportion of patients benefiting with ibuprofen and placebo varies wildly, but the relative proportions stay the same.

This shows that the relative risk can stay exactly the same in the face of huge changes in NNT and absolute percentages of patients benefiting. It explains why statistical outputs like relative risk may be great for measuring statistical significance, but lack utility in everyday practice.

This table could be criticised because these are clearly different trials or conditions, where the event rate with placebo varies between 1% and 36% in 1000 patients. Indeed, this would be an obvious case

Table 1.7.2 Hypothetical trials with 1000 patients using different outputs each given ibuprofen or placebo

Trial	At least 50% pain relief		EER (%)	CER (%)	Relative risk	NNT
	Analgesic	Placebo				
1	800	360	80	36	2.2	2.3
2	400	180	40	18	2.2	4.6
3	200	90	20	9	2.2	9.1
4	100	45	10	5	2.2	18.2
5	50	23	5	2	2.2	37.0
6	20	9	2	1	2.2	90.9

where we would expect clinical heterogeneity in condition, its severity, patients recruited, or outcomes or duration. What is interesting is that using statistical tests for heterogeneity, this is a 'perfect' result. It underlines the fact that most statistical tests for heterogeneity are usually wrong, and even the one that is right is useless at detecting whether a group of trials is homogeneous or not [1].

A real example

Finally let us look at a real example, a single-patient meta-analysis of all the randomised single-dose trials of rizatriptan compared with placebo in acute migraine [2]. This is interesting because it looks at the four outcomes for migraine discussed in sections 1.2 and 1.3, and because it allows us to compute all the different outputs (Table 1.7.3).

In migraine, the absolute risk increase (ARI) is also called therapeutic gain. It really is difficult to know what to say about the first two columns, in that both odds ratios and relative risk tell us that rizatriptan 10 mg is better than placebo, but the numerical values are not helpful. ARI is a bit more helpful, but NNT is useful, and best of all is the absolute percentage of patients who will get each outcome if given 10 mg rizatriptan when they have a migraine.

Comment

We have found it most useful to follow the following procedures when looking at outputs from systematic reviews and meta-analyses:

1. First check on the statistical result.

2. If statistically significant, proceed to calculate an NNT. Use NNT to estimate the *treatment specific therapeutic effort* needed for one outcome and put some clinical relevance on the result.

3. If this seems sensible, look at what percentage of patients benefit (or are harmed) with treatment, and use this figure for every day work because this is immediately clinically relevant every time.

Table 1.7.3 Outputs of meta-analysis of rizatriptan 10 mg versus placebo for acute migraine [2]

Outcome	Odds ratio	Relative risk	ARI	NNT	Per cent
Headache response at 2 h	3.9 (3.4–4.5)	1.9 (1.7–2.0)	33	3.0 (2.8–3.4)	71
Pain free at 2 h	4.5 (3.8–5.2)	4.1 (3.4–4.9)	31	3.2 (3.0–3.5)	41
Sustained headache response over 24 h	2.5 (2.1–2.9)	2.1 (1.8–2.3)	19	5.3 (4.6–6.2)	37
Sustained pain free over 24 h	3.4 (2.8–4.0)	3.6 (2.9–4.5)	18	5.5 (4.9–6.4)	25
Bigger or smaller numbers better	Bigger	Bigger	Bigger	Smaller	Bigger

It seems to work, if only because we can remember and use percentages quite easily, and because that is what is relevant in everyday practice. It is also worth noting that the knowledge base of busy ordinary professionals may just not be up to other outputs. For example, a number of GPs in Wessex were asked about their knowledge of evidence-based terms in 1996 [3].

The questionnaire asked some penetrating questions about GPs' knowledge of technical terms used in evidence-based medicine (things like odds ratios, heterogeneity and the like). They used a very high hurdle – whether respondents understood the term and could explain it to others. Of all the terms, the one which came out top of this stiff test was the number needed to treat (NNT), with 35% of GPs being able to understand it and explain it to others (Figure 1.7.1).

What is also interesting is that GPs were able to spot that heterogeneity tests were not worth thinking about, that odds ratios lack intuitive utility, and that publication bias is something best left to academic pointy heads to argue about because it can never be proved or disproved. All we can say is that tests to detect publication bias do not work [4].

There is no one answer to what output works best for everyone, or anyone. The main thing is to be sure that you know and understand whatever output you choose, and especially not to be swayed by things like relative risk, or odds ratios, or relative risk reduction, or whatever, when some of these can be highly statistically significant but clinically irrelevant.

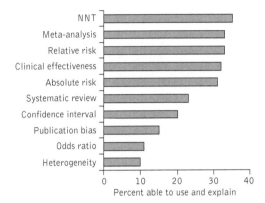

Figure 1.7.1 GPs' ability to explain and used evidence-based medicine terms.

References

1. Gavaghan, D. J. *et al.* (2000). An evaluation of homogeneity tests in meta-analyses in pain using simulations of individual patient data, *Pain* 85: 415–24.

2. Ferrari, M. D. *et al.* (2001). Meta-analysis of rizatriptan efficacy in randomised controlled clinical trials, *Cephalalgia* 21: 129–36.

3. McColl, A. *et al.* (1998). General practitioners' perceptions of the route to evidence based medicine: a questionnaire survey, *BMJ* 316: 361–5.

4. Sterne, J. A. *et al.* (2000). Publication and related bias in meta-analysis: Power of statistical tests and prevalence in the literature, *Journal of Clinical Epidemiology* 53(11): 1119–29.

1.8 **Adverse events**

One of the problems with adverse events is that they can be various things at various times. Some of the properties of adverse events are shown in Figure 1.8.1. There are at least three dimensions – common or rare, minor or major, reversible or permanent.

By and large, though, they fall into two distinct groups: they tend to be common, minor and reversible on the one hand, or rare, major and permanent on the other. Examples might be dry mouth with antidepressants, and upper gastrointestinal bleeding on the other.

We need to recognise the importance of adverse events. In the USA adverse drug reactions (ADR) have been found to be involved with large numbers of deaths, with fatal ADRs ranking in the fourth to sixth leading cause of death after heart disease, cancer, and stroke, and similar to pulmonary disease and accidents [1]. In hospitals, analgesics are associated with the single largest number, with opioids particularly a concern [2]. As well as the human dimension, adverse events are expensive. Studies of the cost of gastrointestinal bleeding due to NSAIDs across countries are consistent, and in the UK the estimate was a conservative £250 million (€410 million, $353 million) a year [3], and estimates from other countries confirm this size of expenditure.

Common, minor, reversible adverse events

Information on these may be present in clinical trial reports, but these are frequently matters of secondary importance to efficacy, and consequently they are poorly reported [4]. In a review of adverse event reporting in 192 randomised trials in seven clinical areas, the number of discontinuations was most commonly reported in 75% of trials, though the reason in only 46% [5]. Inadequate reporting was found in a full half of all the randomised trials (Table 1.8.1) [5].

A similar picture can be seen in acute pain trials from systematic reviews of paracetamol and ibuprofen [4]. Table 1.8.2 shows that full

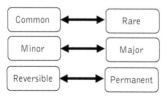

Figure 1.8.1 Properties of adverse events.

Table 1.8.1 Adequacy of reporting of adverse events in 192 randomised trials

Reporting of safety	Percent of trials	Range
Discontinuations because of harm		
Number per arm given	75	30–100
Reasons per arm given	46	20–68
Clinical adverse events		
Adequate reporting	39	0–62
Partially adequate reporting	11	0–20
Inadequate reporting	50	22–100
Laboratory defined toxicity		
Adequate reporting	29	0–62
Partially adequate reporting	8	0–20
Inadequate reporting	63	25–100

Range refers to the limits found in each of seven clinical areas.

Table 1.8.2 Adverse event assessment and reporting methods in 55 paracetamol and ibuprofen acute pain trials

	Number	Percent
Method of Assessment		
Spontaneous	7	13
Patient diaries	18	33
Direct questioning	6	11
Not stated	19	35
Adverse effects not reported	2	4
Reporting of adverse events		
Adverse effect information not reported	2	4
No adverse effects occurred	6	11
No difference as only mention	2	4
No details on frequency and type	8	15
Full details on frequency and type	34	62

details on frequency and type of adverse events were seen in just over a half of all trials.

Adverse events can be collected in systematic reviews, and some systematic reviews do this, though many unfortunately ignore adverse effects of treatment. Because reporting is commonly not done in any standard way in clinical trials, we usually make do with one of several ways of reporting adverse events:

• Patients reporting any adverse event: This collects information on all patients who had any complaint, of any severity.

• Particular adverse events: This collects patient information about specific (hopefully well defined) adverse events.

◆ Severe adverse events: If there is a definition of an adverse event that has a clinically evident severe consequence.

If reported, information can be dealt with in the same way as with efficacy, using L'Abbé plots, statistical tests, numbers needed to harm, and finally percentage of patients with the event. The biggest problem is that adverse events often occur less frequently than do efficacious ones, and that means amounts of information available are often inadequate for a sensible answer. Adverse events are more complicated to assess and analyse because there may be several different types of adverse events with different severity. The importance of an adverse event also depends on the patient (cannot possibly do with a dry mouth or inability to drive a car) and his/her condition (constipation after bowel surgery). How should all these different measures be taken into account? In addition, different methods of collecting common adverse events produces different results, and right now we just do not have a clue whether any one method is better than any other [4].

The method of assessment (spontaneous report, checklist and patient diary) and data provided by the informed consent form affects the incidence of adverse events, and that complicates the comparison of results across trials. This was shown by Edwards [4] who sought and analysed for adverse events all RCTs of single oral doses of paracetamol and ibuprofen in postoperative pain. In 55 trials, 33% used patient diaries, 13% spontaneous reporting, and 11% direct questioning, but a third did not mention the method used (Table 1.8.2). This was important, because for both paracetamol and ibuprofen patient diaries were more sensitive in reporting adverse events compared with spontaneous reporting or direct questioning. Adverse event rates were very similar in the active and control (placebo) groups indicating that most 'adverse events' were probably not due to the analgesic itself but could have been caused by the intervention or anaesthesia given. This makes identifying an adverse event that is solely due to the analgesic being used difficult because circumstances create background noise.

Adverse events are uncommon with single doses of analgesics and the statistical power of the trial is usually calculated for efficacy and not adverse events. Information from several studies can produce more useful information about adverse events though numbers can be low. The meta-analysis of tramadol in postoperative pain [6] showed that increasing the dose of tramadol also increased the incidence of adverse events.

Rare, major and permanent adverse events

This is even more tricky territory, because by their very rarity these are unlikely to be seen in randomised trials, and therefore in systematic reviews. There are exceptions. For instance, because there were a large number of randomised trials of propofol used for the induction of anaesthesia it was possible to discern a relationship between the use of propofol, bradycardia, asystole, and cardiac death [7]. This is so unusual, however, that it is unlikely to be repeated.

More often information on rare and serious adverse events will be found in epidemiological studies. Examples are those that examined the relationship between NSAID use and upper gastrointestinal bleeding [8,9], and NSAID use and renal failure [10] and heart failure [11]. Sometimes using information from different study architectures we will be able to turn relative risks into absolute risks, as has been done with NSAIDs and upper gastrointestinal bleeding [12].

Because gastrointestinal safety is a major issue when comparing COX-2-selective drugs with non-selective NSAIDs studies have been specifically designed and powered to analyse adverse events. This approach has been attempted for the COX-2-selective drugs in the CLASS- [13] and VIGOR-studies [14], as well as meta-analyses of randomised trials [15,16]. A total of 8000 patients were enrolled in both large randomised trials and they and the meta-analyses showed that COX-2-selectivity decreased the risk for GI-complications by about 50%.

These large studies do provide an estimate of the incidence of rare but serious events; they tell us that the annual risk of a gastrointestinal bleed may be 1–2%, but give no indication of the severity, which could include death. Tramèr *et al.* [12] used a new model to quantitatively estimate rare adverse events which follow a biological progression. They searched systematically for any report of chronic (≥ 2 months) use of NSAIDs which gave information on gastroduodenal ulcer, bleed or perforation, death due to these complications, or progression from one level of harm to the next. In addition to 15 RCTs (nearly 20,000 patients exposed to NSAIDs), three cohort studies (over 215,000 patients), six case-control studies (about 3000 cases) and 20 case series (7400 cases), and about 4450 case reports were analysed. In RCTs the incidence of bleeding/perforation was 0.69% with two deaths. Of the over 11,000 patients with bleeding/perforation with or without NSAID exposure across all reports an average of 12% died. The risk was lowest in RCTs and highest in case reports. Death from bleeding/perforation in all controls not exposed to NSAIDs occurred in 0.002%. From these numbers the authors calculated the NNT for one patient to die due to gastroduodenal complications with chronic NSAIDs as $1/[0.69 \times (12–0.002\%)] = 1220$. On average one in 1200 patients taking NSAIDs for at least two months will die from gastroduodenal complications who would not have died had they not taken NSAIDs.

Balancing benefit and harm

Balancing benefit and harm by comparing NNTs and NNHs is justified only if both values are reliable. Single dose analgesic studies (2898 patients, 1606 receiving ibuprofen, and 1292 placebo) in postoperative pain suggest an NNT of about 3 for 50% pain relief after 400 mg of oral ibuprofen. The respective NNH for any patient experiencing any adverse event is about 25. We know that roughly 16% of the patients have at least 50% pain relief with placebo (control event rate is 16%) and that most common analgesics have experimental event rates (proportion of patients having at least 50% pain relief with the active drug) in the range of 40–60%. The group size required to obtain a probability of 0.95 would be >500 if the EER is 40% [17]. The control event rate for adverse events is 15% and the common analgesics cause an adverse event in 19% of the patients. The group size to obtain a probability of 0.95 would be >2000 [18]. With sufficient information, plots of NNT versus NNH might be useful aides in making clinical or policy decisions.

Knowledge of the absolute risk of an event is important for patient and professional. Older patients might trade a 1 in 1000 risk for good pain relief, while younger patients might not (Edwards *et al.*, unpublished observations). Paradoxically most prescribing advice for Cox-2 inhibitors is that they be given preferentially to people older than 65 years, but not younger people unless there is an increased risk.

Patient withdrawal from a study due to adverse events is considered as major harm and is most commonly reported [5]. The dropout figures in clinical trials may not reflect the real-life situation, as patient compliance may be good during short clinical trials but not thereafter. One way to achieving more realistic estimates of patient preference may be to ask the patient to balance benefit and harm: how much and what adverse events are an acceptable price for a certain amount of pain relief? Studies on drugs affecting the CNS (e.g. antidepressants and anticonvulsants) often have to use a design where the patient titrates him/herself to the dose that gives adequate pain relief or the highest tolerated dose even if pain relief is not adequate.

Comment

Adverse events represent a challenge. The first is that patients are all too infrequently asked their views on adverse events and the balance between harm and benefit of treatment. Even young, well educated, modern women who might be expected to understand an important personal life event like use of oral contraceptives could completely misunderstand this [19]. It is not helped when we have inadequate information on the harms that can attend treatment.

There is a raft of problems in defining adverse events, in measuring them, and in reporting them. Very few studies set out specifically to collect information on adverse events. This is a disgrace. It makes it very difficult when we try and establish whether a group of drugs have a class effect [20] or whether two drugs are equivalent [21].

Finally we should never forget the inverse rule of three. This says that if we have seen no serious adverse event in 1500 exposed patients, we can be 95% sure that they do not occur more frequently than 1 in

500 patients. Few new drugs have been tested in more than a few thousand patients when they first become commercially available. This makes case reports, yellow cards, and properly done postmarketing surveillance important.

References

1. Lazarou, J. *et al.* (1998). Incidence of adverse drug reactions in hospitalized patients, *JAMA* 279: 1200–5.
2. Bates, D. W. *et al.* (1995). Incidence of adverse drug events and potential adverse drug events, *JAMA* 274: 29–34.
3. Moore, R. A. and Phillips, C. J. (1999). Cost of NSAID adverse effects to the UK National Health Service, *Journal of Medical Economics* 2: 45–55.
4. Edwards, J. E. *et al.* (1999). Reporting of adverse effects in clinical trials should be improved. Lessons from acute postoperative pain, *Journal of Pain Symptom Management* 81: 289–97.
5. Ioannidis, J. P. A. and Lau, J. (2001). Completeness of safety reporting in randomized trials: an evaluation of 7 medical areas, *JAMA* 285: 437–43.
6. Moore, R. A. and McQuay, H. J. (1997). Single-patient data meta-analysis of 3453 postoperative patients: Oral tramadol versus placebo, codeine and combination analgesics, *Pain* 69: 287–94.
7. Tramèr, M. *et al.* (1997). Propofol and bradycardia: causation, frequency and severity, *British Journal of Anaesthesia* 78: 642–51.
8. Henry, D. *et al.* (1993). Variability in the risk of major gastrointestinal complications from nonaspirin nonsteroidal anti-inflammatory drugs, *Gastroenterology* 105: 1078–88.
9. Hernandez-Diaz, S. and Rodridguez, L. A. G. (2000). Association between nonsteroidal anti-inflammatory drugs and upper gastrointestinal tract bleeding/perforation, *Archives of Internal Medicine* 160: 2093–9.
10. Henry, D. *et al.* (1997). Consumption of non-steroidal anti-inflammatory drugs and the development of functional renal impairment in elderly subjects. Results of a case-control study, *British Journal of Clinical Pharmacology* 44: 85–90.
11. Page, J. and Henry, D. (2000). Consumption of NSAIDs and the development of congestive heart failure in elderly patients, *Archives of Internal Medicine* 160: 777–84.
12. Tramer, M. R. *et al.* (2000). Quantitative estimation of rare adverse events which follow a biological progression: a new model applied to chronic NSAID use, *Pain* 85: 169–82.
13. Silverstein, F. E. *et al.* (2000). Gastrointestinal toxicity with celecoxib vs nonsteroidal anti-inflammatory drugs for osteoarthritis and rheumatoid arthritis. The CLASS study: a randomised controlled trial, *JAMA* 284: 1247–55.
14. Combardier, B. *et al.* (2000). Comparison of Upper Gastrointestinal Toxicity of Rofecoxib and Naproxen in Patients with Rheumatoid Arthritis, *NEJM* 343: 1520–8.

15. Langman, M. J. *et al.* (1999). Adverse upper gastrointestinal effects of rofecoxib compared with NSAIDs, *JAMA* 282: 1929–33.

16. Bensen, W. G. *et al.* (2000). Upper gastrointestinal tolerability of celecoxib, a COX-2 specific inhibitor, compared to naproxen and placebo, *Journal of Rheumatology* 27: 1876–83.

17. Moore, R. A. *et al.* (1998). Size is everything—large amounts of information are needed to overcome random effects in estimating direction and magnitude of treatment effects, *Pain* 78: 209–16.

18. Edwards, J. E. (2000). Determination of analgesic efficacy and harm in acute postoperative pain using systematic review methods, DPhil Thesis, University of Oxford.

19. Edwards, J. E. *et al.* (2000). Women's knowledge of, and attitudes to, contraceptive effectiveness and adverse health effects, *British Journal of Family Planning* 26: 73–80.

20. McAlister, F. A. *et al.* (1999). Users' Guides to the Medical Literature. XIX. Applying clinical trial results B. Guidelines for determining whether a drug is exerting (more than) a class effect, *JAMA* 282: 1371–7.

21. McAlister, F. A. and Sackett, D. L. (2001). Active-control equivalence trials and antihypertensive agents, *American Journal of Medicine* 111: 553–8.

1.9 **Placebo**

This is perhaps one of the most difficult of all topics, especially with a subjective outcome like pain. If we were discussing a topic like myocardial infarction and our outcome were death, then we might be reasonably sure that a placebo would have no effect on the outcome. But with pain, we might surmise that patients would feel better, and consequently have less pain, if the doctor or nurse was nice to them, or appeared authoritative, or the placebo were given as a big red capsule instead of a tiny white pill, or as an injection and not a tablet. Whatever we think, proving it will be difficult because of the problems of size, as discussed in section 1.6.

Table 1.9.1 summarises effects that we might expect to find in various control groups [1].

It's all very complicated, and made more so by difficulty in proving that 'negativity', or 'interaction', or 'expectation' contribute anything at all to the actual perception of pain as it is measured. We don't help ourselves by lax, if understandable, shorthand. When we want to discuss the effect that we observe when patients are given a placebo, we call it the 'placebo effect'. Immediately that can be retranslated as 'the effect *caused by* placebo'. The simple fact is that this causation is not proven, and possibly unprovable given the huge numbers of patients we would need to demonstrate a small difference.

Common misconceptions

There are a number of misconceptions about placebo, and they are worth examining because they are highly instructive.

Misconception 1. *For every intervention, a fixed fraction of the population, usually a third responds to placebo, whatever the outcome.* This just is not so. In Table 1.9.2 is listed rates of response with placebo in a number of clinical conditions in acute and chronic pain conditions.

Table 1.9.1 Effects in control groups

Control	Effects
Waiting list	Natural course of disease *minus* the negativity from nothing being done
Visits without treatment	Natural course of disease *plus* doctor/nurse/patient interaction
Placebo	Natural course of disease *plus* interaction *plus* expectation that there will be an effect
Active control	Natural course of disease *plus* interaction *plus* expectation *plus* actual effect

Table 1.9.2 Response rates with placebo in acute and chronic pain conditions

Pain condition	Treatment	Outcome	Duration	Number given placebo	Per cent with pain relief with placebo
Acute postoperative pain	Oral analgesics	At least 50% pain relief	4–6 h	12,000	18
Strains and sprains	Topical NSAID	At least 50% pain relief	7 days	3239	39
Migraine	Oral triptan	No pain or mild pain	2 h	3148	28
Migraine	Oral triptan	Pain free	2 h	2661	7
Dysmenorrhoea	Oral analgesics	At least 50% pain relief	About 1 day	1607	22
Trigeminal neuralgia	Antiepileptics	At least 50% pain relief	3–7 months	224	18
Diabetic neuropathy	Tricyclic antidepressant	At least 50% pain relief	3–7 months	200	36
Diabetic neuropathy	Topical capsaicin	Pain at least much better	4–8 weeks	165	49
Atypical facial pain	Tricyclic antidepressant	At least 50% pain relief	3–7 months	85	35
Postherpetic neuralgia	Tricyclic antidepressant	At least 50% pain relief	3–7 months	68	12

Despite different sizes, there is a wide range of response from 7% for the response of freedom from pain 2 h after a pain of moderate or severe intensity with a migraine, to 49% of patients with diabetic neuropathy saying their pain is at least much better after eight weeks of treatment with a topical placebo. For some of the chronic painful conditions we have pitifully little information and the estimates may just be wrong, but even where we have large amounts of data there is wide variation. Why are we surprised? Would we not expect a large response if we do nothing in strains and sprains over a week, when a fair proportion are going to get better anyway? People with a migraine will rarely have it next week, at least not the same attack.

The real issue here is how hard the outcome is to attain. In section 1.2 we looked at measurement of pain in migraine, with outcomes of:

- no pain or mild pain at 2 h;
- no pain at 2 h;
- no pain or mild pain at two hours and pain not returned and no analgesics over 24 h;
- no pain at two hours and pain not returned and no analgesics over 24 h.

We might guess that no pain is harder to achieve than mild pain, and that no return of pain plus no additional analgesics over 24 h is more difficult to achieve than outcomes over only two hours. Not surprisingly, we find 35–40% of people can obtain no pain or mild pain at two hours, but that only about 10% have no pain. Fewer people have a favourable outcome over 24 h than over two hours (Figure 1.9.1). No surprise there, then.

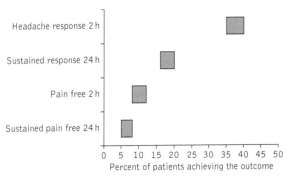

Figure 1.9.1 Responses to placebo in migraine using different outcome measures. Bars represent the 95% confidence interval of the response.

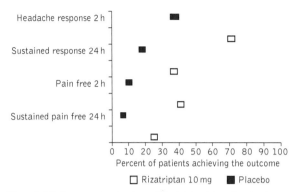

Figure 1.9.2 Responses to placebo and rizatriptan 10 mg in migraine using different outcome measures. Bars represent the 95% confidence interval of the response.

Misconception 2. *The placebo response is a fixed fraction (about a third) of the maximum effect of treatment – the bigger the treatment effect the bigger the placebo response.* This idea came from an analysis of five randomised trials [2]. It has been shown that this relationship held in acute pain studies only when mean values of skewed TOTPAR data were used, and could not be demonstrated when median values were used [3]. It was an artefact of incorrect use of data.

Of course it may be the case that when the outcome is easier to attain, both the response to placebo and the response to treatment are likely to be higher. Figure 1.9.2 is a replotting of Figure 1.9.1 with the addition of the response from rizatriptan 10 mg. There is a general relationship based on degree of difficulty of the outcome, but it is not a fixed fraction.

Misconception 3. *The more invasive the method of delivering a treatment, the higher will be the response to placebo – injection will give bigger response than tablets.* Again this is not so. Table 1.9.3 shows that while we have relatively small numbers of patients given intramuscular placebo, the proportion of patients having at least 50% pain relief is no bigger than with oral administration of tablets. The same complete lack of any difference can be seen in an analysis of responses to placebo with different routes of administration in migraine (Table 1.9.4). Though injection has been claimed to give higher response rates to placebo in migraine [4], this was based on an analysis of a limited data set.

Misconception 4. *Randomisation of different numbers of patients to active and placebo can affect the response to placebo.* This final

Table 1.9.3 Response to placebo in acute postoperative pain by oral and injection administration of placebo

Active intervention	Route	Number given placebo	Per cent with at least 50% pain relief
All placebo	**Oral + IM**	**>12,000**	**18**
Aspirin 600/650 mg	Oral	2562	16
Ibuprofen 400 mg	Oral	2183	14
Paracetamol 600/650 mg	Oral	613	22
Paracetamol 600/650 mg plus codeine 60 mg	Oral	432	20
Tramadol 100 mg	Oral	414	8
Morphine 10 mg	IM	460	16
Ketorolac 30 mg	IM	183	23

Table 1.9.4 Response to placebo in acute migraine by oral and injection administration of placebo

Route of administration	Number of trials	2-h headache response with placebo (number/total)	Per cent responders (95% CI)
Oral	30	875/3148	28 (26 to 29)
Subcutaneous	14	382/1257	30 (28 to 33)
Intranasal	6	205/650	32 (28 to 35)

Data are from patients given placebo in randomised, double blind trials of migraine diagnosed using IHS criteria and with initial pain of moderate or severe intensity

misconception comes again from the migraine field. It has been claimed that randomisation to different proportions of active treatment and placebo can affect the response with placebo. This was on the basis of one trial in which 16 patients were randomised to active treatment for every one randomised to placebo. Fifty-six patients were randomised to placebo, and the response rate at 2 h for no pain or mild pain, or just no pain, was high (Figure 1.9.3). The answer, though, was that with 56 patients the 95% confidence interval of the response rate included that of the overall response rate from all randomisation schedules.

Comment

Placebo is important, especially in the ethical context in any trial investigating pain and analgesia. It has to be taken seriously, but mainly

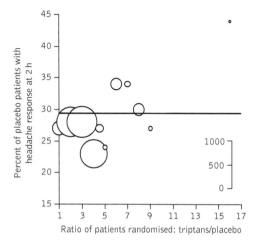

Figure 1.9.3 Different randomisation rates in migraine trials. Two hour headache response, with black horizontal line showing overall response with placebo.

from the point that it tells us what happens without treatment. Claims that the placebo response can be manipulated – that is by doing things differently patients get more pain relief from doing nothing – have to be taken with a large pinch of salt. If based on any observation, it will either be a non-randomised observation, or a tiny population or both.

References

1. Kalso, E. and Moore, R. A. (2000). Five easy pieces on evidence-based medicine (2), *European Journal of Pain* 4: 321–4.
2. Evans, F. J. (1974). The placebo response in pain reduction. In: Bonica, J. J. (ed.), *Advances in neurology* (vol. 4) New York, Raven Press, pp. 289–96.
3. McQuay, H. *et al.* (1996). Variation in the placebo effect in randomised controlled trials of analgesics: All is as blind as it seems, *Pain* 64: 331–5.
4. de Craen, A. J. *et al.* (2000). Placebo effect in the acute treatment of migraine: subcutaneous placebos are better than oral placebos, *Journal of Neurology* 247: 183–8.

1.10 **Being sure of a result**

This section could better be described as 'bullshit detection'. It aims to draw together ideas about bias and error from preceding sections and use them with examples of how systematic reviews can mislead. This is more important than most of us realise. Entire countries have changed medical policy on the basis of flawed research. An uncritical acceptance of results of systematic reviews and meta-analysis is almost as bad as not using them at all. Many of the sources we think of as being or aiming to be impeccable, like government agencies, academics or even the Cochrane Collaboration, produce reports that are just plain rubbish.

First steps in bullshit detection – scoring systems

Section 1.5 outlined many sources of bias. The major ones are randomisation and blinding. Examples were given of results of systematic reviews where sensitivity analysis in the report or subsequently demonstrated that results were completely different between randomised and non-randomised, or blind and unblind trials.

Scoring trials for bias. These are the major sources of bias in clinical trials of efficacy, and the frequently used Oxford five-point scoring system [1] uses three criteria (for details see section 1.5):

1. Is the trial randomised (1 point)? Additional point if method is given and appropriate.
2. Is the trial double-blind (1 point)? Additional point if method given and appropriate.
3. Were withdrawals and dropouts described and assigned to different treatments (1 point)?

Trials that scored 3 or more were relatively free of bias and could be trusted. Lower scores were shown to be associated with increased treatment effects – they were biased (section 1.5).

Scoring trials for validity. The Oxford pain validity scale (OPVS; for details see section 6.1) was designed specifically to examine issues regarding validity in pain trials [2]. It uses eight criteria (16 points total) in randomised trials, including blinding, size, statistics, dropouts, credibility of statistical significance and authors' conclusions, baseline measures and outcomes to examine whether a trial might be considered valid or not.

The scale was applied in a systematic review of back and neck pain. In 13 trials the conclusions of the original authors were found to be incorrect in two cases (and as an aside, this is not an uncommon

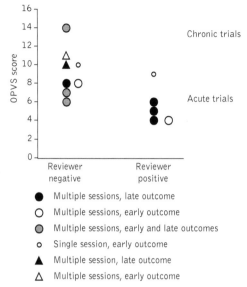

Figure 1.10.1 Validity scores of positive and negative trials of acupuncture for back and neck pain based on reviewer conclusions.

problem in clinical trial reporting, or even systematic reviews, where frank errors change the results). Using reviewers' conclusions, more valid trials were significantly more likely to have a negative conclusion (Figure 1.10.1).

Scoring systematic reviews for believability. There is also the excellent Oxman & Guyatt guide for evaluating the scientific quality (i.e. adherence to scientific principles) of research overviews (review articles) published in the medical literature [3]. It is not intended to measure literary quality, importance, relevance, originality, or other attributes of overviews, but is very useful as a guide to whether a review has the quality you need to use it. Details are in Section 9.2. Like all such guides, it will never stop all bad reviews, but few should get through.

The guide has been applied to systematic reviews of pain topics [4]. And the results are worth noting because they teach us much about the need for scepticism when reading systematic reviews. Seventy reports were included in the quality assessment. The earliest report was from 1980. Over two thirds appeared after 1990. Reviews considered between two and 196 primary studies (median 28). Sixty reviews reached positive conclusions, 7 negative, 12 uncertain and one

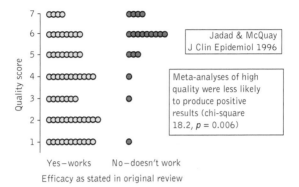

Figure 1.10.2 Oxman & Guyatt guide applied to reviews of pain topics.

did not manage any conclusion. All were based on published data only (no individual patient data analysis), without validity checks with the study investigators.

The median agreed overall Oxman & Guyatt score for the systematic reviews was 4 (range 1–7). Systematic reviews of high quality were significantly less likely to produce positive results (Figure 1.10.2). Sixteen of the 19 systematic reviews with negative or uncertain results had overall quality scores above the median, compared with only 20 of the 60 with positive results. Systematic reviews restricted to RCTs were significantly less likely to produce positive conclusions (19 of the 31) than those which included other study architectures (41 of the 49). All conclusions from systematic reviews of psychological interventions were positive. In only one of those reviews was quality scored above the median. All abstracts scored below the median, and 6 out of the 8 abstracts received the minimum possible score.

Second steps in bullshit detection – subtle influences

Many people are quite rightly exercised by the possibility of overt and covert influence of pharmaceutical companies over prescribing influences, especially academic links when so much funding for basic and clinical research comes from industry. Much thought has gone into declarations of interest by authors of papers, and many trees sacrificed for people to air their views. For the record, the single best declaration of interest ever is from David Sackett in a paper why randomised trials fail but need not [5].

What is often overlooked is the differing but important interests in the groves of what passes for academia, and in government. An example may help. We have made it up, but very similar ones can be found in many reviews, including places like the Cochrane Library.

You read a review on voodoo from the voodoo research fellow at the voodoo research institute. The acknowledgement says that the research fellow is supported by the voodoo society of Great Britain, representing all voodoo practitioners and setting standards for the practice of voodoo. Does this give you confidence in the results expressed, or are you doubly or even triply sceptical?

The point is this, whether we are talking voodoo, or acupuncture , or advice from prescribing advisors, or whatever. We all have our biases, sometimes overt, sometimes subconscious, sometimes the product of ignorance. When we examine systematic reviews of evidence we have to find ways to try and ensure that those biases are excluded or minimised.

Bullshit detection – simple suggestions

When faced with a systematic review we need to be able to pick the bones out of it. There are many, many things to look for, but it comes down to the following:

- *Searching*: Was the search strategy sensible and comprehensive?

- *Inclusion and exclusion*: Were the reasons for including studies or excluding them sensible?

- *Architecture*: Was the study architecture of included studies robust? Were they randomised and double blind as a minimum?

- *Validity*: Even when randomised and double blind, were the studies included valid? In acute pain, for instance, did patients have moderate or severe initial pain?

- *Outcomes*: Was the outcome chosen for the systematic review a clinically sensible one that you recognise as being of value to your patients?

- *Combining data*: In a meta-analysis were the trial results that were combined clinically homogeneous in terms of interventions used, doses of drugs, types of patients, severity of disease, duration of treatment or of observation?

- *Outputs*: Do you understand the output? Is it clinically relevant as well as being statistically significant?

- *Size*: Were there sufficient numbers of patients or outcomes to make sense of it even if everything else was perfect?

- *Conclusions*: Was the conclusion drawn by the authors of the review a sensible one based on the data they provide? If it was not, can you trust any of it?

- *And even then*: Still be a bit sceptical, because systematic review and meta-analysis is not the answer to everything, because your clinical appreciation is valid and you should not be stampeded into changing practice without good reason. You need to feel convinced.

Bullshit detection – some examples

In the next few pages systematic reviews will be selected for criticism. They may bear heavily on some complementary therapies because these reviews so often have problems, but we will try not to concentrate exclusively on this. Also, we will look at this from the point of view of the ordinary healthcare professional trying to decide whether these interventions make sense for our practice. Often the problems pointed out will have been pointed out by the authors of the original reviews, so let's say in advance that no slight is intended on the original authors' ability or intent. Their reviews just make good examples, but we begin with a *Bandolier* review of acupuncture for stroke because it shows how to use some of the scoring systems and suggestions.

Acupuncture for stroke

A full version of this review [6], with all references, can be found as HTML or PDF versions on the *Bandolier* Internet site.

Full published reports of RCTs of traditional and non-traditional acupuncture treatment for stroke rehabilitation were sought. Different search strategies were used to identify eligible reports and searching was comprehensive. Inclusion criteria were RCTs comparing acupuncture, with or without electrical stimulation, or laser acupuncture with a control group; patients had an acute stroke diagnosed by standard neurological tests; group size ≥10 and physical function outcomes.

There were seven studies with 505 patients that met the inclusion criteria. All seven included studies examined the effects of acupuncture on patients following a first stroke, using a parallel group design, where acupuncture plus a standard treatment was compared with standard treatment alone. None used sham acupuncture as a control. In all cases electrical stimulation of the acupuncture needles was used, and three studies reported that the stimulation intensity was sufficient to cause muscle contraction. The stimulation frequencies used in the studies ranged from 2 Hz to at least 25 Hz. Three studies were conducted in Scandinavia, and four in China or Taiwan.

A wide range of outcomes was described, and no study defined a primary outcome measure for effectiveness. Typically outcomes included some measure of motor function, some assessment of activities of daily living (Barthel's index), and frequently a patient assessed quality of life assessment (Nottingham Health Profile). No study was double blind. Three were single blind and used an observer blinded to the treatment given. The other studies made no attempt to blind the observations. Reporting quality overall was poor. One study had a quality score of

Table 1.10.1 Trials of acupuncture in stroke

Potential source of bias	Conclusion of original authors		Conclusion of reviewers	
	Positive	Negative	Positive	Negative
No source of bias considered	6	1	2	5
Double-blind trials	0	0	0	0
Observer-blind trials	2	1	0	3
Non-blind trials	4	0	2	2
Reporting quality 3 or more	0	1	0	1
Reporting quality 2 or less	6	0	2	4
Validity score 9 or more	1	1	0	2
Validity score 8 or less	5	0	2	3
European studies	2	1	1	2
Far east studies	4	0	1	3

Reporting quality using 0–5 scale (Jadad *et al.*, 1996); Validity scoring using 0–16 scale (Smith *et al.*, 2000); Geographical definitions (Vickers *et al.*, 1998)

three and all others were two or below. Validity scores were nine or above in two studies and the others ranged from four to eight.

In only one study did the original authors conclude that acupuncture was ineffective. In four studies reviewers did not agree with the authors' conclusions. The reason for the difference was because the data presented in the paper did not support their conclusion. Typically some derivative index (change from baseline) was compared between acupuncture and control and found to be better with acupuncture, while there remained no difference in the absolute values at either baseline or at the time of assessment. One study had results which were unbelievable, including identical control scores in 59 patients for seven different outcomes.

Overall, reviewers concluded that two studies had a positive result and five a negative (Table 1.10.1). The three observer-blind trials were judged to be negative. The single trial with a quality score of three was negative. The two trials with a validity score of nine or more we judged to be negative. Two of the three European studies we judged to be negative.

What is clear is that while there may be seven trials available, the judgement on those with least likelihood of bias was that acupuncture was ineffective. A particular problem was that the original authors overstated the efficacy of acupuncture, a good example of that bias from belief referred to above.

Acupuncture in dental pain

A review of the evidence for the effectiveness of acupuncture in treating acute dental pain [7] reported 'a positive result'. Based on

16 clinically controlled trials they concluded the data 'suggest that acupuncture is effective in alleviating pain during dental operations, postoperatively and during experimentally induced dental pain'. This was refuted in a letter [8]. The original review has been used to support acupuncture in a report on acupuncture from the Centre for Reviews and Dissemination, with the backing of the National Institute of Clinical Excellence.

Of the 16 trials included in the Ernst and Pittler review, five were not randomised. Of the remaining 11 trials, two made no attempt to blind patients. A further three trials were simply too small to provide meaningful data (group size <10). Of the remaining six trials, two were on experimental dental pain, and are therefore not appropriate to determine whether acupuncture is useful in alleviating clinical dental pain. One trial had an inadequate placebo condition, in that it looked at acupuncture versus acupuncture plus d-phenylalanine. We are then left with three trials, with a total of 110 patients, from which we may draw conclusions.

What of the randomised, double-blind trials? One trial with only 10 patients per group reported significantly better pain relief with 15 min of Ho-Ku acupuncture administered after surgery compared with placebo. Two trials looked at pain caused by drilling into the dentine. Both compared 30 min of Ho-Ku electro-acupuncture carried out during surgery with placebo (although a small number of patients received traditional acupuncture). Patients in one trial also received additional pre-surgery acupuncture. Both trials reported on a number of pain outcomes, and it was possible to pool data on three of these and the results are in Table 1.10.2.

Table 1.10.2 Analgesic effectiveness of acupuncture compared with placebo during dental restoration [8]

Efficacy measure	No. of trials	Success/total patients		
		Acupuncture	Placebo	Relative benefit (95% CI)
Pain reduction – patient rating*	2	40/46	33/44	1.2 (0.96–1.4)
Local anaesthetic required**	2	45/46	42/44	1.0 (0.94–1.1)
Dentist rating of procedure as successful	2	44/46	39/44	1.1 (0.96–1.2)
Patient rating of no pain	1	13/26	11/25	1.1 (0.63–2.1)
Pain reduction – dentist rating*	1	18/26	20/25	0.87 (0.63–1.2)

*success = pain reduction excellent or good; **success = no anaesthetic required

Not a single one of these trials would be regarded as valid for registration purposes if this were a new analgesic drug rather than acupuncture. So even though a prestigious document from a prestigious centre backed by a major government agency tells us that acupuncture works for dental pain, the evidence is just not there.

Perioperative mortality and anaesthetic technique

A systematic review and meta-analysis of anaesthetic technique concluded that [9] the risk of perioperative death was lower with neuraxial blockade than with general anaesthesia. On the basis of this review whole countries have changed their guidance on how anaesthesia should be conducted.

The review was exemplary in the way it searched for papers, found additional information, contacted authors, and extracted data. The aim was to find all trials where patients were randomised to neuraxial blockade or not. Patients receiving neuraxial blockade could also have general anaesthesia. Considerable effort went into extracting all useful data, but here we concentrate on mortality within 30 days of randomisation.

There were 141 trials with 9559 patients. There were 247 deaths within 30 days, recorded in 35 trials. There were nine trials with at least 10 deaths per trial, and these are shown in Figure 1.10.3 as a L'Abbé plot. For only three of these smaller trials was there a large effect of neuraxial blockade, and in these three there was an extraordinary high

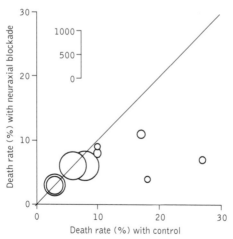

Figure 1.10.3 L'Abbé plot of perioperative mortality with neuraxial blockade or general anaesthesia.

Table 1.10.3 Sensitivity analysis of perioperative mortality according to the number and rate of deaths

Condition	Number of trials	Number of patients (% total)	Deaths/total (%)		Relative risk (95% CI)	NNT (95% CI)
			With neural blockade	Without neural blockade		
All trials	141	9559 (100)	103/4871 (2.1)	144/4688 (3.1)	0.7 (0.5–0.9)	98 (60–265)
Trials with fewer than 10 deaths	132	7067 (74)	32/3537 (0.9)	44/3530 (1.2)	0.7 (0.5–1.2)	n/c
Trials with more than 10 deaths	9	2492 (26)	71/1334 (5.3)	100/1158 (8.6)	0.6 (0.5–0.8)	30 (19–77)
Trials with more than 10 deaths 'AND with more than 100 patients (death rate in control less than 10%)	4	1889 (20)	49/1054 (4.6)	48/835 (5.7)	0.9 (0.6–1.4)	n/c
Trials with more than 10 deaths and with fewer than 100 patients (death rate in control more than 10%)	5	603 (6)	22/280 (7.9)	52/323 (16.1)	0.5 (0.3–0.8)	12 (7.5–32)
All trials with a death rate with control of less than 10%	136	8956 (94)	81/4591 (1.8)	92/4365 (2.1)	0.8 (0.6–1.1)	n/c

n/c = NNT not calculated because no significant difference

death rate with control of over 15%. For six other trials in which the death rate with control was below 15%, the death rates with neuraxial blockade and control were about the same.

This could be interpreted as some form of heterogeneity, and the L'Abbé plot was first suggested as an aid to detecting that all trials in a meta-analysis were giving the same sort of result [10]. Clearly here they were not homogeneous.

So some sensitivity analysis would seem in order. Much sensitivity analysis according to methodological issues had been done in the original paper, but not one according to event rates. Table 1.10.3 shows the results obtained for all 141 trials, and for those with more or fewer than 10 deaths. Clearly the latter show the largest treatment effect.

In those trials with more than 10 deaths, four with more than 100 patients per group have a death rate of below 10% and show no statistically significant effect of neuraxial blockade. Five trials had fewer than 100 patients per group and a death rate with control of over 10%, and show a very large effect.

If we exclude all trials with death rates of over 10% from the combined analysis, then the effect of neuraxial blockade is very small, perhaps reducing the death rate from 2.1% to 1.8%, a reduction that is not statistically significant, but in 136 trials with 94% of the patients.

Now this sensitivity analysis was not presented in the original paper, but had to be done by a thoughtful reader. The overall impression was that there was a statistically significant and important result. Clinically it may not have been regarded as so significant with a NNT (or NNH) of 98. But the review misled because it combined information from trials with death rates as high as 25%, and all the effect was in trials in death rates above 10%. Is this level of evidence worth changing a whole country's anaesthetic technique for?

Comment

Being sure of a result is one of the most difficult things. Even large, randomised trials are often subject to debate about their validity. There is no simple way in which we can defend ourselves. There is a complicated way. It involves vigilance, plus a working knowledge of things known likely to give an incorrect result, plus a large dose of scepticism.

References

1. Jadad, A. R. *et al.* (1996). Assessing the quality of reports of randomized clinical trials: is blinding necessary? *Controlled Clinical Trials* 17: 1–12.
2. Smith, L. A. *et al.* (2000). Teasing apart quality and validity in systematic reviews: an example from acupuncture trials in chronic neck and back pain, *Pain* 86: 119–32.
3. Oxman, A. and Guyatt, G. H. (1992). Index for the scientific quality of research overviews: Instructions and forms, obtained from the authors.

4. Jadad, A. R. and McQuay. H. J. (1996). Meta-analyses to evaluate analgesic interventions: a systematic qualitative review of their methodology, *Journal of Clinical Epidemiology* 49: 235–43.

5. Sackett, D. L. (2001). Why randomized controlled trials fail but needn't: 2. Failure to employ physiological statistics, or the only formula a clinician-trialist is ever likely to need (or understand!), *Canadian Medical Association Journal* 165: 1226–37.

6. Smith, L. A. *et al.* Assessing the evidence of effectiveness of acupuncture for stroke rehabilitation: stepped assessment of likelihood of bias. Bandolier Extra (www.jr2.ox.ac.uk/bandolier/booth/alternat/ACstroke.html).

7. Ernst, E. and Pittler, M. H. (1998). The effectiveness of acupuncture in treating acute dental pain: a systematic review, *British Dental Journal* 184: 443–7.

8. Smith, L. and Oldman, A. (1999). Acupuncture and dental pain, *British Dental Journal* 186: 158–9.

9. Rodgers, A. *et al.* (2000). Reduction of postoperative mortality and morbidity with epidural or spinal anaesthesia: results from overview of randomised trials, *BMJ* 321: 1493.

10. L'Abbé, K. A. *et al.* (1987). Meta-analysis in clinical research, *Annals of Internal Medicine* 107: 224–33.

Section 2
Acute pain

2.1 **Introduction**

Acute pain is not always well treated. For instance, a survey of UK hospitals [1] showed that many patients (medical and surgical) had moderate or severe pain in hospital (Table 2.1.1). The problem is not that we have ineffective treatments, but that the delivery of effective treatments is often ineffective. Dealing with acute pain is not just a question of doling out analgesics effectively, and there are many other features to dealing with acute pain in hospital [2] and elsewhere. This section is not a comprehensive survey of everything that might be done in any particular circumstance, but a look at the evidence behind what might commonly be used in many circumstances.

Acute pain trials

Measuring the efficacy of analgesics in acute pain is done in clinical trials that have been standardised over many years. These trials have to be randomised and double blind.

Typically, patients in the first few days after an operation will develop pain that is moderate or severe in intensity (Figure 1.4.1) and will then be given an analgesic or placebo. Pain will then be measured using standard pain intensity or pain relief scales (section 1.2) over 4 to 6 h. After a delay of usually 60–90 min, those who do not have adequate pain relief will be given additional analgesia (often called 'escape' analgesia), and for these patients it is usual to make no additional pain measurements, but for all subsequent pain intensity measures to revert to the initial pain intensity, and for all subsequent pain relief measures to revert to zero. This process ensures that analgesia from the escape analgesic is not wrongly ascribed to the test intervention.

A variety of pain outcomes can be chosen as the outcomes of the trial (section 1.3), and commonly several are reported, like summed pain intensity difference (SPID) or total pain relief (TOTPAR), or their visual analogue equivalents. For the purposes of meta-analysis the most commonly used outcome has become the percentage of

Table 2.1.1 Survey on inpatients in UK hospitals [1]

Problem	Number/total	Percent
Pain was present all or most of the time	1042/3162	33
Pain was severe or moderate	2755/3157	87
Pain was worse than expected	182/1051	17
Had to ask for drugs	1085/2589	42
Drugs did not arrive immediately	455/1085	41

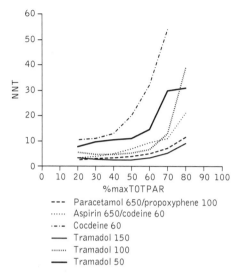

Figure 2.1.1 Numbers needed to treat (NNT) calculated at cut points of %maxTOTPAR between 20% and 80%.

patients in a treatment arm who achieve at least 50% of the maximum available pain relief (%maxTOTPAR). Methods have been developed and validated that reliably allow conversion of a variety of outcomes measures to %maxTOTPAR [3–5].

Half pain relief over 4 to 6 h is a high hurdle, and has been shown to distinguish between more and less effective analgesics (Figure 2.1.1) [6]. Although the outcome of half pain relief was chosen merely because it is half way between 0% and 100%, similar discrimination can be seen over a wide range of cut points from about 20% to 60% of maximum pain relief (Figure 2.1.1). Lower and higher values lose discrimination because all or none of the treatments can meet the outcome.

Acute pain trials usually have sufficient numbers of patients to be able to detect a difference between a test analgesic and placebo, which means using about 40 patients in each arm of the trial (section 1.6). This gives rise to much discrepancy between individual trials, and in, for instance, response rates with placebo. This becomes consistent at about 18% of patients given placebo in acute pain trials having at least 50% pain relief (Figure 1.6.5).

Pain models

A number of different clinical situations have been used to measure the efficacy of analgesics in acute pain, including third molar dental extraction, orthopaedic or general surgery. We know [7] that analgesics do not behave differently in different acute pain models.

Study design and validity

Even in the early days of pain measurement it was understood that the design of studies contributed directly to the validity of the result obtained. Trial designs lacking validity produce information that is at best difficult to use, and at worst is useless.

Placebo. People in pain respond to placebo treatment. Some patients given placebo obtain 100% pain relief (Figure 2.1.2), not because placebo 'gives' pain relief, but rather because these are patients whose pain, though initially moderate or severe, was not long lasting. The effect is reproducible, and some work has been done to try and assess the characteristics of the 'placebo responder', by sex, race and psychological profile. None has succeeded, but we do know that women have better responses to some analgesics than men, getting more analgesia from the same plasma concentration of drug.

Sensitivity. Particularly for a new analgesic, a trial should prove its internal sensitivity – the study was an adequate analgesic assay. This can be done in several ways (Figure 2.1.3). For instance, if a known analgesic (paracetamol) can be shown to have statistical difference from placebo, then the analgesic assay should be able to distinguish another analgesic of similar effectiveness. Alternatively, two different doses of a standard analgesic (e.g. morphine) could be used – showing the higher dose to be statistically superior to the lower dose again provides confidence that the assay is sensitive.

Failure to demonstrate sensitivity in one assay invalidates the results from that particular assay. The results could still be included in meta-analysis.

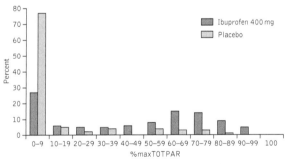

Figure 2.1.2 Analgesic responses to placebo and ibuprofen 400 mg in about 800 individuals.

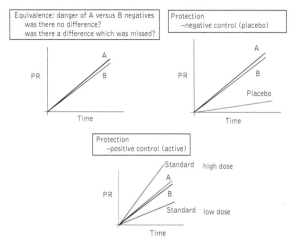

Figure 2.1.3 Using placebo or active comparators to protect against A versus B negative results.

Studies of analgesics of an A versus B design are notoriously difficult to interpret. If there is a statistical difference, then that suggests sensitivity. Lack of a significant difference means nothing – there is no way to determine whether there is an analgesic effect which is no different between A and B, or whether the assay lacks the sensitivity to measure a difference that is actually present.

Equivalence. A more difficult problem, if only because of the large variations that occur in pain studies [8,9]. Equivalence studies might take the form of two doses of a new analgesic compared with two doses of a standard analgesic, plus placebo to establish sensitivity. Simple calculations could show what dose of the new analgesic was equivalent to the usual dose of the standard analgesic.

Problems

The correct design of an analgesic trial is situation dependent. In some circumstances very complicated designs have to be used to ensure sensitivity and validity.

No gold standard. There may be circumstances in which there is no established analgesic treatment of sufficient effectiveness to act as a gold standard against which to measure a new treatment, often the case in chronic pain. Clearly, the use of placebo or non-treatment controls is of great importance, especially when effects are to be examined over prolonged periods of weeks or months.

But it is paradoxically these very circumstances in which ethical constraints act against using placebo or non-treatment controls because of the need to do *something*. In acute pain studies, conversely, there is little problem with using placebos, since the failure of placebo (or any treatment) can be dealt with by prescribing additional analgesics that should work.

When there is no pain to begin with. Clearly, where there is no pain it is difficult to measure an analgesic response. Yet a number of studies seek to do this by pre-empting pain, or using an intervention where there is no pain (intraoperatively, for instance) to produce analgesia when pain is to be expected.

These are difficult, but not impossible, circumstances in which to conduct research. Meticulous attention to trial design is necessary to be able to show differences.

Comment

For the purposes of this chapter, many of the intricacies of acute pain studies will be relegated to the sidelines, and we will concentrate on the effectiveness of single doses of analgesics or analgesic combinations when compared with placebo, and some other common procedures in acute pain.

References

1. Bruster, S. *et al.* (1994). National survey of hospital patients, *BMJ* 309: 1542–6.
2. McQuay, H. J. *et al.* (1997). Treating acute pain in hospital, *BMJ* 314: 1531–5.
3. Moore, A. *et al.* (1996). Deriving dichotomous outcome measures from continuous data in randomised controlled trials of analgesics, *Pain* 66: 229–37.
4. Moore, A. *et al.* (1997). Deriving dichotomous outcome measures from continuous data in randomised controlled trials of analgesics: Verification from independent data, *Pain* 69: 127–30.
5. Moore, A. *et al.* (1997). Deriving dichotomous outcome measures from continuous data in randomised controlled trials of analgesics: Use of pain intensity and visual analogue scales, *Pain* 69: 311–5.
6. Moore, R. A. and McQuay, H. J. (1997). Single-patient data meta-analysis of 3453 postoperative patients: Oral tramadol versus placebo, codeine and combination analgesics, *Pain* 69: 287–94.
7. Edwards, J. E. *et al.* (1999). Oral aspirin in postoperative pain: a quantitative systematic review, *Pain* 81: 289–97.
8. Jones, B. *et al.* (1996). Trials to assess equivalence: the importance of rigorous methods, *BMJ* 313: 36–9.
9. McQuay, H. and Moore, A. (1996). Placebos are essential when extent and variability of placebo response are unknown, *BMJ* 313: 1008.

2.2 League table of analgesics in acute pain

This league table was constructed for analgesics in acute pain. Data were taken from systematic reviews of randomised, double-blind, single-dose studies in patients with moderate to severe pain. For each review the outcome was identical – that is at least 50% pain relief over 4–6 h. The pain measurements were standardised, and have been validated.

The league table works because it only has apples, and is not a fruit salad. Only like is compared with like, and there is a common comparator throughout, namely placebo. Information is presented in a number of formats, but the definitive source is Table 2.2.1, which has

Table 2.2.1 The Oxford league table of analgesic efficacy

Analgesic	Number of patients in comparison	Percent with at least 50% pain relief	NNT	Lower confidence interval	Higher confidence interval
Ibuprofen 800	76	100	1.6	1.3	2.2
Ketorolac 20	69	57	1.8	1.4	2.5
Ketorolac 60 (intramuscular)	116	56	1.8	1.5	2.3
Diclofenac 100	411	67	1.9	1.6	2.2
Piroxicam 40	30	80	1.9	1.2	4.3
Paracetamol 1000 + Codeine 60	197	57	2.2	1.7	2.9
Oxycodone IR 5 + Paracetamol 500	150	60	2.2	1.7	3.2
Bromfenac 25	370	51	2.2	1.9	2.6
Rofecoxib 50	675	54	2.3	2.0	2.6
Diclofenac 50	738	63	2.3	2.0	2.7
Naproxen 440	257	50	2.3	2.0	2.9
Oxycodone IR 15	60	73	2.3	1.5	4.9
Ibuprofen 600	203	79	2.4	2.0	4.2
Ibuprofen 400	4703	56	2.4	2.3	2.6
Aspirin 1200	279	61	2.4	1.9	3.2

Table 2.2.1 (continued)

Analgesic	Number of patients in comparison	Percent with at least 50% pain relief	NNT	Lower confidence interval	Higher confidence interval
Bromfenac 50	247	53	2.4	2.0	3.3
Bromfenac 100	95	62	2.6	1.8	4.9
Oxycodone IR 10 + Paracetamol 650	315	66	2.6	2.0	3.5
Ketorolac 10	790	50	2.6	2.3	3.1
Ibuprofen 200	1414	45	2.7	2.5	3.1
Oxycodone IR 10 + Paracetamol 1000	83	67	2.7	1.7	5.6
Piroxicam 20	280	63	2.7	2.1	3.8
Diclofenac 25	204	54	2.8	2.1	4.3
Dextropropoxyphene 130	50	40	2.8	1.8	6.5
Bromfenac 10	223	39	2.9	2.3	4.0
Pethidine 100 (intramuscular)	**364**	**54**	**2.9**	**2.3**	**3.9**
Tramadol 150	561	48	2.9	2.4	3.6
Morphine 10 (intramuscular)	**946**	**50**	**2.9**	**2.6**	**3.6**
Naproxen 550	169	46	3.0	2.2	4.8
Naproxen 220/250	183	58	3.1	2.2	5.2
Ketorolac 30 (intramuscular)	**359**	**53**	**3.4**	**2.5**	**4.9**
Paracetamol 500	561	61	3.5	2.2	13.3
Paracetamol 1500	138	65	3.7	2.3	9.5
Paracetamol 1000	2759	46	3.8	3.4	4.4
Oxycodone IR 5 + Paracetamol 1000	78	55	3.8	2.1	20.0
Paracetamol 600/ 650 + Codeine 60	1123	42	4.2	3.4	5.3
Ibuprofen 100	396	31	4.3	3.2	6.3
Paracetamol 650 + Dextropropoxyphene (65 mg hydrochloride or 100 mg napsylate)	963	38	4.4	3.5	5.6
Aspirin 600/650	5061	38	4.4	4.0	4.9
Paracetamol 600/650	1886	38	4.6	3.9	5.5

Table 2.2.1 (continued)

Analgesic	Number of patients in comparison	Percent with at least 50% pain relief	NNT	Lower confidence interval	Higher confidence interval
Ibuprofen 50	316	31	4.7	3.3	7.9
Tramadol 100	882	30	4.8	3.8	6.1
Tramadol 75	563	32	5.3	3.9	8.2
Aspirin 650 + Codeine 60	598	25	5.3	4.1	7.4
Oxycodone IR 5 + Paracetamol 325	149	24	5.5	3.4	14.0
Ketorolac 10 (intramuscular)	142	48	5.7	3.0	53.0
Paracetamol 300 + Codeine 30	379	26	5.7	4.0	9.8
Bromfenac 5	138	20	7.1	3.9	28.0
Tramadol 50	770	19	8.3	6.0	13.0
Codeine 60	1305	15	16.7	11.0	48.0
Placebo	>10,000	18	N/A	N/A	N/A

NNT are calculated for the proportion of patients with at least 50% pain relief over 4–6 h compared with placebo in randomised, double-blind, single-dose studies in patients with moderate to severe pain. Drugs were oral, unless specified, and doses are milligrams. Bold rows are intramuscular administration.

the number of patients in the comparison, the percent with at least 50% pain relief with analgesic, the number needed to treat (NNT) and the high and low 95% confidence interval.

Also presented is a simplified table (Table 2.2.2) with information on common doses of common analgesics. Two figures (Figures 2.2.1 and 2.2.2) present information on common analgesic doses giving NNTs, and in terms of percentages of patients achieving at least 50% pain relief.

Understanding the league table

Effective relief can be achieved with oral non-opioids and non-steroidal anti-inflammatory drugs (NSAIDs). Analgesic efficacy is expressed as the NNT, the number of patients who need to receive the active drug for one to achieve at least 50% relief of pain compared with placebo over a 4–6 h treatment period. The most effective drugs have a low NNT of just over 2. This means that for every two patients who receive the drug one patient will get at least 50% relief because of

Table 2.2.2 The Oxford league table of analgesic efficacy
(commonly used analgesic doses)

Analgesic	Number of patients in comparison	Percent with at least 50% pain relief	NNT	Lower confidence interval	Higher confidence interval
Diclofenac 100	411	67	1.9	1.6	2.2
Paracetamol 1000 + Codeine 60	197	57	2.2	1.7	2.9
Rofecoxib 50	675	54	2.3	2.0	2.6
Diclofenac 50	738	63	2.3	2.0	2.7
Naproxen 440	257	50	2.3	2.0	2.9
Ibuprofen 600	203	79	2.4	2.0	4.2
Ibuprofen 400	4703	56	2.4	2.3	2.6
Ketorolac 10	790	50	2.6	2.3	3.1
Ibuprofen 200	1414	45	2.7	2.5	3.1
Piroxicam 20	280	63	2.7	2.1	3.8
Diclofenac 25	204	54	2.8	2.1	4.3
Pethidine 100 (intramuscular)	364	54	2.9	2.3	3.9
Morphine 10 (intramuscular)	946	50	2.9	2.6	3.6
Naproxen 550	169	46	3.0	2.2	4.8
Naproxen 220/250	183	58	3.1	2.2	5.2
Ketorolac 30 (intramuscular)	359	53	3.4	2.5	4.9
Paracetamol 500	561	61	3.5	2.2	13.3
Paracetamol 1000	2759	46	3.8	3.4	4.4
Paracetamol 600/ 650 + Codeine 60	1123	42	4.2	3.4	5.3
Paracetamol 650 + Dextropropoxyphene (65 mg hydrochloride or 100 mg napsylate)	963	38	4.4	3.5	5.6
Aspirin 600/650	5061	38	4.4	4.0	4.9
Paracetamol 600/650	1886	38	4.6	3.9	5.5
Tramadol 100	882	30	4.8	3.8	6.1
Tramadol 75	563	32	5.3	3.9	8.2
Aspirin 650 + Codeine 60	598	25	5.3	4.1	7.4
Paracetamol 300 + Codeine 30	379	26	5.7	4.0	9.8
Tramadol 50	770	19	8.3	6.0	13.0
Codeine 60	1305	15	16.7	11.0	48.0

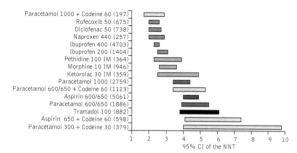

Figure 2.2.1 Common analgesics – NNTs (number in parenthesis is total in comparison).

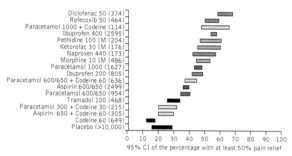

Figure 2.2.2 Common analgesics – percent of patients with at least 50% pain relief (number in parenthesis is total given analgesic).

the treatment (the other patient may or may not obtain relief but it does not reach the 50% level).

The NNT is treatment-specific, and is drug, dose, and context specific. In these special circumstances NNT is useful for comparison of relative efficacy. Because the NNT comparisons here are against placebo, the best NNT of 2 means that 50 of 100 patients will get at least 50% relief specifically because of the treatment who would not have done with placebo. Another ten to twenty will have had adequate pain relief with placebo giving them at least 50% relief. With ibuprofen 400 mg, therefore, about 60 of 100 in total will have effective pain relief. For comparison, with 10 mg intramuscular morphine about 50% of patients get more than 50% pain relief. Because the effect of placebo is added in when looking at percentages with the outcome of at least 50% pain relief, the comparisons between analgesics are not as stark as with NNT.

For many of the doses or drugs, a real problem is small numbers, resulting in wide confidence intervals, and low confidence in the result. Some analgesics may not appear in the league table because they were not effective.

For paracetamol 1 g the NNT is nearly 4. Combination of paracetamol 1000 mg with codeine 60 mg improves the NNT to 2. Ibuprofen 400 mg is better at 2.4 and diclofenac 50 mg at about 2.3. NSAIDs generally do well with lower (better) NNTs.

It is clear that the oral NSAIDs do extremely well in this single-dose postoperative comparison. Many doses of NSAIDs have NNT values of between 2 and 3, and the point estimate of the mean is below that of (i.e. better than) 10 mg of intramuscular morphine, even though the confidence intervals overlap. The simple analgesics, aspirin and paracetamol are significantly less effective than 10 mg intramuscular morphine. The point estimates of the NNT are higher, and there is no overlap of the confidence intervals. Weak opioids perform poorly in single doses on their own. Combining them with simple analgesics improves analgesic efficacy.

Drawbacks of the league table

The most important drawback is size. Small trials (or small data sets) cannot accurately estimate the magnitude of the analgesic effect. To know that the NNT of an analgesic is 3.0 with a confidence interval of 2.5–3.5 we need at least 1000 patients in a comparative trial. So as you contemplate the numbers, be conscious of the amount of information upon which NNTs and percent of patients with at least 50% pain relief are based. In practice any comparison with more than 250 or so patients is probably adequate.

For instance, ibuprofen 800 mg is at the top of the league, with an NNT of 1.6 and with 100% of patients achieving at least 50% pain relief. But only 76 patients have ever been involved in comparative trials with placebo. This makes the apparent wonderful result less so, and you should treat it cautiously.

The information is presented here, warts and all, so that professionals and public can make their own assessments.

What is missing?

Adverse effect data from single-dose analgesic trials are rarely helpful with simple analgesics and NSAIDs, though they may be much more helpful with opioids.

Some analgesics used commonly outside the UK may not be represented. Again work is ongoing to plug these gaps, but so often the randomised trials (placebo-controlled, randomised, double-blind and with proper outcome measures and entry criteria), have not been done. New analgesics are becoming available (like the COX-2 inhibitors) and not all completed trials are published in their full form yet, making judgement of their efficacy difficult.

2.3 **Aspirin in postoperative pain**

Clinical bottom line. A single oral dose of aspirin is effective in the relief of postoperative pain (doses 600–1200 mg). A dose of 600/650 mg had an NNT of 4.4 (4.0–4.9) for at least 50% pain relief over 4–6 h compared with placebo in pain of moderate to severe intensity with information on over 5000 patients. It was associated with increased adverse effects (gastric irritation and nausea).

Aspirin (acetylsalicylic acid) is an important analgesic. It is widely available, and prescriptions of 300 mg tablets total approximately three quarters of a million annually in England alone (1996).

Systematic reviews

Edwards, J. E., Oldman, A., Smith, L., Wiffen, P. J., Carroll, D., McQuay, H. J. and Moore, R. A. (1999). Oral aspirin in postoperative pain: a quantitative systematic review, *Pain* 81: 289–97.

Edwards, J. E., Oldman, A., Smith, L., Collins, S. L., Carroll, D., Wiffen, P., McQuay, H. J. and Moore, R. A. (2000). Single dose aspirin in acute pain, The Cochrane Library, Update Software, Oxford (updated with no additional results 2002).

Date review completed: January 2002

Number of trials included: 72 (88 aspirin versus placebo comparisons)

Number of patients: 6550 (3253 active/3297 control)

Control group: Placebo

Main outcomes: Main outcomes: pain relief at 4–6 h (TOTPAR/ SPID), NNT (with 95% confidence intervals), relative benefit and relative risk (with 95% confidence intervals)

Inclusion criteria were full journal publication; randomised placebo-controlled trials of aspirin; postoperative oral administration; adult patients; group size $\geqslant 10$; double blind; standard pain outcomes; baseline pain moderate to severe.

Mean TOTPAR and SPID values for each trial were converted to %maxTOTPAR and %maxSPID, and then the proportion of patients achieving at least 50%maxTOTPAR were calculated. This information was used to calculate NNT and relative. Adverse effects frequency data were used to calculate numbers needed to harm (NNH) and relative risk.

Findings

Aspirin was significantly superior to placebo with single oral doses of 600/650 mg, 1000 mg and 1200 mg. A dose of 600/650 mg (Figure 2.3.1)

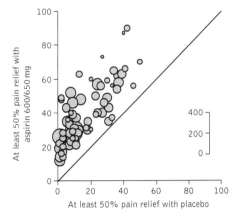

Figure 2.3.1 Comparisons of aspirin 600/650 mg with placebo in postoperative pain.

Table 2.3.1 NNTs for at least 50% pain relief over 4–6 h for aspirin at different doses compared with placebo

Aspirin dose (mg)	Number of trials	At least 50% pain relief, number/total (%)		Relative benefit (95% CI)	NNT (95% CI)
		Aspirin	Placebo		
500	3	45/135 (34)	32/115 (28)	1.2 (0.8–1.8)	–
600/650	68	950/2499 (40)	404/2562 (17)	2.0 (1.8–2.2)	4.4 (4.0–4.9)
1000	8	153/337 (44)	64/359 (20)	2.2 (1.4–3.4)	4.0 (3.2–5.4)
1200	5	85/140 (62)	27/139 (19)	3.3 (1.8–6.3)	2.4 (1.9–3.2)

had an NNT of 4.4 (4.0–4.9). Aspirin 500 mg was not effective for pain relief (Table 2.3.1).

There was a dose response for aspirin (Figure 2.3.2), with higher doses producing lower (better) NNTs. With aspirin 600/650 mg 40% of patients with initial pain of moderate or severe intensity had at least 50% pain relief over 4–6 h, as did 44% with aspirin 1000 mg and 62% with aspirin 1200 mg.

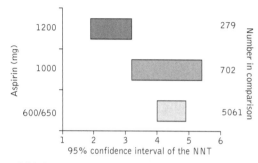

Figure 2.3.2 Dose response of aspirin compared with placebo.

Table 2.3.2 Adverse effects: aspirin 600/650 mg compared with placebo

	Dose	Number of trials	Patients with adverse effects with aspirin	Patients with adverse effects with placebo	Relative risk (95% CI)	NNH (95% CI)
All doses	Total adverse effects	60	313/2619	261/2660	1.3 (0.9–1.5)	nc
Aspirin 600/ 650 mg	Total adverse effects	53	257/1976	229/2088	1.2 (1.03–1.4)	44 (23–345)
	Dizziness	30	41/1429	27/1557	1.6	nc (0.9–2.6)
	Drowsiness	33	103/1542	56/1672	1.9 (1.4–2.5)	28 (19–52)
	Gastric irritation	11	20/546	6/562	2.5 (1.2–5.1)	38 (22–174)
	Headache	29	34/1237	56/1363	0.7 (0.4–1.02)	nc
	Nausea	34	54/1563	68/1683	0.8 (0.6–1.2)	nc
	Vomiting	21	12/835	18/927	0.7 (0.4–1.6)	nc

nc: Not calculated because relative risk not statistically significant

Adverse effects

A meta-analysis was carried out for aspirin 600/650 mg versus placebo (Table 2.3.2). All patients with at least one adverse effect generated a relative risk of 1.2 (1.03–1.4), and an NNH of 44 (23–345) for aspirin compared with placebo. At this dose, there was a significantly higher incidence of drowsiness, NNH 28 (19–52) and gastric irritation, NNH 38 (22–174), but not of nausea, vomiting, dizziness or headache.

Comment

Aspirin is an effective analgesic at standard doses, but not as effective as standard doses of other analgesics. There is considerable information on over 5000 patients for aspirin 600/650 mg. In chronic use it is associated with gastric erosions and ulcers, and it is interesting that gastric irritation was found to be significantly higher with aspirin than with placebo in these single dose studies.

2.4 **Ibuprofen in postoperative pain**

Clinical bottom line. Ibuprofen is an effective analgesic. A single dose administration of 400 mg had an NNT of 2.4 (2.3–2.6) for at least 50% pain relief over 4–6 h compared with placebo in pain of moderate to severe intensity. This is as effective as 10 mg intramuscular morphine.

Ibuprofen is an NSAID with prominent anti-inflammatory, antipyretic and analgesic actions. Analgesic effects are due to both peripheral and central effects. It is a potent inhibitor of cyclooxygenase, which results in marked reductions in prostaglandin synthesis. In 1996 ibuprofen accounted for nearly 5.5 million prescriptions in England.

Systematic reviews

Collins, S. L., Moore, R. A., McQuay, H.J. and Wiffen, P. J. (1998). Oral ibuprofen and diclofenac in postoperative pain: a quantitative systematic review, *European Journal of Pain* 2: 285–91.

Collins, S. L., Moore, R. A., McQuay, H. J., Wiffen, P. J. and Edwards, J. (2000). Single dose oral ibuprofen and diclofenac for postoperative pain, The Cochrane Library, Update Software, Oxford.

Barden, J., Ewards, J. E., Collins, S. L., McQuay, H. J. and Moore, R. A. (2002). Single dose ibuprofen for postoperative pain, The Cochrane Library, Update Software, Oxford.

Date review completed: February 2002

Number of trials included: 52

Number of patients: 6358 (3789 active/2569 control)

Control group: Placebo

Main outcomes: 4–6 h TOTPAR or SPID; NNT for 50% pain relief (with 95% confidence intervals); relative benefit (with 95% confidence intervals).

Inclusion criteria were full journal publication of trials of ibuprofen in acute postoperative pain; single oral dose; randomised; placebo-controlled; double-blind; moderate to severe baseline pain; adult populations; group sizes $\geqslant$10.

For each trial the mean TOTPAR or SPID values for ibuprofen and placebo groups were converted to the percent of maximum total pain relief based on the categorical pain scales (%maxTOTPAR or %max SPID). These values were then converted to dichotomous information

Table 2.4.1 NNTs for at least 50% pain relief over 4–6 h for ibuprofen at different doses compared with placebo

Ibuprofen dose (mg)	Number of trials	At least 50% pain relief, number/total (%)		Relative benefit (95% CI)	NNT (95% CI)
		Ibuprofen	Placebo		
50	3	50/159 (31)	17/157 (10)	2.9 (1.8–4.8)	4.7 (3.3–7.9)
100	4	60/192 (31)	16/204 (8)	3.7 (2.2–6.0)	4.3 (3.2–6.3)
200	16	365/805 (45)	52/609 (9)	5.0 (3.9–6.6)	2.7 (2.5–3.1)
400	49	1454/2595 (56)	302/2108 (14)	3.9 (3.5–4.3)	2.4 (2.3–2.6)
600	3	90/114 (79)	38/89 (43)	1.9 (1.4–2.4)	2.4 (2.0–4.2)
800	1	39/39 (100)	14/37 (38)	2.6 (1.8–4.0)	1.6 (1.3–2.2)

on the proportion, and then the number of patients, who achieved at least 50%maxTOTPAR. A NNT for at least 50% pain relief and the relative benefit of the treatment were then calculated.

Findings

Ibuprofen 50, 100, 200, 400, 600 and 800 mg were significantly superior to placebo (Table 2.4.1) and then there was a lower NNT (more effect) with increasing doses. A 400-mg dose (Figure 2.4.1) had an NNT of 2.4 (2.3–2.6). Data from standard and soluble formulation trials were pooled as there was no difference in the NNTs generated by different formulations at 400 mg.

There was a clear dose response with ibuprofen (Figure 2.4.2), with higher doses producing lower (better) NNTs. With ibuprofen 200 mg 45% of patients with initial pain of moderate or severe intensity had at least 50% pain relief over 4–6 h, as did 56% with ibuprofen 400 mg and 79% with ibuprofen 600 mg.

Adverse effects

Single dose oral studies showed no difference in adverse effects between ibuprofen and placebo. Reported adverse effects were mild and transient. Four patients withdrew after ibuprofen and two after placebo, mainly for vomiting soon after the dose was given.

Comment

Ibuprofen is an effective analgesic in postoperative pain, and there is considerable information on over 4600 patients to support ibuprofen 400 mg.

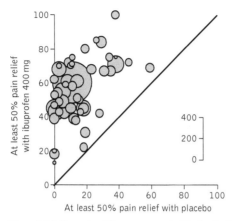

Figure 2.4.1 Ibuprofen 400 mg compared with placebo in postoperative pain.

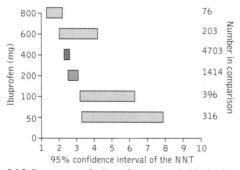

Figure 2.4.2 Dose response for ibuprofen compared with placebo.

2.5 **Paracetamol (acetaminophen) in acute postoperative pain**

Clinical bottom line. Paracetamol is an effective analgesic. A single dose of 1000 mg paracetamol had an NNT of 3.8 (3.4–4.4) for at least 50% pain relief over 4–6 h in patients with moderate or severe pain compared with placebo based on information from 2759 patients. Paracetamol 600/650 mg had an NNT of 4.6 (3.9–5.5) based on information from 1886 patients. Paracetamol is not associated with increased adverse effects in single dose administration.

Paracetamol (acetaminophen) is an important non-opiate analgesic. It accounts for over 5 million prescriptions in England alone (1995), as well as being widely available without prescription.

Systematic reviews

Moore, R. A., Collins, S., Carroll, D. and McQuay, H. J. (1997). Paracetamol with and without codeine in acute pain: a quantitative systematic review, *Pain* 70: 193–201.

Moore, R. A., Collins, S. L., Carroll, D., McQuay, H. J. and Edwards, J. (2000). Single dose paracetamol (acetaminophen), with and without codeine, for postoperative pain, The Cochrane Library, Update Software, Oxford.

Barden, J., Edwards, J. E., Moore, R. A., Collins, S. L. and McQuay, H. J. (2002). Single dose paracetamol (acetaminophen) for postoperative pain, The Cochrane Library, Update Software, Oxford.

Date review completed: 2002

Number of trials included: 46

Number of patients: 4124 (2530 paracetamol/1594 placebo)

Control group: Placebo

Main outcomes: 4–6 h TOTPAR (predominantly); NNT for 50% pain relief (with 95% confidence intervals); relative benefit (with 95% confidence intervals)

Inclusion criteria were full journal publication of trials of paracetamol in acute postoperative pain; single oral dose; randomised; placebo-controlled; double-blind; moderate to severe baseline pain; adult populations; group sizes ⩾10; sufficient data to calculate the area under the curve for pain relief (TOTPAR).

For each trial the mean TOTPAR values for paracetamol and placebo groups were converted to the percent of maximum total pain relief based on the categorical pain scales (%maxTOTPAR). These values were then converted to dichotomous information on the proportion, and then the number of patients, who achieved at least 50%maxTOTPAR. A NNT for at least 50% pain relief and the relative benefit of the treatment were then calculated.

Findings

All doses of paracetamol between 325 and 1500 mg were statistically superior to placebo (Table 2.5.1). Compared with placebo a single dose of 1000 mg paracetamol had an NNT of 3.8 (3.4–4.4) for at least 50% pain relief over 4–6 h in patients with moderate or severe pain compared with placebo (Figure 2.5.1). A 600/650-mg dose had an NNT of 4.6 (3.9–5.5).

The dose-response of paracetamol against placebo was rather flat (Figure 2.5.2), although there were few patients and trials in the comparisons at extremes of dose. With paracetamol 600/650 mg 38% of patients with initial pain of moderate or severe intensity had at least 50% pain relief over 4–6 h, as did 46% with paracetamol 1000 mg and 65% with paracetamol 1500 mg.

Adverse effects

No study reported a significant difference in number of adverse effects between paracetamol and placebo. Adverse effects in studies of paracetamol against placebo were variable, mild and transient and there were no significant differences between paracetamol and placebo for drowsiness/somnolence/sleepiness, dizziness, headache, nausea or

Table 2.5.1 NNTs for at least 50% pain relief over 4–6 h for paracetamol at different doses compared with placebo

Paracetamol dose (mg)	Number of trials	At least 50% pain relief, number/total (%)		Relative benefit (95% CI)	NNT (95% CI)
		Paracetamol	Placebo		
325	1	34/49 (69)	22/51 (43)	1.6 (1.1–2.3)	3.8 (2.2–13.3)
500	6	179/290 (61)	86/271 (32)	1.9 (1.6–2.3)	3.5 (2.7–4.8)
600/650	19	358/954 (38)	145/932 (16)	2.4 (2.0–2.8)	4.6 (3.9–5.5)
1000	24	746/1627 (46)	222/1132 (20)	2.1 (1.8–2.3)	3.8 (3.4–4.4)
1500	1	53/81 (65)	22/57 (39)	1.7 (1.2–2.5)	3.7 (2.3–9.5)

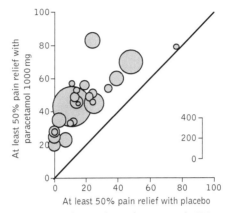

Figure 2.5.1 Randomised comparisons of paracetamol 1000 mg versus placebo.

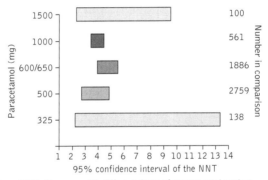

Figure 2.5.2 Response with different doses of paracetamol against placebo.

vomiting. There were four withdrawals with paracetamol and one with placebo in these trials.

Comment

Paracetamol is an effective analgesic, but somewhat less effective than others. For paracetamol 1000 mg (the usual UK and European dose) there was information on over 2700 patients and for 600/650 mg information on nearly 1900 patients.

Further reading

These are two very good reviews addressing similar questions about the effectiveness of paracetamol with and without codeine, but in slightly different ways, and without NNTs.

de Craen, A. J. M., Di Giulio, G., Lampe-Schoenmaeckers, A. J. E., Kessels, A. G. H. and Kleijnen, J. (1996). Analgesic efficacy and safety of paracetamol-codeine combinations versus paracetamol alone: A systematic review, *BMJ* 313: 321–5.

Zhang, W. Y. and Li Wan Po, A. (1996). Analgesic efficacy of paracetamol and its combination with codeine and caffeine in surgical pain – A meta-analysis, *Journal of Clinical Pharmacy and Therapeutics* 21: 261–82.

2.6 **Paracetamol (acetaminophen) with codeine in acute postoperative pain**

Clinical bottom line. Paracetamol with codeine is an effective analgesic. The NNT for at least 50% pain relief with a single dose of paracetamol 1000 mg plus codeine 60 mg was 2.2 (1.7–3.9) based on infomation on 197 patients. Paracetamol 600/650 mg plus codeine 60 mg had an NNT of 4.2 (3.4–5.3) for at least 50% pain relief over 4–6 h in patients with moderate to severe pain compared with placebo based on information from 1136. Paracetamol plus codeine produced significantly more pain relief than paracetamol alone.

Paracetamol is an important non-opiate analgesic, accounting for over 5 million prescriptions in England alone (1995). In combination with codeine it accounts for a further 6.4 million prescriptions (1996). Paracetamol/codeine combinations are also widely available without prescription.

Systematic reviews

Moore, R. A., Collins, S., Carroll, D. and McQuay, H. J. (1997). Paracetamol with and without codeine in acute pain: a quantitative systematic review, *Pain* 70: 193–201.

Moore, R. A., Collins, S. L., Carroll, D., McQuay, H. J. and Edwards, J. (2000). Single dose paracetamol (acetaminophen), with and without codeine, for postoperative pain. The Cochrane Library, Update Software, Oxford.

Smith, L. A., Moore, R. A., McQuay, H. J. and Gavaghan, D. (2001). Using evidence from different sources: an example using paracetamol 1000 mg plus codeine 60 mg. BMC Medical Research Methodology, 1:1 (http://www.biomedcentral.com/1471-2288/1/1).

Barden, J., Edwards, J. E., Moore, R. A., Collins, S. L. and McQuay, H. J. (2002). Single dose paracetamol (acetaminophen) plus codeine for postoperative pain. The Cochrane Library, Update Software, Oxford.

Date review completed: 2002

Number of trials included: 25 paracetamol plus codeine versus placebo/13 paracetamol plus codeine versus paracetamol

Number of patients: 1385 paracetamol + codeine versus placebo/794 paracetamol + codeine versus paracetamol

Control groups: Placebo and paracetamol

Main outcomes: 4–6 h TOTPAR (predominantly); NNT for 50% pain relief (with 95% confidence intervals); relative benefit (with 95% confidence intervals)

Inclusion criteria were full journal publication of trials of paracetamol and paracetamol plus codeine in acute postoperative pain; single oral dose; randomised; placebo-controlled; double-blind; moderate to severe baseline pain; adult populations; group sizes at least 10; sufficient data to calculate the area under the curve for pain relief (TOTPAR).

For each trial the mean TOTPAR values for paracetamol and placebo groups were converted to the percent of maximum total pain relief based on the categorical pain scales (%maxTOTPAR). These values were then converted to dichotomous information on the proportion, and then the number of patients, who achieved at least 50%max-TOTPAR. A NNT for at least 50% pain relief and the relative benefit of the treatment were then calculated.

Findings

A single oral dose of paracetamol 600/650 mg plus codeine 60 mg generated an NNT of 4.2 (3.4–5.3) for at least 50% pain relief over 4–6 h in patients with moderate to severe pain compared with placebo. Paracetamol 1000 mg plus codeine 60 mg (Figure 2.6.1; Table 2.6.1) had an NNT of 2.2 (1.7–3.9) compared with placebo.

Higher doses of both paracetamol and codeine led to increased efficacy and lower NNTs (Figure 2.6.2). With paracetamol 600/650 mg plus codeine 60 mg 42% of patients with initial pain of moderate or severe intensity had at least 50% pain relief over 4–6 h, as did 57% with paracetamol 1000 mg plus codeine 60 mg.

Addition of 60 mg of codeine was associated with significant extra analgesic effect when compared directly with paracetamol alone.

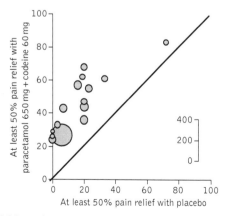

Figure 2.6.1 Randomised comparisons of paracetamol 600/650 mg plus codeine 60 mg versus placebo.

Table 2.6.1 NNTs for at least 50% pain relief over 4–6 h for paracetamol plus codeine at different doses compared with placebo

Paracetamol + Codeine dose (mg)	Number of trials	At least 50% pain relief, number/total (%)		Relative benefit (95% CI)	NNT (95% CI)
		Paracetamol + Codeine	Placebo		
300 + 30	4	56/215 (26)	14/164 (8)	3.0 (1.8–5.3)	5.7 (4.0–9.8)
500 + 30	1	13/49 (27)	7/45 (16)	0.7 (0.7–3.9)	9.1 (3.7–18.7)
600/650 + 60	17	261/636 (42)	83/487 (18)	2.4 (1.9–2.9)	4.2 (3.4–5.3)
800 + 60	1	16/44 (36)	0/21 (0)	15.6 (1.0–249)	2.7 (2.0–4.5)
1000 + 60	3	65/114 (57)	8/83 (9)	4.8 (2.6–8.8)	2.2 (1.7–2.9)

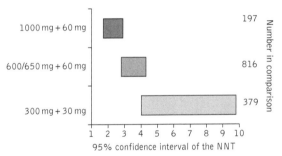

Figure 2.6.2 95% confidence intervals of NNTs with paracetamol/codeine combinations.

An additional 13–22% of patients had at least 50% pain relief when codeine 60 mg was added to paracetamol (Figure 2.6.3; Table 2.6.2).

Adverse effects

There were no serious adverse effects which necessitated withdrawal from any study. For paracetamol 600/650 mg there was significantly higher levels of drowsiness (NNH 11 (7–18)) and dizziness (NNH 19 (11–50)) with paracetamol plus codeine compared with placebo.

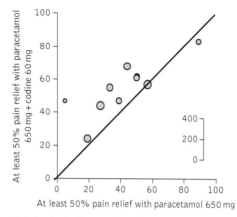

Figure 2.6.3 Randomised comparisons of paracetamol 600/650 mg plus codeine 60 mg versus paracetamol 650 mg.

Table 2.6.2 NNTs for at least 50% pain relief over 4–6 h for paracetamol plus codeine at different doses compared with paracetamol

Paracetamol + Codeine dose (mg)	Number of trials	At least 50% pain relief, number/total (%)		Relative benefit (95% CI)	NNT (95% CI)
		Paracetamol + Codeine	Paracetamol		
600/650 + 60	10	165/309 (54)	129/313 (41)	1.3 (1.1–1.5)	8.2 (5.0–22.7)
1000 + 60	3	74/109 (68)	52/108 (46)	1.4 (1.1–1.8)	5.1 (3.1–14.5)

Comment

Paracetamol plus codeine is an effective analgesic combination, with low NNTs for at least half pain relief over 4–6 h at doses of paracetamol 600/650 mg plus codeine 60 mg and paracetamol 1000 plus 60 mg. Though there was limited information for the combination of paracetamol 1000 mg plus codeine 60 mg, there was considerable supporting evidence from other combinations. In addition, three trials lacking a placebo had similar event rates for paracetamol 1000 mg plus codeine 60 mg as did those with a placebo. Six other trials with some design issues like the use of different pain measures that meant that they could not be combined showed the combination to be better than placebo or comparators.

Further reading

These are two very good reviews addressing similar questions about the effectiveness of paracetamol with and without codeine, but in slightly different ways, and without NNTs.

de Craen, A. J. M., Di Giulio, G., Lampe-Schoenmaeckers, A. J. E., Kessels, A. G. H. and Kleijnen, J. (1996). Analgesic efficacy and safety of paracetamol-codeine combinations versus paracetamol alone: A systematic review, *British Medical Journal* 313: 321–5.

Zhang, W. Y. and Li Wan Po, A. (1996). Analgesic efficacy of paracetamol and its combination with codeine and caffeine in surgical pain – A meta-analysis, *Journal of Clinical Pharmacy and Therapeutics* 21: 261–82.

2.7 **Diclofenac in postoperative pain**

Clinical bottom line. Diclofenac is an effective analgesic. A single dose administration of 50 mg had an NNT of 2.3 (2.0–2.7) for at least 50% pain relief over 4–6 h compared with placebo in pain of moderate to severe intensity based on information from 738 patients.

Diclofenac is an NSAID, which accounted for nearly 6 million prescriptions in England in 1996.

Systematic review

Collins, S. L., Moore, R. A., McQuay, H. J. and Wiffen, P. J. (1998). Oral ibuprofen and diclofenac in postoperative pain: a quantitative systematic review, *European Journal of Pain* 2: 285–91.

Collins, S. L., Moore, R. A., McQuay, H. J., Wiffen, P. J. and Edwards, J. (2000). Single dose oral ibuprofen and diclofenac for postoperative pain, The Cochrane Library, Update Software, Oxford.

Barden, J., Ewards, J. E., Collins, S. L., McQuay, H. J. and Moore, R. A. (2002). Single dose diclofenac for postoperative pain, The Cochrane Library, Update Software, Oxford.

Date review completed: January 2002

Number of trials included: 7

Number of patients: 982 (618 active/304 control)

Control group: Placebo

Main outcomes: 4–6 h TOTPAR or SPID; NNT for 50% pain relief (with 95% confidence intervals); relative benefit (with 95% confidence intervals)

Inclusion criteria were full journal publication of trials of diclofenac in acute postoperative pain; single oral dose; randomised; placebo-controlled; double-blind; moderate to severe baseline pain; adult populations; group sizes ⩾10.

For each trial the mean TOTPAR or SPID values for diclofenac and placebo groups were converted to the percent of maximum total pain relief based on the categorical pain scales (%maxTOTPAR or %maxSPID). These values were then converted to dichotomous information on the proportion, and then the number of patients, who achieved at least 50%maxTOTPAR. A NNT for at least 50% pain relief and the relative benefit of the treatment were then calculated.

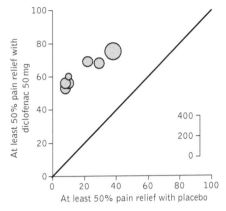

Figure 2.7.1 Diclofenac 50 mg compared with placebo in postoperative pain.

Table 2.7.1 NNTs for diclofenac at different doses over 4–6 h

Diclofenac dose (mg)	Number of trials	At least 50% pain relief, number/total (%)		Relative benefit (95% CI)	NNT (95% CI)
		Diclofenac	Placebo		
25	2	55/102 (54)	19/102 (19)	5.7 (2.1–15.4)	2.8 (2.1–4.3)
50	7	237/374 (63)	72/364 (20)	3.4 (2.7–4.4)	2.3 (2.0–2.7)
100	4	137/205 (67)	28/206 (14)	7.7 (4.5–13.1)	1.9 (1.6–2.2)

Findings

Single oral doses of diclofenac 25, 50 and 100 mg were all significantly superior to placebo (Figure 2.7.1; Table 2.7.1). A 50-mg dose generated an NNT of 2.3 (2.0–2.7).

There was a dose response for diclofenac with higher doses producing lower (better) NNTs (Figure 2.7.2). With diclofenac 25 mg 54% of patients with initial pain of moderate or severe intensity had at least 50% pain relief over 4–6 h, as did 63% with diclofenac 50 mg and 67% with diclofenac 100 mg.

Adverse effects

Single dose oral studies showed no difference in adverse effects between diclofenac and placebo. Reported adverse effects were mild

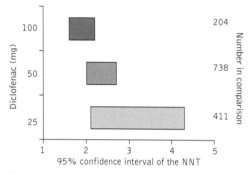

Figure 2.7.2 Dose-response for diclofenac versus placebo.

and transient. One patient withdrew after diclofenac and one after placebo in these trials.

Comment

Diclofenac at standard doses is an effective analgesic based on information from 738 patients for the 50-mg dose.

2.8 **Injected morphine in postoperative pain**

Clinical bottom line. A 10-mg intramuscular dose of morphine is an effective analgesic. It has an NNT of 2.9 (2.6–3.6) for at least 50% pain relief over 4–6 h compared with placebo in pain of moderate to severe intensity. The incidence of minor adverse effects is significantly higher with 10 mg intramuscular morphine compared with placebo.

Few trials of acceptable quality have been carried out. This is especially true for subcutaneous and intravenous studies.

Morphine is the archetypal analgesic for use in moderate or severe pain. It is the principle alkaloid of opium, and is given by many different routes. Morphine is the 'gold standard' against which other injected analgesics are tested.

Systematic review

McQuay, H. J., Carroll, D. and Moore, R. A. (1999). Injected morphine in postoperative pain: a quantitative systematic review, *Journal of Pain and Symptom Management* 17: 164–74.

Date review completed: March 1997

Number of trials included: 20

Number of patients: 1259 (696 active/563 control; 494 treated patients for 10-mg dose)

Control group: Placebo

Main outcomes: 4–6 h TOTPAR or SPID; NNT for 50% pain relief (with 95% confidence intervals); relative benefit (with 95% confidence intervals)

Inclusion criteria were full journal publication of trials of injected morphine in acute postoperative pain; single dose treatment of injected morphine and placebo (intravenous, intramuscular or subcutaneous); randomised; blinded design; moderate to severe baseline pain; adult populations.

For each trial the mean TOTPAR or SPID values for intramuscular morphine and placebo groups were converted to the percent of maximum total pain relief based on the categorical pain scales (%maxTOTPAR or %maxSPID). These values were then converted to dichotomous information on the proportion, and then the number of patients, who achieved at least 50%maxTOTPAR. A NNT for at least 50% pain relief and the relative benefit of the treatment were then calculated. Adverse effects frequency data were used to calculate NNH and relative risk.

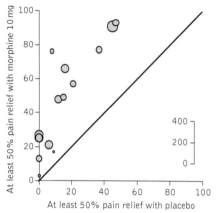

Figure 2.8.1 At least 50% pain relief with intramuscular morphine 10 mg compared with placebo.

Findings

Morphine was given by intramuscular injection in all trials except one intravenous trial. Sufficient data for meta-analysis was available for 10 mg intramuscular morphine trials only (Figure 2.8.1). The NNT for 10 mg intramuscular morphine was 2.9 (2.6–3.6). Overall 50% of patients given 10 mg morphine had at least 50% pain relief over 4–6 h.

Adverse effects

Minor adverse effects occurred in 34% of patients given intramuscular morphine compared with 23% with placebo. This was significantly higher than placebo, with an NNH of 9.1 (5.6–27). There was no difference between morphine and placebo with major adverse effects (drug-related study withdrawal).

Comment

Morphine 10 mg intramuscularly was shown to be an effective analgesic in 946 patients.

2.9 **Dihydrocodeine in postoperative pain**

Clinical bottom line. A single 30 mg oral dose of dihydrocodeine does not provide effective analgesia. A 60-mg dose is significantly less effective than ibuprofen 400 mg. Quality data do not exist for a placebo comparison. Patients should be offered a more effective analgesic in the treatment of postoperative pain.

Dihydrocodeine is a synthetic opioid analgesic which was developed in the early 1900s. Its structure and pharmacokinetics are similar to codeine, and it is used for the treatment of postoperative pain and as an antitussive. Nearly one tenth of all analgesic preparations issued in England were for dihydrocodeine in 1995.

Systematic review

McQuay, H. J. and Moore, R. A. (1998). An evidence-based resource for pain relief, Oxford University Press March 1998, ISBN 0-19-262718-X.

Date review completed: February 1997

Number of trials included: 4

Number of patients: (97 active versus 97 placebo; 80 active versus 80 active control)

Control group: Placebo (3 trials)/ibuprofen (1 trial)

Main outcomes: 4–6 h TOTPAR or SPID; NNT for 50% pain relief (with 95% confidence intervals); relative benefit (with 95% confidence intervals)

Inclusion criteria were full journal publication of trials of dihydrocodeine in acute postoperative pain; single oral dose; postoperative administration; randomised; placebo-controlled; double-blind; moderate to severe baseline pain; adult populations.

For each trial the mean TOTPAR or SPID values for dihydrocodeine and placebo groups were converted to the percent of maximum total pain relief based on the categorical pain scales (%maxTOTPAR or %maxSPID). These values were then converted to dichotomous information on the proportion, and then the number of patients, who achieved at least 50%maxTOTPAR. A NNT for at least 50% pain relief and the relative benefit of the treatment were then calculated.

Findings

Oral dihydrocodeine versus placebo

Dihydrocodeine 60 mg data were not available from the included trials. Dihydrocodeine 30 mg (dihydrocodeine tartrate) was not

Table 2.9.1 NNTs for comparisons of dihydrocodeine versus placebo and ibuprofen

Number of trials	Dose of dihydrocodeine (mg)	At least 50% pain relief with		Relative benefit (95% CI)	NNT (95% CI)
		Dihydrocodeine	Placebo		
vs. placebo 3	30	29/97	19/97	1.7 (0.7–4.0)	Not calculated
	Dose of dihydrocodeine (mg)	**Dihydrocodeine >50% pain relief/total**	**Ibuprofen >50% pain relief/ total**	**Relative benefit (95% CI)**	**NNT (95% CI)**
vs. ibuprofen 1	30	3/40	18/40	0.2 (0.1–0.5)	−2.7 (−1.8 to −5)
1	60	6/40	18/40	0.3 (0.2–0.8)	−3.3 (−2.1 to −9)

Negative NNTs in the comparison with ibuprofen mean that ibuprofen is better than dihydrocodeine

significantly different from placebo (Table 2.9.1). Only 30% of patients given dihydrocodeine 30 mg had at least 50% pain relief.

Oral dihydrocodeine versus ibuprofen

Ibuprofen was significantly more effective than dihydrocodeine 30 and 60 mg (Table 2.9.1).

Adverse effects

Single dose oral trials of dihydrocodeine showed no difference in adverse effects compared with placebo. All adverse effects were mild and transient, with no study withdrawals as a result. No single dose adverse effects data were presented in the original ibuprofen trials.

Comment

There is limited information regarding the analgesic efficacy of dihydrocodeine, but what little we have suggests that 30 mg is no better than placebo.

2.10 **Oral codeine in acute postoperative pain**

Clinical bottom line. Codeine 60 mg is not an effective analgesic for postoperative pain. A 60-mg oral dose of codeine had an NNT of 16.7 (11–48) for at least 50% pain relief over 4–6 h compared with placebo in pain of moderate to severe intensity.

Codeine is an opium alkaloid, with activity similar to, but weaker than morphine. It is also widely available in combination with aspirin or paracetamol.

Systematic review

Moore, R. A. and McQuay, H. J. (1997). Single-patient data meta-analysis of 3453 postoperative patients: Oral tramadol versus placebo, codeine and combination analgesics, *Pain* 69: 287–94.

Date review completed: 1995

Number of trials included: 17

Number of patients: 1305 (649 codeine/656 placebo)

Control group: Oral placebo

Main outcomes: Pain relief at 6 h (TOTPAR), NNT (with 95% confidence intervals) and relative benefit with 95% confidence intervals)

Inclusion criteria were single oral dose, randomised, placebo-controlled, double-blind trials of codeine in acute postoperative pain with sufficient data to calculate the area under the curve for pain relief (TOTPAR). Baseline pain was moderate to severe. The 6-h TOTPAR was calculated for each patient, and the data were converted to the percent of maximum total pain relief from categorical pain scales (%maxTOTPAR), and then to dichotomous information to generate a NNT for at least 50% pain relief. Relative benefit was calculated to provide an assessment of how much more likely an individual given a particular treatment is to have at least 50% pain relief than someone given no treatment. Adverse effects frequency data were used to calculate NNH and relative risk.

Findings

The meta-analysis was carried out on eight postsurgical pain trials and nine dental extraction trials.

Codeine 60 mg generated an NNT of 16.7 (11–48).

Table 2.10.1 Adverse effects with codeine 60 mg compared with placebo

Adverse effect	Harmed on active	Harmed on control	Relative risk (95% CI)	NNH (95% CI)
Dizziness	44/666	15/714	3.1 (1.8–5.6)	20 (15–43)
Drowsiness/ somnolence	94/666	48/714	2.1 (1.5–2.9)	14 (9.4–24)
Headache	43/666	41/714	1.1 (0.7–1.7)	Not calculated
Nausea	46/666	31/714	1.6 (1.0–2.5)	Not calculated
Vomiting	14/666	6/714	2.5 (1.0–6.5)	Not calculated

Adverse effects

Dizziness and drowsiness/somnolence were significantly more frequent with codeine 60 mg (Table 2.10.1). Headache, nausea and vomiting were not.

Comment

Oral codeine alone is not an effective analgesic in single doses.

2.11 **Dextropropoxyphene alone and with paracetamol in postoperative pain**

Dextropropoxyphene alone

Clinical bottom line. 65 mg of dextropropoxyphene is not an effective analgesic. Dextropropoxyphene is a relatively weak opioid analgesic that has been widely available since the 1950s. It is used alone and in combination with paracetamol or aspirin.

Systematic review

Collins, S. L., Edwards, J. E., Moore, R. A. and McQuay, H. J. (1998). Single dose dextropropoxyphene in postoperative pain: a quantitative systematic review, *European Journal of Clinical Pharmacology* 54: 107–12.

Date review completed: November 1996

Number of trials included: 6

Number of patients: 490 (239 dextropropoxyphene/251 placebo)

Control group: Oral placebo

Main outcomes: Pain relief at 4–6 h (TOTPAR/SPID), NNT (with 95% confidence intervals), relative benefit and relative risk (with 95% confidence intervals)

Inclusion criteria were full journal publication, single oral dose, randomised, placebo-controlled, double-blind trials of dextropropoxyphene in acute postoperative pain, baseline pain moderate to severe. Mean TOTPAR and SPID values for each trial were converted to %maxTOTPAR and %maxSPID, and then the proportion of patients achieving at least 50%maxTOTPAR were calculated. This information was used to calculate the NNT and relative benefit. Adverse effects frequency data were used to calculate NNH and relative risk.

Findings

Six reports compared dextropropoxyphene hydrochloride 65 mg with placebo, and one trial also compared a dose of 130 mg with placebo.

A single oral dose of dextropropoxyphene 65 mg was no better than placebo for pain of moderate to severe intensity – relative benefit 1.5 (1.2–1.9). The NNT was 7.7 (4.6–22).

Adverse effects

No patient withdrew as a result of adverse effects, and all reported were transient and of mild to moderate severity. Overall, at doses of 65 mg there was no significant difference in adverse effects with dextropropoxyphene compared with placebo.

Dextropropoxyphene with paracetamol

Clinical bottom line. Paracetamol 650 mg plus dextropropoxyphene is an effective analgesic in postoperative pain. A single oral dose had an NNT of 4.4 (3.5–5.6) for at least 50% pain relief over 4–6 h compared with placebo in pain of moderate to severe intensity. This is equivalent to 1000 mg of paracetamol alone. Adverse effects were transient and of mild to moderate severity, mainly dizziness and drowsiness.

Paracetamol (acetaminophen) is an important non-opioid analgesic. It accounts for over 5 million prescriptions in England alone (1995), and is widely available, alone and in combination, without prescription. Dextropropoxyphene is a relatively weak opioid analgesic usually prepared in combination with paracetamol or aspirin. Paracetamol/dextropropoxyphene combinations accounted for over 10 million prescriptions in England (1996).

Systematic review

Collins, S. L., Edwards, J. E., Moore, R. A. and McQuay, H. J. (1998). Single dose dextropropoxyphene in postoperative pain: a quantitative systematic review, *European Journal of Clinical Pharmacology* 54: 107–12.

Date review completed: November 1996

Number of trials included: 4 plus 1 meta-analysis of 18 trials

Number of patients: 963 (478 paracetamol plus dextropropoxyphene/ 485 placebo)

Control group: Oral placebo

Main outcomes: Pain relief at 4–6 h (TOTPAR/SPID), NNT (with 95% confidence intervals), relative benefit and relative risk (with 95% confidence intervals)

Inclusion criteria were full journal publication, single oral dose, randomised, placebo-controlled, double-blind trials of paracetamol plus dextropropoxyphene in acute postoperative pain, baseline pain moderate to severe. Mean TOTPAR and SPID values for each trial were converted to %maxTOTPAR and %maxSPID, and then the proportion of patients achieving at least 50%maxTOTPAR were calculated. This information was used to calculate the NNT and relative benefit. Adverse effects frequency data were used to calculate NNH and relative risk.

Trials of dextropropoxyphene hydrochloride 65 mg and napsylate 100 mg were analysed together.

Findings

Four reports compared dextropropoxyphene napsylate 100 mg plus paracetamol 650 mg with placebo, and one used dextropropoxyphene hydrochloride 65 mg plus paracetamol 650 mg, with a total of about 950 patients. Paracetamol 650 mg plus dextropropoxyphene had an NNT of 4.4 (3.5–5.6) for at least 50% pain relief over 4–6 h compared with placebo for pain of moderate to severe intensity. The analgesic response was significantly more effective than placebo.

Adverse effects

No patient withdrew as a result of adverse effects, and all reported were transient and of mild to moderate severity. Dizziness and drowsiness were the most commonly reported adverse effects (Table 2.11.1). Both were significantly higher in comparison to placebo.

Comment

What information we have, in relatively few patients, is that dextropropoxyphene alone is not effective in single doses, but that in combination with paracetamol it is better.

Table 2.11.1 Adverse effects with dextropropoxyphene 65 mg plus paracetamol 650 mg compared with placebo

Number of trials	Adverse effect	Number of patients with adverse effects		Relative risk (95% CI)	NNH (95% CI)
		Active	Placebo		
3	Nausea	12/405	33/799	0.7 (0.4–1.4)	Not calculated
1	Vomiting	2/323	6/714	1.4 (0.3–6.7)	Not calculated
4	Dizziness	17/435	16/829	2.2 (1.1–4.3)	43 (22–607)
3	Drowsiness/ somnolence	57/405	55/799	2.2 (2.0–2.4)	14 (9.1–30)
4	Headache	14/435	51/829	0.5 (0.4–0.6)	−33 (−170 to −19)

Negative NNTs indicate that fewer headaches occur with dextroropoxyphene plus paracetamol than with placebo

2.12 **Intramuscular pethidine in postoperative pain**

Clinical bottom line. Intramuscular pethidine is an effective analgesic. A single dose of intramuscular pethidine 100 mg had an NNT of 2.9 (2.3–3.9) for at least 50% pain relief over 4–6 h in patients with moderate or severe pain compared with placebo. This is similar to intramuscular morphine 10 mg which has an NNT of 2.9 (2.6–3.6). Based on small numbers of patients, pethidine 50 mg does not appear to offer effective pain relief.

Pethidine 100 mg was associated with significantly more adverse effects than placebo. The NNH for a single intramuscular dose of pethidine 100 mg was 2.6 (2.1–3.6).

Pethidine is a commonly used postoperative opioid analgesic. It has similar properties to morphine, but with a more rapid onset and shorter duration of action.

Systematic review

Smith, L. A., Carroll, D., Edwards, J. E., Moore, R. A. and McQuay, H. J. (2000).
  Single-dose ketorolac and pethidine in acute postoperative pain: a systematic review, *British Journal of Anaesthesia* 84: 48–58.

  Date review completed: July 1998

  Number of trials included: 8 trials (10 comparisons)

  Number of patients: 468 (254 active/214 control)

  Control group: Placebo

  Main outcomes: Pain relief at 4–6 h (TOTPAR/SPID), NNT (with 95% confidence intervals), relative benefit and relative risk (with 95% confidence intervals)

Inclusion criteria were randomised, double-blind, placebo controlled trials of pethidine in postoperative pain; oral, intramuscular, intravenous administration; adult patients; baseline pain of moderate to severe intensity; pain outcome at least 4 h.

Mean TOTPAR and SPID values for each trial were converted to %maxTOTPAR and %maxSPID, and then the proportion of patients achieving at least 50%maxTOTPAR were calculated. This information was used to calculate NNT and relative benefit. Adverse effects frequency data were used to calculate NNH and relative risk.

Findings

No trials of oral or intravenous pethidine met inclusion criteria, and all information refers to intramuscular pethidine.

Pethidine 50 mg

Two trials with 104 patients showed no significant benefit of pethidine over placebo (Table 2.12.1), with relative benefit 1.7 (0.9–3.0).

Pethidine 100 mg

Eight trials of 364 patients showed significant pain relief with pethidine compared with placebo (Table 2.12.1; Figure 2.12.1), with an NNT of 2.9 (2.3–3.9). On average 54% of patients with initially moderate or severe pain had at least 50% pain relief over 4–6 h with pethidine 100 mg.

Adverse effects

Sufficient data were available only for 100 mg doses of pethidine. Pethidine was associated with significantly more adverse effects than

Table 2.12.1 Pethidine 50 and 100 mg compared with placebo

Pethidine dose (mg)	Number of comparisons	Number of patients with at least 50% pain relief (%)		Relative benefit (95% CI)	NNT (95% CI)
		With pethidine	With placebo		
50	2	19/51 (37)	12/53 (23)	1.7 (0.9–3.0)	Not calculated
100	8	109/203 (54)	30/161 (19)	3.2 (2.3–4.6)	2.9 (2.3–3.9)

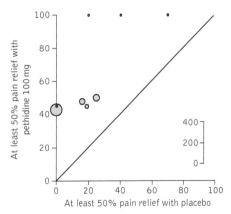

Figure 2.12.1 Proportion of patients in each trial achieving at least 50% pain relief with pethidine 100 mg over 4–6 h compared with placebo.

placebo. The NNH for a single intramuscular dose of pethidine 100 mg was 2.6 (2.1–3.6). The most frequently reported adverse effects were drowsiness or somnolence, dizziness or lightheadedness, and nausea or vomiting. These were significantly different compared with placebo for all but nausea and vomiting. Nine pethidine and four placebo patients withdrew from the trials due to adverse effects.

Comment

Pethidine 100 mg given intramuscularly was an effective analgesic based on evidence from 364 patients.

2.13 **Naproxen in postoperative pain**

Clinical bottom line. Naproxen is an effective analgesic. A single dose of 550 mg naproxen sodium versus placebo had an NNT of 3.0 (2.2–4.8) for at least 50% pain relief over 4–6 h in patients with moderate or severe pain compared with placebo. This is more effective than a 1000 mg dose of paracetamol which has an NNT of 4.6 (3.9–5.4). Naproxen sodium 220 and 440 mg were also more effective than placebo.

The most commonly reported adverse effects were nausea, vomiting, headache, gastric irritation, dizziness and somnolence. These were predominantly of mild to moderate severity.

Naproxen is a non-steroidal anti-inflammatory (NSAID) and antipyretic agent. Naproxen sodium is absorbed more rapidly than naproxen.

Systematic review

Smith, L. A., Moore, R. A. and McQuay, H. J. Oral naproxen in acute postoperative pain: a systematic review (unpublished).

Date review completed: March 1998

Number of trials included: 6

Number of patients: 607 (366 naproxen/241 placebo)

Control group: Placebo

Main outcomes: Pain intensity, pain relief, 4–6 h TOTPAR; NNT for 50% pain relief (with 95% confidence intervals); relative benefit (with 95% confidence intervals)

Inclusion criteria were full journal publication of trials of naproxen in acute postoperative pain; single oral dose; randomised; placebo-controlled; double-blind; moderate to severe baseline pain; adult populations; group sizes at least 10; sufficient data to calculate the area under the curve for pain relief (TOTPAR).

For each trial the mean TOTPAR values for naproxen and placebo groups were converted to the percent of maximum total pain relief based on the categorical pain scales (%maxTOTPAR). These values were then converted to dichotomous information on the proportion, and then the number of patients, who achieved at least 50% maxTOTPAR. A NNT for at least 50% pain relief and the relative benefit of the treatment were then calculated. Adverse effects frequency data were used to calculate NNH and relative risk.

Table 2.13.1 Numbers-needed-to-treat and relative benefits for naproxen versus placebo

Naproxen dose (mg)	Number of comparisons	Number of patients with at least 50% pain relief with		Relative benefit (95% CI)	NNT (95% CI)
		Naproxen	Placebo		
220/250	2	63/109 (58)	18/72 (25)	2.3 (1.5–3.6)	3.1 (2.2–5.2)
440	2	86/173 (50)	5/84 (6)	8.4 (3.5–20)	2.3 (2.0–2.9)
550	2	39/84 (46)	5/85 (7)	3.6 (2.0–6.5)	3.0 (2.2–4.8)

All naproxen sodium apart from naproxen 250 mg.

Trials of naproxen and naproxen sodium were pooled if the doses were pharmacokinetically equivalent.

Findings

Five trials of naproxen sodium were found, and one of naproxen. Naproxen 250 mg was pooled with naproxen sodium 220 mg, as they were regarded as being pharmacokinetically equivalent. All doses (220/250, 440 and 550 mg) were superior to placebo (Table 2.13.1).

In two trials of 169 patients given a single dose of 550 mg naproxen or placebo, naproxen had an NNT of 3.0 (2.2–4.8) for at least 50% pain relief over 4–6 h in patients with moderate or severe pain compared with placebo (Figure 2.13.1).

In two trials of 257 patients given a single dose of 440 mg naproxen or placebo, naproxen had an NNT of 2.3 (2.0–2.9) for at least 50% pain relief over 4–6 h in patients with moderate or severe pain compared with placebo (Figure 2.13.1).

In two trials of 181 patients given a single dose of 220/250 mg naproxen or placebo, naproxen had an NNT of 3.1 (2.2–5.2) for at least 50% pain relief over 4–6 h in patients with moderate or severe pain compared with placebo (Figure 2.13.1).

Adverse effects

Five of the six trials reported on adverse effects. Nausea, vomiting, headache, gastric irritation, dizziness and somnolence were the most commonly reported adverse effects, and were predominantly of mild to moderate severity. There were no trial withdrawals that were attributed to trial medications. For all doses and all adverse effects analysed together, there were significantly more adverse effects with naproxen

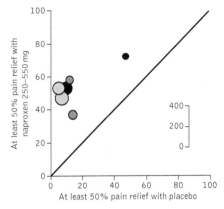

Figure 2.13.1 Randomised comparisons of naproxen versus placebo.

compared with placebo: relative risk was 1.5 (1.0–2.1) and NNH was 16 (8.2–350).

Comment

Based on limited information naproxen, like other NSAIDs, appears to be an effective analgesic in acute pain.

2.14 **Oral tramadol in postoperative pain**

Clinical bottom line. Tramadol is an effective analgesic in postoperative pain. A single 100 mg oral dose of tramadol is equivalent to 1000 mg paracetamol. A dose of 100 mg had an NNT of 4.6 (3.6–6.4) for at least 50% pain relief over 4–6 h in patients with moderate to severe pain compared with placebo.

At doses of 50 and 100 mg incidence of adverse effects (headache, nausea, vomiting, dizziness and somnolence) was similar to comparator drugs. In dental trials there was increased incidence of vomiting, nausea, dizziness and somnolence.

Tramadol (tramadol hydrochloride) has been in use in Europe since the 1970s for a range of pain conditions, and in the US since the late 1980s. It is a weak opioid receptor agonist with a number of other properties including serotonin release and inhibition of noradrenaline uptake. Tramadol is produced as a racemic mixture.

Systematic review

Moore, R. A. and McQuay, H. J. (1997). Single-patient data meta-analysis of 3453 postoperative patients: Oral tramadol versus placebo, codeine and combination analgesics, *Pain* 69: 287–94.

Date review completed: 1995

Number of trials included: 18

Number of patients: 3453 (1486 tramadol/695 placebo)

Control group: Oral placebo

Main outcomes: Pain relief at 6 h (TOTPAR), NNT (with 95% confidence intervals) and relative benefit (with 95% confidence intervals).

Inclusion criteria were single oral dose, randomised, placebo-controlled, double-blind trials of tramadol in acute postoperative pain with sufficient data to calculate the area under the curve for pain relief (TOTPAR). Baseline pain was moderate to severe. The 6 h TOTPAR was calculated for each patient, and the data were converted to the percent of maximum total pain relief from categorical pain scales (%maxTOTPAR), and then to dichotomous information to generate a NNT for at least 50% pain relief. Relative benefit was calculated to provide an assessment of how much more likely an individual given a particular treatment is to have at least 50% pain relief than someone given no treatment. Adverse effects frequency data were used to calculate NNH and relative risk.

Table 2.14.1 Oral tramadol in acute postoperative pain (data for all analgesics in the review)

	Number (%) with at least 50% pain relief		Relative benefit (95% CI)	NNT (95% CI)
	Treatment	Placebo		
Codeine 60 mg	99/649 (15)	63/656 (10)	1.6 (1.2–2.1)	16.7 (11–48)
Tramadol 50 mg	79/409 (19)	26/361 (7)	2.7 (1.8–4.1)	8.3 (6.0–13)
Tramadol 75 mg	90/281 (32)	37/282 (13)	2.4 (1.7–3.5)	5.3 (3.9–8.2)
Tramadol 100 mg	140/468 (30)	35/414 (8)	3.5 (2.5–5.0)	4.8 (3.8–6.1)
Tramadol 150 mg	135/279 (48)	37/282 (13)	3.7 (2.7–5.1)	2.9 (2.4–3.6)
Paracetamol 650 mg & propoxyphene 100 mg	114/316 (38)	40/322 (12)	2.9 (2.1–4.0)	4.2 (3.3–5.8)
Aspirin 650 mg & codeine 60 mg	76/305 (25)	17/293 (6)	4.3 (2.6–7.1)	5.3 (4.1–7.4)

Dental trials and postsurgical trials were also analysed separately to establish whether this had an effect on the NNTs and relative benefits of the drug conditions. Comparisons with codeine and combination analgesics were also made.

Findings

The meta-analysis was carried out on nine postsurgical pain trials and nine dental extraction trials. All trials showed a significantly superior analgesia to placebo (Table 2.14.1), with a clear dose response for tramadol (higher doses associated with higher benefit and lower NNTs, Figure 2.14.1). Tramadol 100 mg had an NNT of 4.6 (3.6–6.4).

With the exception of tramadol 100 mg, NNTs were lower in postsurgical pain than in dental extraction models. This was not due to differences in baseline pain intensity.

Adverse effects

The most commonly reported effects were headache, vomiting, nausea, dizziness and somnolence, though predominantly of mild intensity. In dental trials only, this was significantly different to placebo for vomiting, nausea, dizziness and somnolence, and there was a distinct dose-response, particularly in dental patients, with higher doses producing greater incidence of adverse events.

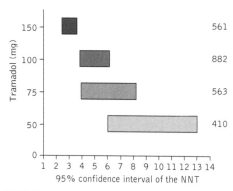

Figure 2.14.1 Dose response for oral tramadol.

Comment

Tramadol was an effective analgesic in single oral doses, but these were associated with a higher risk of adverse effects especially after dental extraction.

2.15 **Paracetamol plus tramadol for acute pain**

Clinical bottom line. Based on somewhat limited information, a combination of paracetamol plus tramadol is an effective analgesic in acute postoperative pain. The NNT compared with placebo over 6 h was about 2.7.

The combination of tramadol with paracetamol is not commonly available for prescription, but has recently (2002) become available in the USA. The exact dosage strengths in the combinations may vary from country to country, so affecting its efficacy.

Systematic review

Edwards, J. E. *et al.* (2002). Combination analgesic efficacy: Individual patient data meta-analysis of single dose oral tramadol plus acetaminophen in acute postoperative pain, *Journal of Pain and Symptom Management* 23: 121–30.

Date review completed: 2001

Number of trials included: 7

Number of patients: Various, because different combination strengths

Control group: Oral placebo

Main outcomes: Pain relief at 6 h (TOTPAR), NNT (with 95% confidence intervals) and relative benefit (with 95% confidence intervals). Duration of analgesia through time to remedication

Inclusion criteria were single oral dose, randomised, placebo-controlled, double-blind trials of paracetamol plus tramadol in acute postoperative pain with sufficient data to calculate the area under the curve for pain relief (TOTPAR). Baseline pain was moderate to severe. The 6- and 8-h TOTPAR was calculated for each patient (this was an individual patient analysis), and the data were converted to the percent of maximum total pain relief from categorical pain scales (%maxTOTPAR), and then to dichotomous information to generate a number-needed-to-treat for at least 50% pain relief.

Relative benefit was calculated to provide an assessment of how much more likely an individual given a particular treatment is to have at least 50% pain relief than someone given no treatment. Adverse effects frequency data were used to calculate numbers-needed-to-harm and relative risk.

Findings

Paracetamol plus tramadol was an effective analgesic in dental and postsurgical pain, based on limited information (Table 2.15.1),

Table 2.15.1 NNTs for paracetamol plus tramadol for half pain relief over 6 h compared with placebo

Pain model/dosage	At least half pain relief, number/total (%)		NNT (95% CI)
	Paracetamol + Tramadol	Placebo	
Dental pain:			
Paracetamol 650 mg	145/340	14/339	2.6 (2.3–3.0)
+ Tramadol 75 mg	(43)	(4)	
Postsurgical pain:			
Paracetamol 975 mg	61/101	25/100	2.8 (2.1–4.4)
+ Tramadol 112.5 mg	(60)	(25)	

with NNTs between 2 and 3. NNTs over 8 h were similar to those over 6 h.

More patients reported adverse events with paracetamol plus tramadol than with placebo in an analysis of dental pain patients. There were more patients experiencing any adverse effect (NNH 5.4), and dizziness (NNH 23), nausea (NNH 7) and vomiting (NNH 6) with paracetamol plus tramadol.

Comment

The paper calculates results based on pain intensity, pain relief and patient global evaluation of treatment, based on individual patient data. All produced very similar NNTs, confirming findings from other studies, and underpinning the methods used in meta-analysis in acute pain.

2.16 **Oral rofecoxib in postoperative pain**

Clinical bottom line. Rofecoxib is an effective analgesic in acute pain. The NNT for rofecoxib 50 mg for at least 50% pain relief over 6 h was 2.3 (95% confidence interval 2.0–2.6). The weighted mean remedication time was 1.9 h for placebo (126 patients), 7.4 h for ibuprofen 400 mg (97 patients) and 13.6 h for rofecoxib 50 mg (322 patients).

Rofecoxib is a COX-2 inhibitor that has been shown to be an effective analgesic in osteoarthritis and rheumatoid arthritis at single daily doses of 12.5 or 25 mg. At these (and higher) doses it has also been shown to reduce the incidence of gastrointestinal bleeding on chronic use for arthritis compared with NSAIDs, in both a systematic review and a separate large randomised trial.

Systematic review

Barden, J., Edwards, J. E., McQuay, H. J. and Moore, R. A. (2002). Rofecoxib for acute postoperative pain: a quantitative systematic review, *BMC Anesthesiology* 2: 4 (http://www.biomedcentral.com/1471–2253/2/4).

Date review completed: 2002

Number of trials included: 5

Number of patients: 1118 (464 rofecoxib/ 211 placebo)

Control group: Oral placebo

Main outcomes: Pain relief at 6 h (TOTPAR), NNT (with 95% confidence intervals) and relative benefit (with 95% confidence intervals). Duration of analgesia through time to remedication

Inclusion criteria were single oral dose, randomised, placebo-controlled, double-blind trials of rofecoxib in acute postoperative pain with sufficient data to calculate the area under the curve for pain relief (TOTPAR). Baseline pain was moderate to severe. The 6 h TOTPAR was calculated for each patient, and the data were converted to the percent of maximum total pain relief from categorical pain scales (%maxTOTPAR), and then to dichotomous information to generate a NNT for at least 50% pain relief. Relative benefit was calculated to provide an assessment of how much more likely an individual given a particular treatment is to have at least 50% pain relief than someone given no treatment. Adverse effects frequency data were used to calculate NNH and relative risk.

Findings

There were five placebo-controlled trials that also had active comparators. All showed statistical benefit of rofecoxib 50 mg over placebo

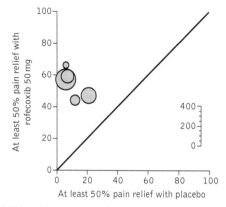

Figure 2.16.1 Trials comparing rofecoxib 50 mg with placebo in acute postoperative pain.

(Figure 2.16.1). Overall 252/464 patients (54%) given rofecoxib 50 mg had at least 50% maxTOTPAR over 6 h, compared with 24/211 patients (11%) with placebo. The NNT for one patient to have at least half pain relief over 6 h was 2.3 (2.0–2.6).

Median time to remedication was given in three studies allowing calculation of a weighted mean. For placebo the weighted mean time to remedication from 126 patients in three trials was 1.9 h. For rofecoxib 50 mg the weighted mean time to remedication from 322 patients in three trials was 13.6 h. For ibuprofen 400 mg the weighted mean time to remedication from 97 patients in two trials was 7.4 h.

Adverse events

Two trials reported the proportion of patients having any adverse event. An adverse event was reported by 33% of patients on placebo and 28% of those on rofecoxib 50 mg. There was limited evidence based on few events that nausea and vomiting were slightly less likely with rofecoxib.

Comment

Rofecoxib was an effective analgesic in single oral doses about twice those given for arthritis. Good analgesia over 6 h may be accompanied by good long-duration analgesia, but the evidence on this is not yet conclusive.

2.17 Transcutaneous electrical nerve stimulation (TENS) in acute postoperative pain and labour pain

Clinical bottom line. TENS is not effective in the relief of postoperative pain. Patients should be offered effective methods of pain relief. TENS neither alleviates labour pain nor reduces the use of additional analgesics. Women should be offered effective interventions for relief of labour pain.

TENS was originally developed as a way of controlling pain through the 'gate' theory. There is conflicting professional opinion about the use of TENS in acute postoperative pain. For example, the Agency for Health Care Policy and Research recommend TENS as effective in reducing pain and improving physical function, whilst the UK College of Anaesthetists' working party states that TENS is not effective as the sole treatment of moderate or severe pain after surgery.

Systematic reviews

Carroll, D., Tramer, M., McQuay, H., Nye, B. and Moore, A. (1996). Randomization is important in studies with pain outcomes: systematic review of transcutaneous electrical nerve stimulation in acute postoperative pain, *British Journal of Anaesthesia* 77: 798–803.

Carroll, D., Moore, R. A., Tramèr, M. R. and McQuay, H. J. (1997). Transcutaneous electrical nerve stimulation does not relieve labour pain: updated systematic review, *Contemporary Reviews in Obstetrics and Gynecology* Sept: 195–205.

Postoperative pain

Date review completed: January 1996

Number of trials included: 17

Number of patients: 786

Control groups: Conventional postoperative analgesia (intramuscular opioid)/disabled (sham) TENS

Main outcomes: Include analgesic consumption, pain ratings

Labour pain

Date review completed: April 1997

Number of trials included: 10

Number of patients: 877 (436 active/441 control)

Control group: 'No treatment' or 'sham TENS'

Main outcomes: Prospective measurements of pain at time of labour and when TENS was in use

Inclusion criteria were full journal publication; randomised, controlled trials; TENS; postoperative pain with pain outcomes; group size ≥10.

Statistically significant findings were extracted from the original reports, and then qualitatively summarised. *Post-hoc* subgroup analysis in the original reports was not considered in reviewer judgements of overall effectiveness.

Findings in postoperative pain

TENS versus sham TENS. Fourteen trials were included. None found any difference. One trial reported improved pain ratings with TENS, but reviewers regarded statistical analysis as inappropriate.

TENS versus opioid control. Seven trials compared opioid plus TENS with opioid alone, four of which also included sham TENS. Five of seven trials reported no difference between groups. Of the two significant trials, one reported significantly fewer pethidine injections and higher global ratings of treatment scores on the first postoperative day. The second trial reported improved pain scores with TENS used for 20 min three times a day. Reviewers agreed with these findings.

Adverse effects in postoperative pain

Data on adverse effects were not systematically collected in any trials, and none were reported.

Findings in labour pain

No study recorded any difference in pain intensity or pain relief scores between TENS and control during labour. Eight of the 10 reports recorded additional analgesic interventions. Two of the 10 studies reported on the total number of interventions per group. Figures suggested a decrease in total interventions with TENS, but group sizes were very modest.

Five of the 10 studies reported on numbers of women per group receiving additional analgesic intervention (Figure 2.17.1). There was no difference between active and sham TENS in the three largest of these studies. The final study reported on all interventions other than epidurals.

The combined result of these five studies generated a relative benefit of 0.88 (0.72–1.07). It was not effective and this lack of significance obviated the need to calculate a NNT.

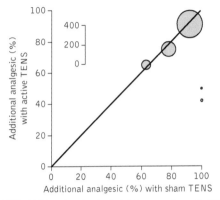

Figure 2.17.1 Additional analgesics in trials comparing active TENS with sham TENS.

Adverse effects in labour pain

There were no reports of adverse effects in any of the 10 studies.

Comment

Information from randomised controlled studies where the control has been inactive or sham TENS shows conclusively that it is ineffective for acute or labour pain.

2.18 **Topically applied non-steroidal anti-inflammatory drugs in acute pain**

Clinical bottom line. Topical NSAIDs are effective in the relief of pain caused by soft tissue injury, sprains, strains and trauma. Ketoprofen, felbinac, ibuprofen and piroxicam have proven efficacy. The NNT was 3.9 (3.4–4.3) for at least 50% pain relief after one week of topical NSAID use compared with placebo. Benzydamine and indomethacin did not appear to be effective. No significant local or systemic adverse effects are associated with topical NSAID use.

Oral NSAIDs are associated with increased risk of adverse effects such as gastrointestinal problems. The question arises therefore whether topical NSAIDs, which are widely available without prescription, are more suitable for a number of conditions. However, it has also been argued that topical NSAIDs have no action other than as rubefacients.

Systematic review

Moore, R. A., Carroll, D., Wiffen, P. J., Tramer, M. and McQuay, H. J. (1998).
  Quantitive systematic review of topically-applied non-steroidal
  anti-inflammatory drugs, *BMJ* 316: 333–8.

  Date review completed: September 1996

  Number of trials included: 40 placebo controlled/24 active controlled

  Number of patients: 3239 in placebo-controlled trials plus 4171 in active-controlled trials

  Control group: Topically applied placebo, other topical NSAIDs, other formulations or route of administration

  Main outcomes: At least 50% pain relief using standard pain scales at approximately one week after start of treatment. NNT, relative risk and relative benefit (with 95% confidence intervals)

Inclusion criteria were randomised, controlled trials of NSAIDs with pain outcomes; acute pain conditions (strains, sprains, sports injuries); full journal publication and unpublished drug company trials. Trials in vaginitis, oral and buccal conditions, thrombophlebitis and experimental pain were excluded.

Dichotomous data on pain outcomes were extracted from trials for analysis. At least 50% pain relief was regarded as a clinically relevant outcome. From the dichotomous data, information on the

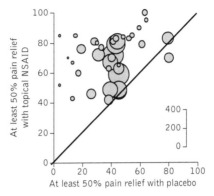

Figure 2.18.1 At least 50% pain relief with topical NSAID versus placebo.

proportion, and then the number of patients who achieved at least 50% pain relief were calculated. A NNT for at least 50% pain relief and the relative risk and benefit of the treatment were then calculated.

Findings

Included trials were in recent soft tissue injury, sprains, strains and trauma.

Twenty-seven of 37 trials with dichotomous outcomes showed significant improvement with topical NSAIDs compared with placebo (Figure 2.18.1). This was also true for the three trials with no dichotomous outcomes. For all 37 comparisons the NNT was 3.9 (3.4–4.3). However, this NNT was increased (i.e. drug less effective) when large trials were analysed separately (Table 2.18.1).

Based on pooled data of a minimum of three trials per drug, ketoprofen, felbinac, ibuprofen and piroxicam were statistically superior to placebo. Indomethacin and benzydamine were not (Table 2.18.1).

Three trials compared topical with oral NSAIDs. In all cases topical NSAIDs were as effective as oral doses.

Adverse effects

There was no significant difference in the frequency of local or systemic adverse effects or drug-related withdrawals (Table 2.18.1).

Comment

Topical NSAIDs were effective in relieving pain of strains and sprains over about a week. The comparison with placebo shows that this was not just the rubbing.

Table 2.18.1 Combined data and for particular topical NSAIDs

	Trials	Patients	Average number of treated patients	Response with placebo (%)	Response with active (%)	Relative benefit (95% CI)	NNT (95% CI)
Combined data for efficacy							
Combined efficacy data	37	3239	47	39	71	1.7 (1.5–1.9)	3.9 (3.4–4.4)
Trials of quality score 3–5	30	2834	52	38	72	1.7 (1.5–1.9)	3.9 (3.4–4.4)
Trials with treatment groups >40 patients	17	2306	75	43	67	1.6 (1.3–1.9)	4.8 (4.0–5.7)
Trials with treatment groups <40 patients	20	933	24	35	76	1.9 (1.6–2.2)	2.6 (2.3–3.1)
Effect of particular topical NSAID							
Ketoprofen	9	724	43	36	74	2.0 (1.5–2.6)	2.6 (2.3–3.2)
Felbinac	3	413	70	32	66	2.0 (1.5–2.7)	3.0 (2.4–4.1)
Ibuprofen	4	284	36	34	70	1.9 (1.2–3.0)	3.5 (2.5–5.6)
Piroxicam	4	589	74	39	69	1.6 (1.2–2.2)	4.2 (3.1–6.1)
Benzydamine	4	245	31	62	84	1.4 (0.9–2.0)	6.7 (3.8–23)
Indomethacin	3	394	66	32	47	1.3 (0.9–1.8)	10 (5–8)
Combined data for adverse events							
Local adverse effects				3	2.6	1.2 (0.8–1.7)	
Systemic adverse effects				0.7	0.8	1.0 (0.6–1.8)	
Withdrawal due to adverse effects				0.4	0.6	0.8 (0.4–1.4)	

Response is either proportion of patients achieving at least 50% pain relief or percent of patients having an adverse effect

2.19 Analgesics for dysmenorrhoea

Clinical bottom line. NSAIDs are effective for treating dysmenorrhoea, with NNTs of 2–3 compared with placebo. They also reduce restriction on daily living and reduce absence from work or school.

Dysmenorrhoea affects many women of reproductive age, and is a frequent cause of time lost from work or school as well as interfering with daily living. Treatment is usually with NSAIDs and minor analgesics.

Systematic review

Zhang, W. Y. and Li Wan Po, A. (1998). Efficacy of minor analgesics in primary dysmenorrhoea: a systematic review, *British Journal of Obstetrics and Gynaecology* 105: 780–9.

Randomised trials were sought using a number of search strategies, including requests for information from manufacturers. Studies had to be randomised, and primary dysmenorrhoea was defined as a history of painful menstrual cycles and exclusion of organic causes by physical examination. The main outcome was pain relief of at least moderate intensity, and the main comparison was with placebo. Secondary outcomes were women needing rescue analgesics, women experiencing restriction of daily living and women experiencing absence from work or school. Adverse effects were also examined.

Findings

Most trials were double-blind of either parallel or cross-over design, predominantly comparing the test analgesic with placebo.

Pain relief

The results for pain relief are shown in the Figure 2.19.1 and Table 2.19.1.

Compared with placebo, naproxen (550 or 275 mg four times daily), ibuprofen (400 mg four times daily) and mefenamic acid (250–500 mg four times daily) had NNT of between 2.4 and 3.0, with overlapping 95% confidence intervals, indicating no real difference between them. Five trials of aspirin (650 mg four times daily) had a much higher NNT of 9.2, with no overlap of confidence intervals with the NSAIDs. One comparison between paracetamol (650 mg four times daily) and placebo showed no difference between them.

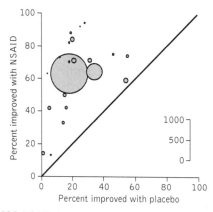

Figure 2.19.1 NSAIDs (not including aspirin) for dysmenorrhoea.

Table 2.19.1 Effectiveness of analgesics for pain relief of primary dysmenorrhoea

Analgesic	Number of trials	Number of patients	Percent improved with analgesic	Percent improved with placebo	Relative benefit (95% CI)	NNT (95% CI)
Naproxen	13	1706	59	17	3.4 (2.9–4.0)	2.4 (2.2–2.7)
Ibuprofen	9	599	70	31	2.2 (1.9–2.7)	2.6 (2.2–3.2)
Mefenamic acid	3	518	64	31	2.1 (1.7–2.6)	3.0 (2.4–4.0)
Aspirin	5	416	29	18	1.6 (1.1–2.2)	9.2 (5.3–35)

Restriction of daily living

Women taking naproxen or ibuprofen were less likely to have restrictions of daily living (Table 2.19.2).

The NNTs were 3.8 (3.2–4.6) for naproxen and 2.4 (1.9–3.2) for ibuprofen. Aspirin did not have this beneficial effect. There were no data on mefenamic acid.

Absence from work or school

Naproxen reduced greatly (by about 70%) the amount of time away from work or school (Table 2.19.2). The NNT was 3.9 (3.3–4.6). One

Table 2.19.2 Effect of NSAIDs on restrictions of daily living and absence from work or school

Analgesic	Number of Trials	Number of patients	Percent affected with analgesic	Percent affected with placebo	Relative benefit (95% CI)	NNT (95% CI)
Restriction of daily living						
Naproxen	7	1341	60	86	0.69 (0.64–0.74)	3.8 (3.2–4.6)
Ibuprofen	3	234	12	55	0.22 (0.14–0.38)	2.4 (1.9–3.2)
Aspirin	3	203	50	62	0.80 (0.62–1.03)	8.0 (3.8–>100)
Absence from work or school						
Naproxen	7	1345	8	34	0.24 (0.18–0.32)	3.9 (3.3–4.6)

study on ibuprofen mirrored this effect, and one study on aspirin did not have this beneficial effect. There were no data on mefenamic acid.

Adverse effects

Adverse effects were mainly nausea, dizziness and headache. There was a suggestion that naproxen caused more adverse effects (mainly nausea), but the power of studies to detect this was low and confidence intervals wide.

Comment

This is a well-done systematic review which demonstrated that naproxen, ibuprofen and mefenamic acid are effective. Aspirin was less effective and paracetamol 650 mg was not effective in a single study. The authors conclude that, based on efficacy and absence of common adverse effects, ibuprofen is probably the treatment of choice.

The only complaint one could have is the issue of dose. It would be helpful to know the NNTs at particular dose levels, though we suspect that the authors reflect what they found in the original reports.

2.20 **Other acute pain interventions with evidence of efficacy**

This section looks at a number of other interventions for acute pain where there is some evidence that they work. What is not included are interventions that could come under the heading of complementary therapy, which are dealt within a later section. The format is a title, clinical bottom line, reference, and a brief commentary for each.

Incisional local anaesthesia for pain after abdominal surgery

Clinical bottom line. Incisional local anaesthetic is effective in relieving postoperative pain after inguinal herniotomy up to about 7 h. For hysterectomy, cholecystectomy and other major/minor surgical procedures, there was a lack of evidence for effectiveness. This may be due in part to inadequate trial design, and further trials are needed before recommendations can be made.

Systematic review

Moiniche, S., Mikkelsen, S., Wetterslev, J. and Dahl, J. B. (1998). A qualitative
systematic review of incisional local anaesthesia for postoperative pain relief
after abdominal operations, *British Journal of Anaesthesia* 81: 377–83.

Comment

A well-done review with 26 trials altogether, showing incisional local anaesthetic to be effective when compared with saline or no treatment.

Pain relief from intra-articular morphine after knee surgery

Clinical bottom line. Intra-articular morphine may have some effect in reducing postoperative pain intensity and consumption of analgesics. The evidence is more consistent for a prolonged analgesic effect than for short term relief. However, the quality of published trials is poor, and it remains unclear whether any analgesia produced is clinically useful.

Systematic review

Kalso, E., Tramer, M., Carroll, D., McQuay, H. and Moore, R. A. (1997). Pain
relief from intra-articular morphine after knee surgery: a qualitative
systematic review, *Pain* 71: 642–51.

For update see also: Kalso, E., Smith, L., McQuay, H. J. and Moore, R. A. (2002). No pain, no gain: clinical excellence and scientific rigour – lessons learned from IA morphine, *Pain*, **98**: 269–75.

Comment

The use of opioids in the knee joint is a hot topic. While there is evidence that it results in longer duration analgesia, there is considerable confusion over why that should be, the mechanism, and dose of morphine required.

Patient-controlled analgesia in postoperative pain

Clinical bottom line. Patient-controlled analgesia produces a modest improvement in pain relief over a 24 h period compared with conventional analgesia. It is preferred by patients, and is not associated with additional side effects.

Patient preference for PCA had an NNT of 1.9 (1.6–2.5) for at least satisfactory analgesia when compared with conventional analgesia at ≤24 h in patients with postoperative pain.

Systematic review

Ballantyne, J. C., Carr, D. B., Chalmers, T. C., Dear, K. B., Angelillo, I. F. and Mosteller, F. (1993). Postoperative patient-controlled analgesia: meta-analyses of initial randomized control trials, *Journal of Clinical Anesthesia* 5: 182–93.

Comment

A famous meta-analysis, showing better analgesic efficacy and patient satisfaction for similar analgesic usage by PCA as by conventional analgesia.

Preoperative information-giving interventions and pain

Clinical bottom line. Preoperative interventions which combine sensory and procedural information significantly reduce postoperative pain, distress and negative affect. This is also true for sensory information given alone, although the effect is not as great.

Preoperatively, patients should be offered information-giving interventions with include explanations of what will be happening to them, and how they can expect to feel.

Systematic review

Suls, J. and Wan, C. K. (1989). Effects of sensory and procedural information on coping with stressful medical procedures and pain: a meta-analysis, *Journal of Consulting Clinical Psychology* 57: 372–9.

Comment

This review is now almost 20 years old and techniques have moved on, but preparation for operation looked useful then. This review should be updated to ensure that it is relevant to contemporary needs.

2.21 **Other acute pain interventions without evidence of efficacy**

This section looks at a number of other interventions for acute pain where there is some evidence that they do not work. What is not included are interventions that could come under the heading of complementary therapy, which are dealt with in a later section. The format is a title, clinical bottom line, reference, and a brief commentary for each.

Analgesic efficacy of NSAIDs: comparison of different routes in acute pain

Clinical bottom line. In renal colic NSAIDs act faster when given intravenously compared with intramuscular or rectal routes. This may be clinically relevant. In all other pain conditions there is no evidence that injected NSAIDs were better than oral. There is, however, increased reporting of adverse effects with intravenous and rectal administration. Where possible, patients should be given NSAIDs orally. Better trials are needed to provide a definitive answer to the question of which routes are the most effective.

Systematic review

Tramèr, M., Williams, J., Carroll, D., Wiffen, P. J., McQuay, H. J. and Moore, R. A. (1998). Comparing analgesic efficacy of non-steroidal anti-inflammatory drugs given by different routes for acute and chronic pain, *Acta Anaesthiologica Scandinavica* **42**: 71–9.

Comment

There were almost 2000 patients included in this review. There was no evidence for faster, better, or longer duration of analgesia from NSAIDs which were injected into muscle or vein, or given rectally.

Analgesic adjuncts for brachial plexus block

Clinical bottom line. There is no convincing evidence from this review that adjunct analgesics are of any benefit.

Systematic review

Murphy, D. B., McCartney, C. J., and Chan, V. W. (2000) Novel analgesic adjuncts for brachial plexus block: a systematic review, *Anesthesia & Analgesia* **90**: 1122–8.

Comment

Though properly randomised and double blind, the trials were predominantly (12/17) methodologically flawed because they lacked a systemic control group and all were small. There is no convincing evidence from this review that adjunct analgesics are of any benefit.

Wound infiltration with local anaesthetic in postoperative pain

Clinical bottom line. Postoperative use of local anaesthetic at the wound site does not appear to be useful in relieving postoperative pain. However, the review did not state the number of patients included, and it is therefore difficult to be certain of the strength of review findings.

Systematic review

Dahl, J. B., Moiniche, S. and Kehlet, H. (1994). Wound infiltration with local anaesthetics for postoperative pain relief, *Acta Anaesthesiolica Scandinavica* 38: 7–14.

Comment

Limited information and diverse outcomes makes this of limited value.

Analgesic efficacy of peripheral opioids

Clinical bottom line. There is no evidence for the efficacy of peripheral opioids either intraoperatively or postoperatively. Trials of a higher quality are needed to provide a definitive answer.

Systematic review

Picard, P. R., Tramèr, M. R., McQuay, H. J. and Moore, R. A. (1997). Analgesic efficacy of peripheral opioids (all except intra-articular): A qualitative systematic review of randomised controlled trials, *Pain* 72: 309–18.

Comment

There were 26 trials with over 900 patients in this review. Though several different blocks were investigated, there was an absence of evidence for any important effect.

Pre-emptive analgesia

Clinical bottom line. Patients do not benefit from pre-emptive analgesia with NSAIDs and paracetamol at conventional dosing. There is weak evidence for local anaesthetic, but trials lack the necessary power. There is some evidence for pre-emptive opioid action, especially with intravenous administration, but trials are not of adequate design.

Trials of adequate design and size are required to assess the role of local anaesthetic and opioids in pre-emptive analgesia.

Systematic reviews

McQuay, H. J. (1995). Pre-emptive analgesia: a systematic review of clinical studies, *Annals of Medicine* 27: 249–56.

Møiniche, S., Kehlet, H. and Dahl, J. B. (2002). A qualitative and quantitative systematic review of preemptive analgesia for postoperative pain, *Anesthesiology* 96: 725–41.

Comment

This is tricky territory where the exact question being asked is often unclear in trials. But two good reviews 7 years apart have now looked at the topic and find absolutely no evidence for any benefit. The later review benefits from using methodological advances, and from having more material to analyse. It finds that using opioids, NSAIDs or NMDA antagonists makes no difference, because they show no benefit. Nor do single-dose epidurals, or continuous epidurals, or local anaesthetic wound infiltration. However the goalposts are moved, these reviews pin down the question and confirm the negative finding. What is astonishing is that so much research has been done, and continues to be done, with so little hope of benefit.

Relaxation techniques for acute pain management

Clinical bottom line. Convincing evidence for the efficacy of relaxation is lacking. More trials of better quality are needed.

Systematic review

Seers, K. and Carroll, D. (1998). Relaxation techniques for acute pain management – a systematic review, *Journal of Advanced Nursing* 27: 466–75.

Comment

There were only 7 trials with 360 patients, and though some trials showed some benefit, others did not, and the clinical relevance of the benefit shown was not obvious.

2.22 **Do NSAIDs inhibit bone healing?**

Clinical bottom line. The only evidence that NSAIDs inhibit bone healing comes from animal experiments (of unknown relevance), and in humans from a retrospective series using high doses of intramuscular ketorolac after spinal fusion, plus a small case control study looking at failure of fractured femurs to heal. NSAIDs are effective in reducing postoperative heterotopic bone formation, with an NNT of 3. NSAIDs do not affect risk of fracture in any significant way.

Some orthopaedic centres do not allow the use of NSAIDs for postoperative analgesia after fractures or orthopaedic surgery because they are thought to interfere with bone healing. The purpose of this section is to examine the evidence we found for the effects of NSAIDs on bone healing.

PubMed was searched using free text terms to detect reviews, RCTs and epidemiological reports relating to bone and fracture healing and the use of NSAIDs. We also had a look at the Cochrane Library.

Background

Bone metabolism has a complex regulatory system that includes prostaglandins, produced abundantly by osteoblasts [1]. The balance of evidence from animal experiments suggests that prostaglandins favour bone formation. NSAIDs might therefore be expected to inhibit bone formation because they inhibit prostaglandin formation. The evidence for this is by no means conclusive, and some NSAIDs in some models have been shown to inhibit bone loss.

Disagreement might be a function of type of NSAID; proprionic acid NSAIDs (ibuprofen, naproxen, ketoprofen) may prevent bone loss in some circumstances while acetic acid NSAIDs (indomethacin, diclofenac) may not. Dose and duration of use may also be factors. Experiments on rabbits (over 20 years ago) have shown that NSAIDs can inhibit fracture healing. Ketorolac has been implicated in failed bone fusion in spinal fusion experiments in rabbits.

Experimental work in animals seems, at best, to leave the role of NSAIDs and bone healing after fracture or operation uncertain.

NSAIDs and bone in orthodontic surgery

Flurbiprofen appeared to increase bone formation in root-form implants in two patients [2], confirmed in a randomised study of 29 patients given flurbiprofen 200 mg a day or placebo for three months [3]. Flurbiprofen was without effect in a small randomised study after periodontal surgery [4] and naproxen did not increase bone healing in another study [5].

In summary there is no convincing evidence that NSAIDs have any major effects on bone in orthodontic surgery.

NSAIDs and heterotopic bone formation

A Cochrane review has examined heterotopic bone formation after hip replacement [6]. It found 12 randomised trials, predominantly relatively small studies of medium to high dose NSAID, plus one large study of low dose aspirin. In 13 studies heterotopic bone formed in 182/806 (23%) patients with medium to high dose NSAID and 430/765 (56%) patients with control (Figure 2.22.1). The relative risk was 0.38 (0.33–0.44) and the number needed to treat to prevent heterotopic bone formation was 3.0 (2.6–3.4).

Most studies recorded heterotopic bone formation at least 6 months after operation. Duration, dose and type of NSAID used were not given, nor was there an analysis according to degree of heterotopic bone. Serious fatal and non-fatal events were small in number (nine reported), but failure of bone healing was not mentioned. This might repay a more thorough review of these papers.

Low dose aspirin (162 mg a day) was without effect in a large (2700 patients) trial [7]. In a detailed analysis that included NSAID use before and after operation (17% needed analgesics after the operation), there was no mention of association of NSAID use and failure of the hip replacement.

Indomethacin has a similar effect on preventing heterotopic bone formation after spinal cord injury [8].

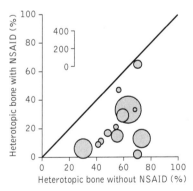

Figure 2.22.1 Heterotopic bone formation with and without NSAID after hip replacement.

NSAIDs and spinal fusion

Ketorolac after spinal fusion was studied in a retrospective review of 288 cases [9] in a single centre. Patients had posterior spinal fusion between 1991 and 1992, and there was a minimum two-year follow up. Ketorolac was administered as a 60 mg intramuscular loading dose followed by 30 mg every 6 h as needed. Seven patients given ketorolac had additional 2–20 (mean 8) 10-mg oral doses as needed.

Ketorolac was given to 167 patients, and no NSAID to 121. Patients having ketorolac received between one and 39 doses of ketorolac after surgery (mean 10). The two groups were demographically similar.

Non-union occurred in 5/121 (4%) of patients having no NSAID and 29/167 (17%) of those receiving ketorolac. The odds ratio was 4.9 (1.8–17). The same degree of increased risk was seen in all subgroups. There was a dose-dependent relationship between non-union rates and ketorolac doses (Figure 2.22.2).

There was an apparent relationship between postoperative use of ketorolac and cigarette smoking. The non-union rate was 2% in those who neither smoked nor had ketorolac, 7% for those who smoked but did not have ketorolac, 10% for non-smokers having ketorolac and 25% for those who both smoked and had ketorolac.

By contrast with these results, Reuben [10] examined non-union rates on 106 patients undergoing posterior spinal fusion with autologous crest bone grafts. All had received 50 mg rofecoxib postoperatively for five consecutive days starting on the morning of surgery. No other NSAIDs were used postoperatively.

Using the same criteria for nonunion as Glassman [9], the one-year non-union rate was 4.7% (5 of the 106 patients). This is the same rate as reported by Glassman for patients not receiving perioperative ketorolac [9].

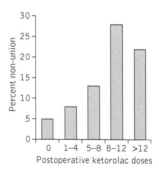

Figure 2.22.2 Non-union rate and postoperative ketorolac doses after spinal fusion surgery.

NSAIDs and Colles fracture

A randomised double-blind study of postmenopausal women with a displaced Colles fracture examined a 8-week regimen of 20 mg daily piroxicam and placebo on recovery [11]. There was no effect on bone mineral density, and no decrease in fracture healing with piroxicam.

Fracture non-union and NSAID

A case-control study from Leeds of 32 patients with non-union of fractured femur and 67 comparable patients whose fracture had united reported an association between non-union and the use of NSAIDs after injury [12], and delayed healing in patients who took NSAIDs and whose fracture had united.

Several other studies of bone healing after fracture make no mention of NSAIDs:

- Nonunion among 67 ankle fusions in Houston was associated with open trauma, and with smoking, alcohol, diabetes or illegal drug use [13].
- A survey of 165 elderly patients with femoral neck fractures in Oslo noted technical issues associated with disturbed healing, but did not mention NSAIDs [14].
- A meta-analysis of the effect of reamed versus nonreamed nailing of lower leg bone fractures [15] examined a number of factors for nonunion, with higher non-union rates being associated with studies of lower quality.
- Risk of nonunion for tibial shaft fractures in 100 consecutive patients from Gothenburg noted that high energy trauma has a relative risk of 2 and open fractures one of 8. NSAID use was not mentioned [16].

NSAIDs and risk of new fractures

Laboratory exploration of the effect of NSAIDs on bone metabolism has demonstrated that bone resorption can be affected through prostaglandin inhibition. One implication is that NSAIDs potentially could reduce bone loss and hence fracture risk. A huge observational study using the UK general practice research database (GPRD) [17] tells us that this hope will not be realised.

Background

A large study of aspirin and NSAID use on bone mineral density in 7768 white women older than 65 years in the USA [18] concluded that bone mineral density was higher in users of these drugs. Risk of fracture was unaffected. The study had the benefit of being large, but aspirin and NSAID users were different from non-users. Osteoarthritis, rheumatoid arthritis, back pain and other conditions were much more common in NSAID users than non-users. Adjustment of results for potential confounding can be difficult in circumstances where subjects and controls differ markedly. NSAID use did not affect the rate of excretion of markers of bone resorption [19], but bone mineral density at some sites was again found to be affected by proprionic acid NSAIDs in 84 older women [20]. The background evidence that NSAIDs reduce fracture risk was thin, but the apparent effects on bone density meant that some reduction in fracture risk might be expected. A very large study would be needed to show this.

Study

A large retrospective cohort study was conducted using the GPRD. It looked at fracture risk in people using NSAIDs and compared that with people who did not use NSAIDs.

NSAID users fulfilling one or more prescriptions for an NSAID from 1987 up to end 1997 were included, and divided arbitrarily into those receiving three or more prescriptions and those receiving one or two prescriptions. A control group of people never having a prescription for NSAIDs was created by matching for sex, age, and practice (where possible). Systemic corticosteroid use was an exclusion criterion for users and controls. Information on about a dozen possible confounding conditions, and about a dozen possible confounding drug treatments was collected for each case and control.

After a prescription was filled follow up was until fracture or 91 days after the last prescription. Nonvertebral fractures were assessed by ICD codes and vertebral by radiography.

Results

NSAIDs were prescribed for 501,000 patients, with 215,000 having three or more prescriptions for a median 3.4 years (regular users), and 287,000 having one or two prescriptions for a mean of 0.7 years (incidental users). There were 215,000 controls. Back pain and rheumatoid arthritis were more common in NSAID users than in controls. Incidental users were about 10 years younger than the mean age of 54 years for regular users and controls.

Non-vertebral fractures occurred more frequently in older women and the oldest men (Figure 2.22.3). For women fracture rates rose substantially after age 64.

Fracture rates with regular NSAID users were certainly not lower than controls. If anything, they were somewhat higher (Table 2.22.1) for vertebral and all non-vertebral fractures. Regular users had fracture rates no different from incidental users.

No NSAID was associated with higher or lower rates of fracture. Restricting analysis to patients with a history of arthopathy reduced the difference between regular users and controls for non-vertebral fractures, with a relative risk of 1.2 (1.1–1.3).

Comment

This beautiful study can tell us that there is no major effect of NSAIDs on risk of fracture. It also shows the problems with confounding.

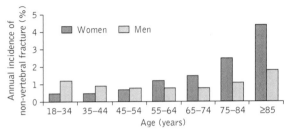

Figure 2.22.3 Fracture rates with age in controls.

Table 2.22.1 Fracture rates in regular users and controls

Fracture type	Regular NSAID user		Control		Relative risk (95% CI)
	Number of fractures	Rate per 100 years	Number of fractures	Rate per 100 years	
Vertebral	808	0.1	192	0.03	2.9 (2.5–3.4)
All non-vertebral	10,505	1.5	5793	1	1.5 (1.4–1.5)
Forearm	2516	0.3	1556	0.3	1.3 (1.2–1.4)
Hip	973	0.1	686	0.1	1.1 (0.98–1.2)

While many confounding factors could be taken into account, others, like diet, exercise or bone density could not. To properly take account of confounding factors you have to know what they are, and how much to adjust for them.

Summary

So far this is the sum of the evidence that appears to be available.

The animal experiments are interesting, but may not be relevant to clinical situations. For instance, the RCT on NSAIDs in Colles fracture [10] was performed by researchers who had shown an inhibitory effect of NSAIDs on fracture healing in rats, but no effect was seen in man.

We have three possible bits of evidence. The first is in spinal fusion surgery [9,10]. The problems with the original retrospective survey [9] include the choice of drug. Ketorolac, especially at the high doses given intramuscularly, is hardly representative of NSAIDs as a class. Intramuscular ketorolac at 30 mg is equivalent to 10 mg orally in analgesic effect [21], but gives a bigger body load of drug. It is particularly effective at producing gastrointestinal bleeding. Then there is the problem that patients needing ketorolac needed more postoperative analgesic, but we do not know whether that itself was a marker for some other pathology. And the synergistic effect with smoking is a puzzle, though this has been examined in a retrospective analysis of 357 patients after spinal fusion [22] (but some of the patients may have been in the earlier analysis [9]). But retrospective analysis of 106 patients given 50 mg of rofecoxib for five days had no increased rate of nonunion using similar nonunion criteria [10].

The second bit of evidence is a case-control study from Leeds suggesting that NSAIDs inhibit healing of fractured femur [12]. The study had only 32 patients with unhealed femur, and small retrospective case-control studies have their problems. No other investigation into failure of fractures to heal mentioned NSAIDs.

So there is not much in the way of top quality evidence for failure to heal. None from randomised controlled trials, and what randomised trials there are show no effect, and no evidence from large good quality observational studies. This latter is important, because it is a dog that does not bark in the night. Given the millions of orthopaedic operations performed and bone fractures every year, plus the frequent use of NSAIDs for postoperative analgesia, and available from pharmacists without prescription, is it credible that a major effect of NSAIDs on bone healing could be missed?

This is borne out to some extent by a huge observational study on fracture rates in 500,000 patients taking NSAIDs and 215,000 controls [17]. The conclusion was that NSAIDs had minimal effects on fracture risk, especially given the large number of possible confounders considered, and some major ones that could not be considered.

So far the evidence that NSAIDs play any major role affecting bone, apart from their important effects on heterotopic bone formation [6], does not stack up.

References

1. Dumont, A. S. *et al.* (2000). Nonsteroidal anti-inflammatory drugs and bone metabolism in spinal fusion surgery. A pharmacological quandary, *Journal of Pharmacology and Toxicology Methods* 43: 31–9.

2. Reddy *et al.* (1990). Assessment of adjunctive flurbiprofen therapy in root-form implant healing with digital subtraction radiography, *Journal of Oral Implantology* XVI: 272–6.

3. Jeffcoat, M. K. *et al.* (1995). The effect of systemic flurbiprofen on bone supporting dental implants, *Journal of the American Dental Association* 126: 305–11.

4. Brägger, U. *et al.* (1997). Effect of the NSAID flurbiprofen on remodelling after periodontal surgery, *Journal of Periodontal Research* 32: 375–82.

5. Bichara, J. *et al.* (1999). The effect of postsurgical naproxen and a bioabsorbable membrane on osseous healing in intrabony defects, *Journal of Periodontology* 70: 869–77.

6. Neal, B. *et al.* (2001). Non-steroidal anti-inflammatory drugs for preventing heterotopic bone formation after hip arthroplasty (Cochrane Review). In: The Cochrane Library, Issue 4, 2001. Oxford: Update Software.

7. Neal, B. C. *et al.* (2000). No effect of low-dose aspirin for the prevention of heterotopic bone formation after total hip replacement, *Acta Orthopaedica Scandinavica* 2: 129–34.

8. Banovac, K. *et al.* (2001). Prevention of heterotopic ossification after spinal cord injury with indomethacin, *Spinal Cord* 39: 370–4.

9. Glassman, S. D. *et al.* (1998). The effect of postoperative nonsteroidal anti-inflammatory drug administration on spinal fusion, *Spine* 23: 834–8.

10. Reuben, S. S. (2001). Considerations in the use of COX-2 inhibitors in spinal fusion surgery, *Anesthesia & Analgesia* 93: 798–804.

11. Adolphson, P. *et al.* (1993). No effects of piroxicam on osteopenia and recovery after Colles' fracture, *Archives of Orthopedics and Trauma Surgery* 112: 127–30.

12. Giannoudis, P. V. *et al.* (2000). Nonunion of the femoral diaphysis. The influence of reaming and non-steroidal anti-inflammatory drugs, *Journal of Bone & Joint Surgery Br* 82: 655–8.

13. Perlman, M. H. and Thordarson, D. B. (1999). Ankle fusion in a high risk population: an assessment of nonunion risk factors, *Foot Ankle International* 20: 491–6.

14. Alho, A. *et al.* (1999). Internally fixed femoral neck fractures. Early prediction of failures in 203 elderly patients with displaced fractures, *Acta Orthopaedica Scandinavica* 70: 141–4.

15. Bhandari, M. *et al.* (2000). Reamed versus nonreamed intramedullary nailing of lower extremity long bone fractures: a systematic overview and meta-analysis, *Journal of Orthopedics and Trauma* 14: 2–9.

16. Karladani, A. H. *et al.* (2001). The influence of fracture etiology and type of fracture healing: a review of 104 consecutive tibial shaft fractures, *Archives Orthopaedics and Trauma Surgery* 121: 325–8.

17. Van Staa, T. P. *et al.* (2000). Use of nonsteroidal anti-inflammatory drugs and risk of fractures, *Bone* 27: 563–8.

18. Bauer, D. C. *et al.* (1996). Aspirin and NSAID use in older women: effect on bone mineral density and fracture risk, *Journal of Bone and Mineral Research*, 11: 29–35.

19. Lane, N. E. *et al.* (1997). Aspirin and nonsteroidal antiinflammatory drug use in elderly women: effects on a marker of bone resorption, *Journal of Rheumatology* 24: 1132–6.

20. Morton, D. J. *et al.* (1998). Nonsteroidal anti-inflammatory drugs and bone mineral density in older women: the Rancho Bernado study, *Journal of Bone and Mineral Research* 12: 1924–31.

21. Smith, L. A. *et al.* (2000). Single-dose ketorolac and pethidine in acute postoperative pain: a systematic review, *British Journal of Anaesthesia* 84: 48–58.

22. Glassman, S. D. *et al.* (2000). The effect of cigarette smoking and smoking cessation on spinal fusion, *Spine* 25: 2608–15.

Section 3
Migraine and headache

3.1 **Introduction**

This chapter is going to deal mainly with migraine, the most common form of headache apart from common headache or headache associated with other illness.

Prevalence of migraine

Migraine *is* common. It affects about 1 adult woman in 5 and 1 adult man in 20.

To investigate the prevalence of migraine, studies were looked for that used International Headache Society (IHS) criteria for migraine in large samples of adults. The results of individual studies are shown in Table 3.1.1 and Figure 3.1.1.

The samples were large, and ranged from 1200 to over 20,000 people (about 58,000 in total), were in adults, were conducted in Europe or North America, and generally used a random sample of a population. The range of results for women was between 11.9% and 21.9%, and for men between 4.0% and 8.2%. The weighted mean prevalence for women was 17% and for men was 6%.

Effect of migraine on personal and work time

On average someone with migraine will have three attacks a month, and lose much time out of their lives. For instance, the amount of time lost to usual activities in a migraine attack was a median 9 h in data collected in a randomised trial (Figure 3.1.2). This reflected a very wide distribution. For example, while half of the patients lost fewer than 9 h, at least 60 patients lost more than 20 h. The mean value was 14.5 h of total time lost. Median work time lost was 4 h [1]. Effective treatment (in this case with 40 mg eletriptan) reduced time lost considerably (Figure 3.1.3).

Statistics from patient surveys show that migraine really does impose negatively on life:

- affects 20% of women aged 20–65;
- affects 7% of men;
- average is 36 attacks in one year;
- average of five days in bed in one year;
- average period of bed rest is 5–6 h.

Yet only a small proportion seek help from the doctors, choosing mostly either to treat with medicines bought from pharmacies, or not to treat at all.

Migraine is also an expensive business. Health economists might argue over how much lost productivity there is in the economy, but

Table 3.1.1 Studies reporting prevalence of migraine over one year or lifetime using IHS criteria

Reference	Type of study	Sample source	Sample size	Age range	Lifetime or one year prevalence (%)		
					Men	Women	Overall
Breslau et al., 1991	Survey, face-to-face interview	HMO population, random sample, USA	1200	21–30	7.0	16.3	12.8
Gobel et al., 1994	Survey, face-to-face interview	General population, random sample, Germany	5000	18+	7.0	15.0	11.0
Henry et al., 1992	Survey, face-to-face interview	General population, stratified quota with random element, France	4204	15+	4.0	11.9	8.1
Linet et al., 1989	Survey, telephone interview	General population, residents of Washington County, Maryland USA	10,000	12–29	5.3	14.0	
O'Brien et al., 1994	Survey, telephone interview	General population, random sample, Canada	4235	18+	7.4	21.9	
Rasmussen et al., 1991	Prospective survey, clinical exam	General population, random sample, Denmark	1000	25–64	6.0	15.0	10.0
Stewart et al., 1992	Survey, PSAQ	General population, random sample, USA	20,468	12–80	5.7	17.6	
Stewart et al., 1996	Survey, telephone interview	General population, USA	12,000	18–65	8.2	19.0	

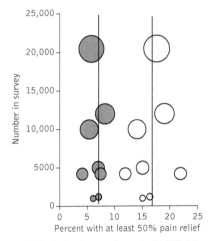

Figure 3.1.1 Individual migraine prevalence studies (filled for men, open for women); vertical lines are the weighted means.

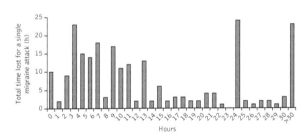

Figure 3.1.2 Total time lost in a single migraine attack.

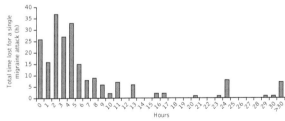

Figure 3.1.3 Total time lost when migraine treated with eletriptan 40 mg.

the costs involved in whatever study one looks at, just because of time lost at home or at work, are large. It has been estimated that the cost of migraine in the USA is $14 billion a year [2] and many other studies confirm the personal, healthcare, employment and societal impact.

A number of studies confirm that migraine is associated with a substantial amount of time lost from work, and a review of health economic studies in migraine is available on the Bandolier migraine site. For instance, in screening 2670 patients for phase III clinical trials, the average estimates for lost work were 8.3 days lost due to absenteeism, and 11.2 days lost because of reduced efficiency [3]. The estimated cost to employers was US$3309 (year 2000 prices), but gives values for a number of countries as well as the USA.

Outcomes in migraine trials

What is it that people who suffer from migraine want from their treatments? A full summary about what people want from migraine treatment comes from a survey of nearly 700 people with migraine in the USA [4]. They want their headache pain relieved, totally, quickly with no adverse effects, and they do not want the pain to come back (Figure 3.1.4).

What happens in migraine trials that can allow us to answer these questions? First, patients have to have pain of moderate or severe intensity when they take a tablet or have an injection. They then score their pain (most migraine trials measure pain as the primary outcome), using the words no pain, mild pain, moderate pain, or severe pain. This is all pretty standard stuff. Pain measurements like this have been used successfully for decades, and we know in other settings like acute pain, that if patients have only mild pain we could have insensitive studies (how can you measure an analgesic effect when there's no pain?).

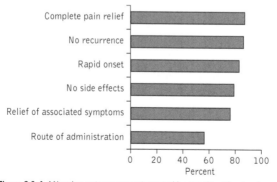

Figure 3.1.4 Migraine outcomes most wanted by people with migraine.

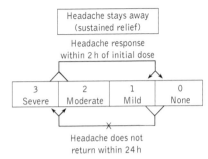

Figure 3.1.5 Migraine trial outcomes.

Pain scores are made by the patient at hourly or half hourly intervals until, say, 6 h, or even as long as 24 h. The outcomes chosen by trialists (rather than patients) has been the headache response at 2 h. This is a headache that starts as moderate or severe but where the pain has declined to mild or no pain by two hours (Figure 3.1.5). The headache response could be measured at any time point. Preferred now is **pain free** at two hours, though pain free at any time could be measured.

Perhaps what we should be measuring is something different – namely the pain gone at 2 h and not returned within the following day. So far this has not been done regularly, but results for headache response within 2 h followed by 22 h during which the headache does not recur (Figure 3.1.5), and when no additional analgesics are taken, is now becoming available. The outcome we really want is that of being pain free at 1 h with no recurrence of headache and no additional analgesics.

The point is that we have a number of possible outcomes from recent trials of high quality and validity, especially for triptans. The results for different outcomes and different doses of different medicines will be gathered together in a later section. Older studies (as with ergotamine) often fail to match up to modern standards, and have many different methods of reporting outcomes.

Results of migraine trials

When we begin to look at migraine trials, using those of high quality and high validity, we find that there are many. Most treatments have been summarised as reviews, or reviewed by us, in our web pages. We can combine the results in league tables (section 3.2), both as numbers needed to treat (NNTs) and simply as percentages of patients having the outcome. Do not take these figures at face value, though, and read the comments in the league table page about the dangers of over-interpreting league tables.

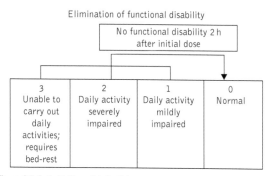

Elimination of functional disability

| 3
Unable to carry out daily activities; requires bed-rest | 2
Daily activity severely impaired | 1
Daily activity mildly impaired | 0
Normal |

No functional disability 2 h after initial dose

Figure 3.1.6 Activities of daily living.

One thing that is worth remembering is that there are many other possible outcomes of benefit in migraine trials, like reduction of nausea and vomiting, or photophobia, or phonophobia, or restrictions of daily living. We do not have reviews of these yet, but they are worth doing and worth reporting when available. An example is for a scale that measures functional disability with migraine (Figure 3.1.6).

Adverse events

These are proving really quite difficult to get to grips with. Part of the problem is the way that adverse events are measured and reported generally. In migraine trials there has been a particular difficulty, in that benefits (pain relief) have been measured over 24 h, while adverse events have been collected over 10 days. The result is that at present it is difficult to find much of interest or value to say.

Ten steps to control your headaches

The US Headache Consortium recently published guidelines for improving migraine treatment. The consortium includes seven organisations: the American Academy of Neurology, the American Academy of Family Physicians, the American Headache Society, the American College of Emergency Physicians, the American College of Physicians–American Society of Internal Medicine, the American Osteopathic Association and the National Headache Foundation. The consortium recommends 10 steps for better migraine management:

1. Know your headache diagnosis. Headache is a symptom that can have many causes. Recurrent, disabling headaches are usually migraine headaches.

2. Find a good clinician. If you are troubled by headaches, find a clinician who understands the problem and is willing to work with you to find appropriate treatment. In most cases, migraine can be diagnosed based on a careful medical history and an examination without the use of expensive diagnostic tests such as magnetic resonance imaging or computed tomography.

3. Tell your doctor how your headaches affect your life. Migraine often causes temporary disability. The frequency and extent of disability are important guides to treatment. These aspects of migraine can be measured using the migraine disability assessment score (MIDAS, at http://www.midas-migraine.net/) questionnaire.

4. Avoid headache triggers. Once migraine is diagnosed, try to avoid or reduce the factors that can trigger your migraine. Possibilities include certain food (especially chocolate, cheese and red wine), changes in sleeping patterns, and changes in the weather.

5. Find appropriate medication for your attacks. The DISC study (section 3.12) shows that degree of disability predicts treatment need. Less severe migraine can be treated successfully with over-the-counter medication or with prescription pain medication. If migraine headaches interfere with your ability to function, as reflected by a high MIDAS score, you may need a migraine-specific medication such as a triptan. Triptans are highly effective for migraine, but not for pain in general. They are available as tablets, pills that melt on your tongue, nasal sprays and injections.

6. Do not overuse pain medication. Overuse of medication, whether over-the-counter or prescription, can make your headaches worse by causing rebound headaches. As the medicine wears off, it can trigger the next headache.

7. Have at least two treatment options available. Ask your doctor to prescribe a 'rescue' medication that you can take if your regular medication fails. This can prevent trips to the emergency room.

8. If one medicine does not work, try another one. Treat several attacks with each treatment to determine if it works. If the medication does not provide satisfactory relief after three attacks, ask for a new medication.

9. Ask your doctor about preventive drugs. If you have two or more headaches a week, ask your doctor about preventive medications that you can take on a daily basis to reduce the number of headaches you get. The benefits of preventive medication may develop over several months.

10. Use treatments other than drugs. Many people find that biofeedback and relaxation training improve their headaches.

Conclusions

Systematic reviews can help us in a number of different ways, especially when thinking about issues like relative efficacy where they provide the best available evidence about prescribing now. As well they help us think about the quality and utility of outcomes, and the validity of trials. Their real place is not only an archaeological rummage through trials of yore, but rather a learning process to ensure that trials and research in the future reach a much higher standard, and are more immediately useful to professionals and to patients.

References

1. Wells, N. E. and Steiner, T. J. (2001). Effectiveness of eletriptan in reducing time loss caused by migraine attacks, *Pharmacoeconomics* 18: 557–66.
2. Hu, X. H. *et al.* (1999). Burden of migraine in the United States, *Archives of Internal Medicine* 159: 813–8.
3. Gert, W. G. *et al.* (2001). The multinational impact of migraine symptoms on healthcare ultization and work loss, *Pharmacoeconomics* 19: 197–206.
4. Lipton, R. B. and Stewart, W. F. (1999). Acute migraine therapy: do doctors understand what patients with migraine want from therapy? *Headache* 39: S20–S26.

3.2 **Diagnosing headache and migraine**

IHS diagnostic criteria

In 1988 the IHS published criteria for the diagnosis of a number of different headache types [1]. Those for some of the common headaches are reproduced below for migraine with and without aura, cluster headache, tension-type headache, and cervicogenic headache.

Migraine without aura (MO) diagnostic criteria

(A) At least five headache attacks lasting 4–72 h (untreated or unsuccessfully treated), which have at least two of the four following characteristics:

1. unilateral location,

2. pulsating quality,

3. moderate or severe intensity (inhibits or prohibits daily activities),

4. aggravated by walking stairs or similar routine physical activity.

(B) During headache at least one of the two following symptoms occur:

1. phonophobia and photophobia,

2. nausea and/or vomiting.

Migraine with aura (MA) diagnostic criteria

(A) At least two attacks fulfilling at least three of the following:

1. One or more fully reversible aura symptoms indicating focal cerebral cortical and/or brain stem functions;

2. At least one aura symptom develops gradually over more than 4 min, or two or more symptoms occur in succession;

3. No aura symptom lasts more than 60 min; if more than one aura symptom is present, accepted duration is proportionally increased;

4. Headache follows aura with free interval of at least 60 min (it may also simultaneously begin with the aura).

(B) At least one of the following aura features establishes a diagnosis of migraine with typical aura:

1. homonymous visual disturbance,

2. unilateral paresthesias and/or numbness,

3. unilateral weakness,

4. aphasia or unclassifiable speech difficulty.

Cluster headache

(A) At least five attacks of severe unilateral orbital, supraorbital and/or temporal pain lasting 15–180 min untreated, with one or more of the following signs occurring on the same side as the pain:

1. conjunctival injection,
2. lacrimation,
3. nasal congestion,
4. rhinorrhoea,
5. forehead and facial sweating,
6. miosis,
7. ptosis,
8. eyelid oedema.

(B) Frequency of attacks from one every other day to eight per day.

Tension-type headache

(A) Headache lasting from 30 min to 7 days.
(B) At least two of the following criteria:

1. pressing/tightening (non-pulsatile) quality;
2. mild or moderate intensity (may inhibit, but does not prohibit activity);
3. bilateral location;
4. no aggravation by walking, stairs or similar routine physical activity.

C. Both of the following:

1. no nausea or vomiting (anorexia may occur);
2. photophobia and phonophobia are absent, or one but not both are present.

Cervicogenic headache

(A) Pain localised to the neck and occipital region. May project to forehead, orbital region, temples, vertex or ears.
(B) Pain is precipitated or aggravated by special neck movements or sustained postures.
(C) At least one of the following:

1. resistance to or limitation of passive neck movements;
2. changes in neck muscle contour, texture, tone or response to active and passive stretching and contraction;
3. abnormal tenderness of neck muscles.

(D) Radiological examination reveals at least one of the following:

1. movement abnormalities in flexion/extension;
2. abnormal posture;

3. fractures, congenital abnormalities, bone tumours, rheumatoid arthritis or other distinct pathology (not spondylosis or osteo-chondrosis).

Evidence on migraine diagnosis

A meta-analysis [2] tells us what clinical features are important, and what irrelevant, in diagnosing migraine. The review used a MEDLINE search up to May 1999 for English language papers with sensitivity and specificity of historical features in patients with primary headaches of migraine, tension-type headaches, or cluster headaches. Headaches caused by other underlying clinical conditions were not examined. Information from studies was pooled to generate overall sensitivity, specificity and likelihood ratios of migraine compared with tension-type headache. The criteria for diagnosis of headache may have been IHS criteria, or similar. Results are given for IHS criteria pooled and all. They were much the same, so the information for all criteria is given in Table 3.2.1 as it represented a larger data set.

The folklore is that factors precipitate a migraine attack. These might be cheese or chocolate, or stress or red wine, or whatever. The finding of this review was that most common precipitating factors were not discriminating for migraine compared with tension-type headache. Positive likelihood ratios were about 1 for stress, alcohol, weather change, menstruation, missing a meal, lack of sleep and perfume or odour.

The only factors with positive likelihood ratios were chocolate, cheese and any food (Table 3.2.2). The negative likelihood ratios for these were not much different from 1, indicating that absence of these features was unhelpful in making a diagnosis.

When compared with patients who had no history of headaches, a family history of migraine, childhood vomiting attacks and motion

Table 3.2.1 Headache features in migraine compared with tension-type headache

| | Likelihood ratios | | | |
| | Positive | | Negative | |
	LR+	95% CI	LR−	95% CI
Nausea	19.2	15–25	0.2	0.19–0.21
Photophobia	5.8	5.1–6.6	0.25	0.24–0.26
Phonophobia	5.2	1.5–5.9	0.38	0.36–0.40
Activity makes it worse	3.7	3.4–4.0	0.24	0.23–0.26
Unilateral	3.7	3.4–3.9	0.43	0.41–0.44
Throbbing/pulsing	2.9	2.7–3.1	0.36	0.34–0.37

Table 3.2.2 Headache precipitants in migraine compared with tension-type headache

| | Likelihood ratios | | | |
| | Positive | | Negative | |
	LR+	95% CI	LR−	95% CI
Chocolate	7.1	4.5–11.2	0.82	0.73–0.93
Cheese	4.9	1.9–12.5	0.68	0.62–0.73
Any food	3.6	2.8–4.6	0.59	0.56–0.62

Table 3.2.3 History in migraine compared with patients with no history of headaches

| | Likelihood ratios | | | |
| | Positive | | Negative | |
	LR+	95% CI	LR−	95% CI
Family history of migraine	5	4.4–5.6	0.47	0.46–0.49
Childhood vomiting attacks	2.4	1.9–2.9	0.79	0.75–0.82
Motion sickness	2.2	1.9–2.5	0.79	0.75–0.82

sickness all had moderate positive likelihood ratios for diagnosis of migraine (Table 3.2.3). Negative likelihood ratios were unhelpful.

Comment

This is all very helpful stuff. IHS guidelines provide a rational basis for diagnosis and the meta-analysis is a rational basis for helping people with migraine understand their disease. Perfume, or a period, or a change in the weather might produce a headache, but they are no guide as to whether that headache is migraine or not. The likelihood ratios are very helpful in this.

First, we know those factors that are not important, and those that are. For those that are important, we know the relevant weights. But we can use the signs, symptoms, predisposing factors and history to make diagnosing a migraine much easier.

For example, suppose a young man complains of unilateral throbbing headaches, made worse by any physical activity. His mother had migraines also, and he thinks that chocolate may bring it on.

We know that the prevalence of migraine in men is about 6%. This is our pre-test probability. By sequentially using the likelihoods for unilateral headache (3.7), throbbing (2.9), exacerbation by physical activity (3.7) and family history (5.0) we arrive at a post-test probability of about 95% that the young man has a migraine.

As well as diagnosing migraine, we need to have some idea about the level of disability the migraines cause. By asking some simple questions

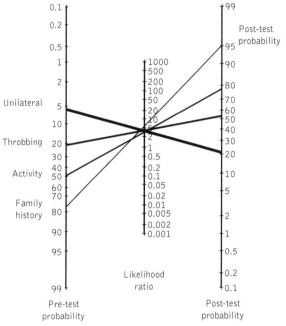

Figure 3.2.1 Likelihood ratio nomogram signs and symptoms for migraine diagnosis.

this can be done using the MIDAS questionnaire (http://www.midas-migraine.net/), which is downloadable from the Internet, then we will have a good idea of how to treat him using data from the DISC study (section 3.12), whether with simple analgesics or triptan.

References

1. Headache classification committee of the IHS (1988). Classification and diagnostic criteria for headache disorders, cranial neuralgias and facial pain, *Cephalalgia* 8: 1–96.
2. Smetana, G. W. (2000). The diagnostic value of historical features in primary headache syndromes, *Archives of Internal Medicine* 160: 2729–37.

3.3 **Migraine: league tables of relative efficacy**

There are a number of treatments available for acute migraine. Choices have to be made about which to prescribe, or even about formularies. Those choices will be influenced by a large number of issues with different resonance in different parts of the world. Policy, patient choice, prescriber preference, cost and experience will all play a part. These league tables allow us to see what is on offer, and make our choices informed by the evidence. The league tables are not there to tell us what to prescribe, or to limit prescribing choice (because there is some evidence that limiting choice is bad for patients and healthcare systems).

This section summarises their efficacy in several ways. The information is drawn predominantly from systematic reviews of comparable trials. The important points that make the treatments comparable are:

- trials enrolled similar patients, with migraine defined according to IHS criteria;
- trials enrolled adults;
- pain had to be moderate to severe intensity before treatments were used;
- the outcome used was headache response at 2 h, so that pain had to be mild or completely gone at 2 h;
- trials were randomised, and double blind;
- an intention-to-treat approach was taken that included all patients randomised and who took the treatment, but not those randomised who never had a migraine;
- only the first attack information was included;
- treatments have all been compared with placebo.

Consequently what we have is a consistent data set. We can tell it is consistent by examining the responses obtained with placebo for the treatments – they are all about 30% for 2 h headache response, about 8% for 2 h pain free, and about 20% for sustained headache response. This does not mean that placebo caused migraine pain to disappear, rather the pain would have faded to mild or no pain in about 30% of patients without treatment – the natural history of migraine pain if you like. Certainly there are no significant differences between responses to placebo between different treatments.

Dangers of over-interpretation

Information from league tables is sometimes over-interpreted. It should not be used to exclude treatments from formularies, for instance. Rather we should celebrate the fact that we have so many effective remedies. Some arguments against over-interpretation follow:

- A league table looks only at one outcome, that of headache response at 2 h, for instance (Figure 3.3.1). Other outcomes may be important, like being pain free at 1 h (a higher hurdle). Patients, when asked, want fast relief that is complete and that does not return. Right now we have no complete answer for that outcome.

- Different outcomes therefore have their own league tables, and here they are given for three outcomes, headache response and pain free at 2 h, and that of sustained response (headache response at 2 h and no return to higher pain level of moderate pain and no additional analgesic over a subsequent 22 h).

- The outcomes used refer only to pain. What about nausea, vomiting, photophobia, phonophobia, or other outcomes important in migraine? This is a deficiency.

- We cannot give information in a league table about adverse effects. Some patients will 'do well' on one treatment but not another.

- We cannot here give a league table for cost. That will differ in different places around the world.

Patient choice, and professional choice, will be influenced by many factors. Analgesic efficacy is only one. Moreover, relative efficacy should be used as a tool to guide personal and professional choice, and

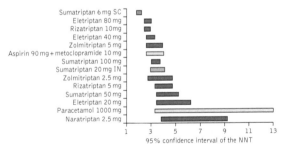

Figure 3.3.1 NNT for headache response at 2 h where bars represent 95% confidence interval of the NNT.

not be used as a rule to exclude certain types of treatment because of cost or convenience.

So use the league table as you would a walking stick. Use it to help you and not to beat others.

Information provided

The information here has been collected from reviews (and for paracetamol 1000 mg from a single large RCT). The tables give all the information thought relevant, including the number of trials and patients from which the table is drawn. The figures show the results graphically for NNTs, and for the percentage of patients given the treatment with the outcome.

Headache response at 2 h
(Figure 3.3.2; Table 3.3.1)

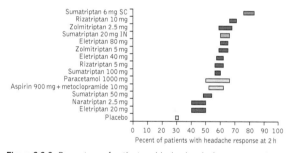

Figure 3.3.2 Percentage of patients achieving headache response at 2 h with each treatment where bars represent the 95% confidence interval.

Table 3.3.1 Headache response at 2 h

Treatment	Route	Number of trials	Treatment Number/total	Percent	Placebo Number/total	Percent	NNT (95% CI)
Sumatriptan 6 mg	Subcutaneous	8	379/477	79	131/461	28	2.0 (1.8–2.2)
Eletriptan 80 mg	Oral	6	763/1221	62	191/779	25	2.6 (2.4–3.0)
Rizatriptan 10 mg	Oral	7	1219/1783	68	303/987	31	2.7 (2.4–2.9)
Eletriptan 40 mg	Oral	6	724/1224	59	191/779	25	2.9 (2.6–3.3)
Zolmitriptan 5 mg	Oral	4	583/943	62	85/285	30	3.1 (2.6–3.9)
Aspirin 900 mg + metoclopramide 10 mg	Oral	3	214/376	57	95/373	25	3.2 (2.6–4.0)
Sumatriptan 100 mg	Oral	13	1346/2311	58	336/1211	28	3.3 (3.0–3.7)
Sumatriptan 20 mg	Intranasal	6	571/907	63	185/546	34	3.4 (2.9–4.1)
Zolmitriptan 2.5 mg	Oral	2	279/438	64	74/213	35	3.5 (2.7–4.7)
Rizatriptan 5 mg	Oral	4	548/933	59	234/713	33	3.9 (3.3–4.7)
Sumatriptan 50 mg	Oral	6	532/1042	51	137/510	27	4.1 (3.4–5.2)
Eletriptan 20 mg	Oral	2	157/349	45	78/353	22	4.4 (3.4–6.2)
Paracetamol 1000 mg	Oral	1	85/147	58	55/142	39	5.2 (3.3–13)
Naratriptan 2.5 mg	Oral	2	154/340	45	61/229	27	5.4 (3.8–9.2)

Pain free at 2 h
(Figures 3.3.3 and 3.3.4; Table 3.3.2)

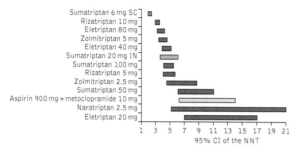

Figure 3.3.3 NNT for pain free at 2 h where bars represent 95% confidence interval of the NNT.

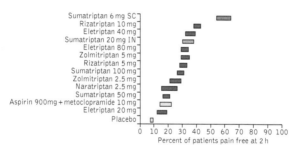

Figure 3.3.4 Percentage of patients pain free at 2 h with each treatment where bars represent the 95% confidence interval.

Table 3.3.2 Pain free at 2 h

Treatment	Route	Number of trials	Treatment		Placebo		NNT (95% CI)
			Number/total	Percent	Number/total	Percent	
Sumatriptan 6 mg	Subcutaneous	6	206/345	60	41/338	12	2.1 (1.9–2.4)
Rizatriptan 10 mg	Oral	7	720/1783	40	83/987	8	3.1 (2.9–3.5)
Eletriptan 80 mg	Oral	6	386/1221	32	38/779	5	3.7 (3.2–4.2)
Zolmitriptan 5 mg	Oral	4	298/943	32	17/285	6	3.9 (3.4–4.6)
Eletriptan 40 mg	Oral	6	335/1224	27	38/779	5	4.5 (3.9–5.1)
Sumatriptan 20 mg	Intranasal	3	182/536	34	33/276	12	4.6 (3.6–6.1)
Sumatriptan 100 mg	Oral	8	415/1461	28	53/744	7	4.7 (4.1–5.5)
Rizatriptan 5 mg	Oral	4	284/933	30	65/713	9	4.7 (4.0–5.7)
Zolmitriptan 2.5 mg	Oral	2	109/438	25	17/213	8	5.9 (4.5–8.7)
Sumatriptan 50 mg	Oral	4	131/711	18	21/372	6	7.8 (6.1–11)
Aspirin 900 mg + metoclopramide 10 mg	Oral	3	69/378	18	25/375	7	8.6 (6.2–14)
Naratriptan 2.5 mg	Oral	1	44/213	21	9/107	8	8.2 (5.1–21)
Eletriptan 20 mg	Oral	2	53/349	15	17/353	5	10 (7–17)

Sustained response over 24 h
(Figures 3.3.5 and 3.3.6; Table 3.3.3)

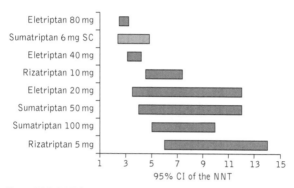

Figure 3.3.5 NNT for sustained response over 24 h where bars represent 95% confidence interval of the NNT.

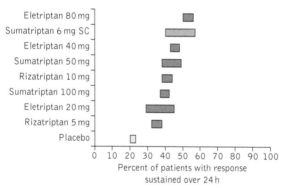

Figure 3.3.6 Percentage of patients achieving sustained response over 24 h with each treatment where bars represent the 95% confidence interval.

Table 3.3.3 Sustained response over 24 h

Treatment	Route	Number of trials	Treatment		Placebo		NNT (95% CI)
			Number/total	Percent	Number/total	Percent	
Sumatriptan 6 mg	Subcutaneous	2	70/144	49	28/160	18	3.2 (2.4–4.8)
Eletriptan 40 mg	Oral	5	526/1157	45	117/662	18	3.6 (3.1–4.2)
Rizatriptan 10 mg	Oral	3	420/1030	41	148/647	23	5.6 (4.5–7.4)
Eletriptan 20 mg	Oral	1	53/144	37	14/56	18	5.4 (3.5–12)
Sumatriptan 50 mg	Oral	2	157/362	43	47/177	27	6.0 (4–12)
Sumatriptan 100 mg	Oral	4	472/1190	40	109/442	25	6.7 (5.0–9.9)
Rizatriptan 5 mg	Oral	3	280/803	35	148/647	23	8.3 (6.0–14)

3.4 **Aspirin plus metoclopramide for acute migraine**

Clinical bottom line. Oral aspirin 900 mg plus metoclopramide 10 mg has been fully tested in three randomised trials with about 750 patients. The NNT for two hour headache response was 3.2 (2.6–4.0). The NNT for 2-h pain free was 8.6 (6.2–14). There was no information for sustained outcomes. Oral aspirin alone has no information yet published in full, though studies have been published in abstract form.

Systematic review

Oldman, A. D., Smith, L. A., McQuay, H. J. and Moore, R. A. (2002). A systematic review of treatments for acute migraine, *Pain* 97: 247–257.

Date review completed: September 2000

Number of trials included: 3

Number of patients: 749 (376 aspirin/metoclopramide; 373 placebo)

Control group: Active and placebo

Main outcomes: Headache intensity and duration

Inclusion criteria were: treatment of acute migraine; randomised allocation to treatment groups; double-blind design; adult population and headache outcomes.

Search

Comprehensive searches of the following databases were made: MEDLINE (1966–July 2000), EMBASE (1980–June 2000), Cochrane Library (Issue 3, 2000) and the Oxford Pain Relief Database (1950–1994). A series of free text searches were undertaken, using generic and trade names. There was no restriction to language. Retrieved reports were searched for additional trials. Neither individual authors nor pharmaceutical companies were contacted for unpublished data.

Findings

The three trials gave consistent results for 2 h headache response (Figure 3.4.1). The main results are in Table 3.4.1.

For oral aspirin 900 mg plus metoclopramide 10 mg, 214/376 patients (57%) had a headache response at 2 h compared with 95/373 (25%) with placebo. The NNT was 3.2 (2.6–4.0). The NNT for 2-h pain free was 8.6 (6.2–14).

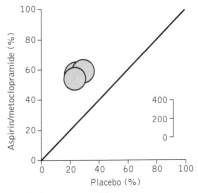

Figure 3.4.1 Headache response at 2 h.

Table 3.4.1 Aspirin 900 mg plus metoclopramide 10 mg

Outcome	Number of trials	Number/total with outcome (%)		NNT (95% CI)
		Treatment	Placebo	
Two hour headache response	3	214/376 (57)	95/373 (25)	3.2 (2.6–4.0)
Two hour pain free	3	69/378 (18)	25/375 (7)	8.6 (6.2–14)
Headache response at 2 h sustained to 24 h		No data		

No useful information on aspirin alone was found.

Adverse effects

Adverse effects are not reported in any way that makes obvious sense.

Comment

Limited data from only three trials, but consistently showing efficacy for the easiest outcome, 2-h headache response. Less effective at producing pain free patients at 2 h, and no information on longer duration outcomes.

3.5 **Paracetamol for acute migraine**

Clinical bottom line. There is good information from only a single high quality trial. For headache response at 2 h, the response rate was 58% for paracetamol 1000 mg and 39% for placebo. The NNT was 5.2 (3.3–13). For pain free at 2 h the response rate was 22% for paracetamol 1000 mg and 11% for placebo. The NNT was 8.9 (5.1–38).

Paracetamol is often recommended as the first line of treatment for acute migraine attacks, and patients frequently self-medicate with over-the-counter drugs. There is only a single study on paracetamol in acute migraine that fulfils IHS criteria for the diagnosis of migraine, and with useful outcomes. The study is described, and a brief review of additional studies on migraine from a systematic review added.

Reference

Lipton, R. B. *et al.* (2000). Efficacy and safety of acetaminophen in the treatment of migraine, *Archives of Internal medicine* 160: 3486–92.

Adults with at least one episode of migraine with at least moderate pain every 2 months were eligible. They were randomised by computer-generated code to 1000 mg of paracetamol or identical placebo. Tablets had to be taken when pain was at least moderate, and rescue medication was to be avoided for at least 2 h. Pain was scored between 0.5 and 6 h. The main outcome measure was pain reduced to mild or none (headache response) at 2 h.

The trial was of high quality and scored 5 of 5 on a quality rating scale. The number randomised who took paracetamol was 147, and 142 took placebo. Migraine was of severe intensity in 40% of patients.

For headache response (pain mild or none) at 2 h, the response rate was 58% for paracetamol 1000 mg and 39% for placebo. The NNT was 5.2 (95% confidence interval 3.3–13).

For pain free at two hours the response rate was 22% for paracetamol 1000 mg and 11% for placebo. The number needed to treat was 8.9 (95% confidence interval 5.1–38).

Rescue medication was taken by 15% of patient on paracetamol, and 32% on placebo. Paracetamol was rated good or excellent by 52% on paracetamol and 28% on placebo. Paracetamol also produced higher rates of patients whose photophobia and phonophobia symptoms were reduced to zero, and more patients whose functional disability was reduced to zero, both at 2 and 6 h. There was no difference between the groups for adverse events.

Systematic review of other trials

Oldman, A. D., Smith, L. A., McQuay, H. J. and Moore, R. A. (2002). A systematic review of treatments for acute migraine, *Pain* 97: 247–257.

Date review completed: December 2000

Number of trials included: 8 randomised controlled trials

Control group: Active and placebo

Main outcomes: Headache severity and duration

Inclusion criteria were treatment of acute migraine with paracetamol by any route; randomised allocation to treatment groups; double-blind design; adult population and headache outcomes.

Search

Comprehensive searches of the following databases were made: MEDLINE (1966–July 2000), EMBASE (1980–June 2000), Cochrane Library (Issue 3, 2000) and the Oxford Pain Relief Database (1950–1994). A series of free text searches were undertaken, using generic and trade names for paracetamol. There was no restriction to language. Retrieved reports were searched for additional trials. Neither individual authors nor pharmaceutical companies were contacted for unpublished data.

Findings

Eight randomised double-blind trials were found with paracetamol given at doses ranging 500–1000 mg. The trials were disparate with respect to dosing regimes, patient diagnosis and outcome measures precluding pooling of data for quantitative analysis. Seven were of oral paracetamol, one of intramuscular (IM). Two were placebo controlled and six used active control groups. One trial scored two, six scored three and one scored four out of a maximum of five using a scale rating trial quality based on randomisation, blinding and withdrawals. However, overall the trials were of low methodological quality based on other aspects of trial design. The trials were all of a crossover design, and many of the authors failed to either report on the absence or presence of carryover effects, or describe a minimum period between attacks to avoid these effects. It was not clear if all patients had sufficient pain at baseline, which is of particular importance in the absence of a placebo group to demonstrate trial assay sensitivity. All of the studies treated multiple attacks, and there is a high proportion of withdrawals and dropouts in many of the trials, data not included in the final analysis. This may bias the results in favour of the responders to treatment. Most of the studies pre-date IHS migraine diagnostic criteria and all use slightly different criteria for migraine diagnosis.

Placebo controlled trials

One trial found no difference between paracetamol 650 mg and placebo for reduction in migraine severity, and the other reported a significant difference between paracetamol 1000 mg and placebo. The NNT for one patient to achieve at least 50% pain relief by two hours with paracetamol 1000 mg over placebo was 7.8 (4.8–21).

Active controlled trials

Based on a vote counting exercise, three of the active controlled trials showed significantly better pain relief with ibuprofen, tolfenamic acid and ketoprofen than paracetamol. Two trials showed no significant difference between paracetamol and tofenamic acid and paracetamol combined with domperidone for the main outcome of headache severity.

Adverse effects

No serious adverse effects were reported.

Comment

This high quality study indicates that 1000 mg of paracetamol is effective in treating migraine attacks, but with limited information from a single high quality study. This is disappointing considering that paracetamol is so often recommended to patients with migraine.

3.6 Ibuprofen for acute migraine

Clinical bottom line. In a large, randomised trial in about 700 patients, done to high standards, ibuprofen 200 and 400 mg each had an NNT for 2-h headache response of 7.5 (4.5–22).

Ibuprofen is sometimes recommended for treatment for acute migraine attacks, and patients frequently self-medicate. There is only a single study on ibuprofen in acute migraine that fulfils IHS criteria for the diagnosis of migraine, and with useful outcomes. The study is described, and a brief review of additional studies on migraine from a systematic review added.

Reference

Codispoti, J. R. *et al.* (2001). Efficacy of nonprescription doses of ibuprofen for treating migraine headache. A randomized controlled trial, *Headache* 41: 665–79.

This randomised controlled trial compared placebo with ibuprofen 200 and 400 mg in adult patients with migraine diagnosed using IHS criteria. Randomisation was computer generated, drugs were identical, and withdrawals and dropouts were described, giving it a quality score of 5/5, and making it a high quality trial. The outcome was pain initially moderate or severe reduced to mild or none at 2 h (headache response).

For ibuprofen 200 mg, 91/216 (42%) had a headache response at 2 h. For ibuprofen 400 mg, 91/223 had a headache response at 2 h. For placebo 62/221 (28%) had a headache response at 2 h. The NNT for each was 7.5 (4.5–22).

Systematic review of other trials

Oldman, A. D., Smith, L. A., McQuay, H. J. and Moore, R. A. (2002). A systematic review of treatments for acute migraine, *Pain* 97: 247–57.

Date review completed: November 2000

Number of trials included: Five randomised controlled trials

Number of patients: 184 patients

Control groups: Active and placebo

Main outcomes: Headache severity and duration

Inclusion criteria were: treatment of acute migraine with ibuprofen by any route; randomised allocation to treatment groups; double-blind design; adult population and headache outcomes.

Search

Comprehensive searches of the following databases were made: MED-LINE (1966–July 2000), EMBASE (1980–June 2000), Cochrane

Library (Issue 3, 2000) and the Oxford Pain Relief Database (1950–1994). A series of free text searches were undertaken, using generic and trade names for ibuprofen. There was no restriction to language. Retrieved reports were searched for additional trials. Neither individual authors nor pharmaceutical companies were contacted for unpublished data.

Findings

Five RCTs were found where 156 patients were randomised to ibuprofen and 126 to placebo. The trials were disparate with respect to dosing regimes, number of attacks studied and outcome measures precluding pooling of data for quantitative analysis. One RCT compared ibuprofen with paracetamol ($n = 30$). All of the trials studied oral ibuprofen at doses from 400 to 1200 mg. One trial studied ibuprofen–arginine 400 mg. Although trials were high quality based on criteria that evaluate randomisation, blinding and withdrawals, they were methodologically flawed in other aspects of trial design.

Only two trials used IHS diagnostic criteria, the other three trials pre-dated IHS criteria and in one of them it did not state which diagnostic criteria were used. In most of the studies it was unclear when the outcomes were assessed, therefore results may have been for more than one dose of study medication. Three of the crossover trials failed to either test for carryover effects or describe a minimum period between attacks to avoid these effects and it was not clear if all patients had sufficient pain at baseline to effectively measure a difference.

Three of the four placebo controlled studies showed significantly better pain relief with ibuprofen than placebo, one showed no difference. Two of these studies also showed a significant reduction in headache duration with ibuprofen. However, mean duration of migraine with ibuprofen was still as much as 4–5 h. The most methodologically sound trial of the five studied ibuprofen–arginine 400 mg, a more rapidly absorbed formulation [5]. All patients had sufficient headache pain when the study drug was given (at least 60 mm VAS), 2 h later, 15/29 patients given ibuprofen-arginine reported considerable or complete headache relief compared with 2/29 patients given placebo. This represents a significant reduction in headache pain and duration with ibuprofen with an NNT of 2.2 (1.5–4.1), albeit on only 29 patients.

One active controlled trial concluded that ibuprofen 400 mg given at 4 to 6-h intervals was significantly better than paracetamol 900 mg at 4 to 6-h intervals for the reduction of severity and duration of attacks.

Adverse effects

Over all studies, ibuprofen was well tolerated. No serious adverse effects were reported, all were of mild to moderate intensity.

Comment

The large, well conducted study was done to strict criteria that make it comparable to studies done on triptans. The result was similar to others found in the systematic review, in that ibuprofen was better than placebo. However, the NNT of 7.5 on nearly 700 patients was far worse than the NNT of 2.2 found in another randomised trial of only 29 patients. This demonstrates the dangers of relying on single small trials.

It is a shame that we do not have better quality studies on ibuprofen in migraine, studies performed with modern entry criteria, and using sensible outcomes. We would then be able to make comparisons with other treatments.

3.7 **Sumatriptan for acute migraine**

Clinical bottom line. Oral sumatriptan 100 mg has been fully tested in thirteen randomised trials with about 3500 patients. The NNT for 2-h headache response was 3.3 (3.0–3.7). Oral sumatriptan 50 mg has been fully tested in six randomised trials with about 5500 patients. The NNT for 2-h headache response was 4.1 (3.4–5.2). Subcutaneous sumatriptan 6 mg has been fully tested in eight randomised trials with about 900 patients. The NNT for 2-h headache response was 2.0 (1.8–2.2). Intranasal sumatriptan 20 mg has been fully tested in six randomised trials with about 1500 patients. The NNT for 2-h headache response was 3.4 (2.9–4.1).

Systematic review

Oldman, A. D., Smith, L. A., McQuay, H. J. and Moore, R. A. (2002). A systematic review of treatments for acute migraine, *Pain* 97: 247–57.

Date review completed: September 2001

Number of trials included: See tables for number of trials and patients for each dose/route combination

Control group: Active and placebo

Main outcomes: Headache intensity and duration

Inclusion criteria were: treatment of acute migraine; randomised allocation to treatment groups; double-blind design; adult population and headache outcomes.

Search

Comprehensive searches of the following databases were made: MEDLINE (1966–July 2001), EMBASE (1980–June 2001), Cochrane Library (Issue 3, 2001), PubMed (to September 2001) and the Oxford Pain Relief Database (1950–1994). A series of free text searches were undertaken, using generic and trade names. There was no restriction to language. Retrieved reports were searched for additional trials. Neither individual authors nor pharmaceutical companies were contacted for unpublished data.

Findings

Oral sumatriptan 100 mg

The results for the 13 trials for oral sumatriptan 100 mg were consistent for all outcomes (Table 3.7.1), and those for 2-h headache response are shown in Figure 3.7.1.

Table 3.7.1 Results for oral sumatriptan 100 mg

Outcome	Number of trials	Number/total with outcome (%)		NNT (95% CI)
		Treatment	Placebo	
Two hour headache response	13	1346/231 (58)	336/1211 (28)	3.3 (3.0–3.7)
Two hour pain free	8	415/1461 (28)	53/744 (7)	4.7 (4.1–5.5)
Headache response at 2 h sustained to 24 h	4	472/1190 (40)	109/442 (25)	6.7 (5.0–9.9)

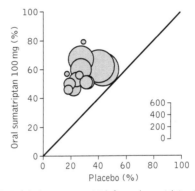

Figure 3.7.1 Headache response at 2 h for oral sumatriptan 100 mg.

For oral sumatriptan 100 mg in 13 trials, 1346/2311 patients (58%) had a headache response at 2 h compared with 336/1211 (28%) with placebo. The NNT was 3.3 (3.0–3.7). The NNT for 2-h pain free was 4.7 (4.1–5.5) in 2205 patients in eight trials. The NNT for two hour headache response sustained for 24 h with no additional analgesic was 6.7 (5.0–9.9) in 1632 patients in four trials.

Oral sumatriptan 50 mg

The results for the eight trials for oral sumatriptan 50 mg were consistent for all outcomes and are given in Table 3.7.2.

For oral sumatriptan 50 mg in six trials, 532/1042 patients (51%) had a headache response at 2 h compared with 137/510 (27%) with placebo. The NNT was 4.1 (3.4–5.2). The NNT for 2-h pain free was 7.8 (6.1–11) in 1083 patients in four trials. The NNT for 2-h headache response sustained for 24 h with no additional analgesic was 6.0 (4.0–12) in 539 patients in two trials.

Table 3.7.2 Results for oral sumatriptan 50 mg

Outcome	Number of trials	Number/total with outcome (%)		NNT (95% CI)
		Treatment	Placebo	
Two hour headache response	6	532/1042 (51)	137/510 (27)	4.1 (3.4–5.2)
Two hour pain free	4	131/711 (18)	21/372 (6)	7.8 (6.1–11)
Headache response at 2 h sustained to 24 h	2	157/362 (43)	47/177 (27)	6.0 (4.0–12)

Table 3.7.3 Results for subcutaneous sumatriptan 6 mg

Outcome	Number of trials	Number/total with outcome (%)		NNT (95% CI)
		Treatment	Placebo	
Two hour headache response	8	379/477 (79)	131/461 (28)	2.0 (1.8–2.2)
Two hour pain free	6	206/345 (60)	41/338 (12)	2.1 (1.9–2.4)
Headache response at 2 h sustained to 24 h	2	71/144 (19)	28/160 (18)	3.2 (2.4–4.8)

Subcutaneous sumatriptan 6 mg

The results for the eight trials for subcutaneous sumatriptan 6 mg were consistent for all outcomes and are given in Table 3.7.3.

For subcutaneous sumatriptan 6 mg in eight trials, 379/477 patients (79%) had a headache response at 2 h compared with 131/461 (28%) with placebo. The NNT was 2.0 (1.8–2.2). The NNT for 2-h pain free was 2.1 (1.9–2.4) in 683 patients in six trials. The NNT for 2-h headache response sustained for 24 h with no additional analgesic was 3.2 (2.4–4.8) in 304 patients in two trials.

Intranasal sumatriptan 20 mg

The results for the eight trials for subcutaneous sumatriptan 6 mg were consistent for all outcomes and are given in Table 3.7.4.

For intranasal sumatriptan 20 mg in six trials, 571/907 patients (63%) had a headache response at 2 h compared with 183/546 (34%) with placebo. The NNT was 3.4 (2.9–4.1). The NNT for 2-h pain free was 4.6 (3.6–6.1)) in 812 patients in three trials. There were no results for 2-h headache response sustained for 24 h with no additional analgesic.

Adverse effects

Adverse effects are not reported in any way that makes obvious sense because efficacy was measured over 24 h and adverse events for up to 10 days.

Table 3.7.4 Results for intranasal sumatriptan 20 mg

Outcome	Number of trials	Number/total with outcome (%)		NNT (95% CI)
		Treatment	Placebo	
Two hour headache response	6	571/907 (63)	183/546 (34)	3.4 (2.9–4.1)
Two hour pain free	3	182/536 (34)	33/276 (12)	4.6(3.6–6.1)
Headache response at 2 h sustained to 24 h		No data		

Comment

Sumatriptan is clearly effective in the treatment of acute migraine, in several doses and by three routes of administration. There is considerable evidence from large, well-conducted randomised trials, with large numbers of patients.

3.8 **Oral naratriptan for acute migraine**

Clinical bottom line. Oral naratriptan 2.5 mg has been tested in two randomised trials with about 550 patients. The NNT for 2-h headache response was 5.4 (3.8–9.2). Two hour pain free was available in only one trial with 320 patients, and the NNT was 8.2 (5–21). There was no information for sustained outcomes.

Systematic review

Oldman, A. D., Smith, L. A., McQuay, H. J. and Moore, R. A. (2002).
   A systematic review of treatments for acute migraine, *Pain* 97: 247–57.

   Date review completed: September 2001

   Number of trials included: Two randomised controlled trials

   Number of patients: 569

   Control group: Active and placebo

   Main outcomes: Headache intensity and duration

Inclusion criteria were: treatment of acute migraine; randomised allocation to treatment groups; double-blind design; adult population and headache outcomes.

Search

Comprehensive searches of the following databases were made: MEDLINE (1966–July 2001), EMBASE (1980–June 2001), Cochrane Library (Issue 3, 2001), PubMed (to September 2001) and the Oxford Pain Relief Database (1950–1994). A series of free text searches were undertaken, using generic and trade names. There was no restriction to language. Retrieved reports were searched for additional trials. Neither individual authors nor pharmaceutical companies were contacted for unpublished data.

Findings

The results for the two trials of oral naratriptan 2.5 mg are shown in Table 3.8.1.

   For oral naratriptan 2.5 mg, 154/340 patients (45%) had a headache response at 2 h compared with 61/229 (27%) with placebo. The NNT was 5.4 (3.8–9.2). Two hour pain free was available in only one trial with 320 patients, and the NNT was 8.2 (5–21). There was no information for sustained outcomes.

Table 3.8.1 Headache response at two hours with oral naratriptan 2.5 mg

Outcome	Number of trials	Number/total with outcome (%)		NNT (95% CI)
		Treatment	Placebo	
Two hour headache response	2	154/340 (45)	61/229 (27)	5.4 (3.8–9.2)
Two hour pain free	1	44/213 (21)	9/107 (8)	8.2 (5.1–21)
Headache response at 2 h sustained to 24 h	No data			

Adverse effects

Adverse effects are not reported in any way that makes obvious sense because efficacy was measured over 24 h and adverse events for up to 10 days.

Comment

Naratriptan outcomes were directed towards 4 h after tablets were taken. This has little relevance, and has been ignored in this review.

3.9 **Oral rizatriptan for acute migraine**

Clinical bottom line. Oral rizatriptan 10 mg has been tested in seven randomised trials with about 2700 patients. The NNT for 2-h headache response was 2.7 (2.4–2.9). For pain free response at 2-h compared with placebo, the NNT was 3.1 (2.9–3.4) in 2770 patients. For sustained headache response the NNT was 5.6 (4.5–7.4) in 1677 patients in three trials.

Oral rizatriptan 5 mg has been tested in four randomised trials with about 1900 patients. The NNT for 2-h headache response was 3.9 (3.3–4.7). For pain free response at two hours compared with placebo, the NNT was 4.7 (4.0–5.7) in 1646 patients. For sustained headache response the NNT was 8.3 (6–14) in 1450 patients in three trials.

Systematic reviews

There are several systematic reviews with rizatriptan, all examining the same trials.

Oldman, A. D., Smith, L. A., McQuay, H. J. and Moore, R. A. (2001). Rizatriptan for acute migraine (Cochrane Review), in: The Cochrane Library, Issue 3, 2001, Oxford, Update Software.

Oldman, A. D., Smith, L. A., McQuay, H. J. and Moore, R. A. (2001). A systematic review of treatments for acute migraine, *Pain* 97: 247–57.

Ferrari, M. D. *et al.* (2001). Meta-analysis of rizatriptan efficacy in randomized controlled clinical trials, *Cephalalgia* 21: 129–36.

Gawel, M. J. *et al.* (2001). A systematic review of the use of triptans in acute migraine, *Canadian Journal of Neurological Science* 28: 30–41.

Date review completed: September 2001

Number of trials included: See tables for number of trials and patients for each dose/route combination

Control group: Active and placebo

Main outcomes: Headache intensity and duration

Inclusion criteria were: treatment of acute migraine; randomised allocation to treatment groups; double-blind design; adult population and headache outcomes.

Search

Comprehensive searches of the following databases were made: MEDLINE (1966–July 2001), EMBASE (1980–June 2001), Cochrane Library (Issue 3, 2001), PubMed (to September 2001) and the Oxford

Pain Relief Database (1950–1994). A series of free text searches were undertaken, using generic and trade names. There was no restriction to language. Retrieved reports were searched for additional trials. Neither individual authors nor pharmaceutical companies were contacted for unpublished data.

Findings

Oral rizatriptan 10 mg

The results for the seven trials for oral rizatriptan 10 mg were consistent for all outcomes (Table 3.9.1), and those for 2-h headache response are shown in Figure 3.9.1.

For oral rizatriptan 10 mg in seven trials, 1219/1783 patients (68%) had a headache response at 2 h compared with 303/987 (31%) with placebo. The NNT was 2.7 (2.4–2.9). For pain free response at 2 h compared with placebo, the NNT was 3.1 (2.9–3.4) in 2770 patients.

Table 3.9.1 Results for oral rizatriptan 10 mg

Outcome	Number of trials	Number/total with outcome (%)		NNT (95% CI)
		Treatment	Placebo	
Two hour headache response	7	1219/1783 (68)	303/987 (31)	2.7 (2.4–2.9)
Two hour pain free	7	720/1783 (40)	83/987 (8)	3.1 (2.9–3.5)
Headache response at 2 h sustained to 24 h	3	420/1030 (41)	146/647 (23)	5.6 (4.5–7.4)

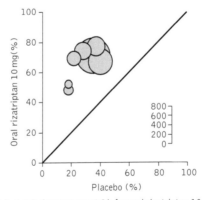

Figure 3.9.1 Headache response at 2 h for oral rizatriptan 10 mg.

For sustained headache response the NNT was 5.6 (4.5–7.4) in 1677 patients in three trials.

Oral rizatriptan 5 mg

The results for the seven trials for oral rizatriptan 5 mg were consistent for all outcomes, and those for 2-h headache response are shown in Figure 3.9.2.

For oral rizatriptan 5 mg in four trials, 548/933 patients (59%) had a headache response at 2 h compared with 234/713 (33%) with placebo. The NNT was 3.9 (3.3–4.7). For pain free response at 2 h compared with placebo, the NNT was 4.7 (4.0–5.7) in 1646 patients. For sustained headache response the NNT was 8.3 (6–14) in 1450 patients in three trials.

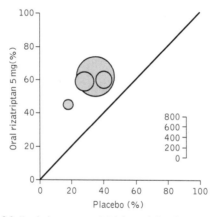

Figure 3.9.2 Headache response at 2 h for oral rizatriptan 10 mg.

Table 3.9.2 Results for oral rizatriptan 10 mg

Outcome	Number of trials	Number/total with outcome (%)		NNT (95% CI)
		Treatment	Placebo	
Two hour headache response	4	548/933 (59)	234/713 (33)	3.9 (3.3–4.7)
Two hour pain free	4	284/933 (30)	65/713 4.7 (4.0–5.7)	4.7 (4.0–5.7)
Headache response at 2 h sustained to 24 h	3	280/803 (35)	148/647 (23)	8.3 (6–14)

Other outcomes

The Ferrari review also reports other outcomes:

• For patients who were pain free at 2 h, and then had no headache recurrence (moderate or severe) and no additional analgesics for 22 h the NNT was 5.5 (4.9–6.4), occurring in 25% on rizatriptan 10 mg and 7% on placebo.

• At 2 h, the NNT with rizatriptan 10 mg compared to placebo to achieve one patient who was not nauseated was 4.8.

• At two hours, the NNT with rizatriptan 10 mg compared with placebo to achieve one patient who did not have photophobia was 3.6.

• At two hours, the NNT with rizatriptan 10 mg compared with placebo to achieve one patient who did not have phonophobia was 3.8.

• At two hours, the NNT with rizatriptan 10 mg compared with placebo to achieve one patient who did not have functional disability was 4.0.

Adverse effects

Adverse effects are not reported in any way that makes obvious sense because efficacy was measured over 24 h and adverse events for up to 10 days.

Comment

Four systematic reviews (one as a dual publication including a Cochrane review) for one treatment (rizatriptan 10 mg) is unusual. It is worth asking the obvious question of whether they all give the same result, especially as two reviews were from published information, and one from a single-patient meta-analysis, and that all took different definitions of intention to treat. Table 3.9.3 shows the results for all the three reviews.

The results for 2 h and sustained outcomes were essentially the same.

Table 3.9.3 Comparison of three reviews for NNT (95% confidence interval) for rizatriptan 10 mg

	At 2 h		Over 24 h	
	Headache response	Pain free	Sustained response	Sustained pain free
Gawel *et al.*	2.8 (2.6–3.2)	3.2 (2.9–3.5)		
Ferrari *et al.*	3.0 (2.8–3.4)	3.2 (3.0–3.5)	5.3 (4.6–6.2)	5.5 (4.9–6.4)
Oldman *et al.*	2.7 (2.4–2.9)	3.1 (2.9–3.4)	5.6 (4.5–7.4)	

Notes: Gawel review used only tablet data from 6 trials. Ferrari review used data from tablets and wafers in 7 trials, but had individual data from trial records. Oldman review combined tablet and wafer from 7 trials, but probably used a different definition of intention to treat as numbers of patients differed.

3.10 Oral zolmitriptan for acute migraine

Clinical bottom line. Oral zolmitriptan 5 mg has been fully tested in four randomised trials with about 1200 patients. The NNT for 2 h headache response was 3.1 (2.6–3.9). The NNT for 2-h pain free was 3.9 (3.4–4.6) in 1228 patients in four trials. In one trial the 2 h headache response sustained for 24 h with no additional analgesic was not significantly different between zolmitriptan 5 mg and placebo.

Oral zolmitriptan 2.5 mg has been fully tested in two randomised trials with about 600 patients. The NNT for 2-h headache response was 3.5 (2.7–4.7). The NNT for 2-h pain free was 5.9 (4.5–8.7) in 651 patients in two trials. There was no information on headache response sustained for 24 h with no additional analgesic.

Systematic review

Oldman, A. D., Smith, L. A., McQuay, H. J. and Moore, R. A. (2002).
  A systematic review of treatments for acute migraine, *Pain* 97: 247–57.

  Date review completed: September 2001

  Number of trials included: Four trials for zolmitriptan 5 mg and two for zolmitriptan 2.5 mg

  Number of patients: 1228 and 651

  Control group: Active and placebo

  Main outcomes: Headache intensity and duration

Inclusion criteria were: treatment of acute migraine with zolmitriptan by any route; randomised allocation to treatment groups; double-blind design; adult population and headache outcomes.

Search

Comprehensive searches of the following databases were made: MEDLINE (1966–July 2001), EMBASE (1980–June 2001), Cochrane Library (Issue 3, 2001), PubMed (to September 2001) and the Oxford Pain Relief Database (1950–1994). A series of free text searches were undertaken, using generic and trade names. There was no restriction to language. Retrieved reports were searched for additional trials. Neither individual authors nor pharmaceutical companies were contacted for unpublished data.

Table 3.10.1 Results for oral zolmitriptan 5 mg

Outcome	Number of trials	Number/total with outcome (%)		NNT (95% CI)
		Treatment	Placebo	
Two hour headache response	4	583/943 (62)	85/285 (30)	3.1 (2.6–3.9)
Two hour pain free	4	298/943 (32)	17/285 (6)	3.9 (3.4–4.6)
Headache response at 2 h sustained to 24 h	1	180/498 (36)	14/56 (25)	No significant benefit

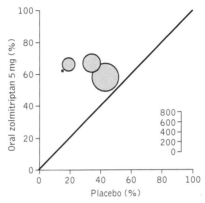

Figure 3.10.1 Headache response at 2 h for oral zolmitriptan 5 mg.

Findings

Oral zolmitriptan 5 mg

The results for the four trials for oral zolmitriptan 5 mg were consistent for all outcomes (Table 3.10.1), and those for 2-h headache response are shown in Figure 3.10.1.

For oral zolmitriptan 5 mg in four trials, 583/943 patients (62%) had a headache response at 2 h compared with 85/285 (30%) with placebo. The NNT was 3.1 (2.6–3.9). The NNT for two hour pain free was 3.9 (3.4–4.6) in 1228 patients in four trials. In one trial the 2-h headache response sustained for 24 h with no additional analgesic was not significantly different between zolmitriptan 5 mg and placebo.

Oral zolmitriptan 2.5 mg

For oral zolmitriptan 2.5 mg in two trials (Table 3.10.2), 279/438 patients (64%) had a headache response at 2 h compared with 74/213

Table 3.10.2 Results for oral zolmitriptan 2.5 mg

Outcome	Number of trials	Number/total with outcome (%)		NNT (95% CI)
		Treatment	Placebo	
Two hour headache response	2	279/438 (64)	74/213 (35)	3.5 (2.7–4.7)
Two hour pain free	2	109/438 (25)	17/213 (8)	5.9 (4.5–8.7)
Headache response at 2 h sustained to 24 h	No data			

(35%) with placebo. The NNT was 3.5 (2.7–4.7). The NNT for 2-h pain free was 5.9 (4.5–8.7) in 651 patients in two trials. There was no information on headache response sustained for 24 h with no additional analgesic.

Adverse effects

Adverse effects are not reported in any way that makes obvious sense because efficacy was measured over 24 h and adverse events for up to 10 days.

Comment

Zolmitriptan is clearly effective in the treatment of acute migraine.

3.11 Oral eletriptan for acute migraine

Clinical bottom line. Oral eletriptan 80 mg has been tested in six randomised trials with about 2000 patients. The NNT for 2-h headache response was 2.6 (2.4–3.0). The NNT for 2-h pain free was 3.7 (3.4–4.2). The NNT for sustained response was 2.8 (2.5–3.2).

Oral eletriptan 40 mg has been tested in six randomised trials with about 2000 patients. The NNT for 2-h headache response was 2.9 (2.6–3.3). The NNT for 2-h pain free was 4.5 (3.9–5.1). The NNT for sustained response was 3.6 (3.1–4.2).

Oral eletriptan 20 mg has been tested in two randomised trials with about 2000 patients. The NNT for 2-h headache response was 4.4 (3.4–6.2). The NNT for 2-h pain free was 9.9 (6.9–17). The NNT for sustained response was 5.4 (3.5–12).

Systematic reviews

Smith, L. A., Oldman, A. D., McQuay, H. J. and Moore, R. A. (2001). Eletriptan for acute migraine (Cochrane Review), in: The Cochrane Library, Issue 3, 2001, Update Software, Oxford.

Oldman, A. D., Smith, L. A., McQuay, H. J. and Moore, R. A. (2002). A systematic review of treatments for acute migraine, *Pain* 97: 247–57.

Date review completed: September 2000

Number of trials included: Six randomised controlled trials – see tables for number of trials and patients for each dose/route combination

Control group: Active and placebo

Main outcomes: Headache intensity and duration

Inclusion criteria were: treatment of acute migraine; randomised allocation to treatment groups; double-blind design; adult population and headache outcomes.

Search

Comprehensive searches of the following databases were made: MEDLINE (1966–July 2000), EMBASE (1980–June 2000), Cochrane Library (Issue 3, 2000) and the Oxford Pain Relief Database (1950–1994). A series of free text searches were undertaken, using generic and trade names. There was no restriction to language. Retrieved reports were searched for additional trials. Pfizer Inc provided data from seven unpublished trials, one of which has subsequently been published.

Findings

Oral eletriptan 80 mg

The results for the six trials for oral eletriptan 80 mg were consistent for all outcomes (Table 3.11.1), and those for 2-h headache response are shown in Figure 3.11.1.

For oral eletriptan 80 mg in six trials, 763/1221 patients (62%) had a headache response at 2 h compared with 191/779 (25%) with placebo. The NNT was 2.6 (2.4–3.0). In six trials, 386/1221 patients (32%) were pain free at 2 h compared with 38/779 (25%) with placebo. The NNT was 3.7 (3.4–4.2). In five trials, 618/1160 patients (53%) had a headache response at 2 h, sustained for 24 hours with no rescue medication and no second dose of study medication compared with 117/662 (18%) with placebo. The NNT was 2.8 (2.5–3.2).

Table 3.11.1 Results for oral eletriptan 80 mg

Outcome	Number of trials	Number/total with outcome (%)		NNT (95% CI)
		Treatment	Placebo	
Two hour headache response	6	763/1221 (62)	191/779 (25)	2.6 (2.4–3.0)
Two hour pain free	6	386/1221 (32)	38/779 (5)	3.7 (3.4–4.2)
Headache response at 2 h sustained to 24 h	5	618/1160 (53)	117/662 (18)	2.8 (2.5–3.2)

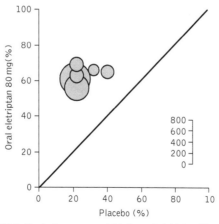

Figure 3.11.1 Headache response at 2 h for oral eletriptan 80 mg.

Table 3.11.2 Results for oral eletriptan 40 mg

Outcome	Number of trials	Number/total with outcome (%)		NNT (95% CI)
		Treatment	Placebo	
Two hour headache response	6	724/1221 (59)	191/779 (25)	2.9 (2.6–3.3)
Two hour pain free	6	335/1221 (27)	38/779 (5)	4.5 (3.9–5.1)
Headache response at 2 h sustained to 24 h	5	526/1160 (45)	117/662 (18)	3.6 (3.1–4.2)

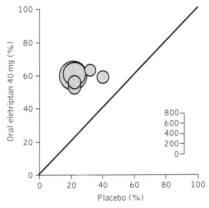

Figure 3.11.2 Headache response at 2 h for oral eletriptan 40 mg.

Oral eletriptan 40 mg

The results for the six trials for oral eletriptan 40 mg were consistent for all outcomes (Table 3.11.2), and those for 2-h headache response are shown in Figure 3.11.2.

For oral eletriptan 40 mg in six trials, 724/1221 patients (59%) had a headache response at 2 h compared with 191/779 (25%) with placebo. The NNT was 2.9 (2.6–3.3). In six trials, 335/1221 patients (27%) were pain free at 2 h compared with 38/779 (5%) with placebo. The NNT was 4.5 (3.9–5.1). In five trials, 526/1160 patients (45%) had a headache response at 2 h, sustained for 24 h with no rescue medication and no second dose of study medication compared with 117/662 (18%) with placebo. The NNT was 3.6 (3.1–4.2).

Oral eletriptan 20 mg

For oral eletriptan 20 mg in two trials (Table 3.11.3), 157/349 patients (45%) had a headache response at 2 h compared with 78/353 (22%)

Table 3.11.3 Results for oral eletriptan 20 mg

Outcome	Number of trials	Number/total with outcome (%)		NNT (95% CI)
		Treatment	Placebo	
Two hour headache response	2	157/349 (45)	78/353 (22)	4.4 (3.4–6.2)
Two hour pain free	2	52/349 (15)	17/353 (5)	10 (7–17)
Headache response at 2 h sustained to 24 h	1	53/144 (37)	26/142 (18)	5.4 (3.5–12)

with placebo. The NNT was 4.4 (3.4–6.2). In two trials, 52/349 patients (15%) were pain free at 2 h compared with 17/353 (25%) with placebo. The NNT was 9.9 (6.9–17). In five trials, 53/144 patients (37%) had a headache response at 2 h, sustained for 24 h with no rescue medication and no second dose of study medication compared with 26/142 (18%) with placebo. The NNT was 5.4 (3.5–12).

Adverse effects

Adverse effects are not reported in any way that makes obvious sense because efficacy was measured over 24 h and adverse events for up to 10 days.

Comment

Eletriptan is clearly effective in the treatment of acute migraine. At present it is not widely available around the world, but it does have good efficacy for the 24-h outcome of sustained relief.

3.12 **Which migraine treatment strategy is most effective?**

A number of strategies can be used to treat acute migraine attacks, each utilising some part of the evidence base.

For instance, the initial attack could be treated with aspirin or simple analgesic, and if or when that fails, a triptan could be used. That is *a step strategy within an attack*.

A different approach may be to try aspirin or simple analgesic for a few attacks. It will work for some, but for those for whom it does not work, a triptan may be an alternative treatment. That is *a step strategy across attacks*, and is probably the strategy most likely to be used in the UK as it is probably seen as the cheapest.

A third way would be to assess the individual patient for the severity of the disorder, and then to treat appropriately: mild disease might be treated with aspirin or simple analgesics, while more severe disease might be treated with a triptan. This would be *stratified care*.

It just so happens that a randomised controlled trial indicates that stratified care produces the best results [1].

Trial

The trial was randomised, but open-label, and examined multiple migraine attacks for patients with established diagnosis of migraine according to IHS criteria. Patients completed the MIDAS questionnaire, that measures lost time in three domains of activity. Patients were assigned a grade of disability from I (little or infrequent disability), grade II (mild or infrequent disability), grade III (moderate disability) to grave IV (severe disability). Patients with grade II–IV disability were included.

Randomisation was done to the following three domains of activity.

Stratified care. Grade II patients received aspirin 800–1000 mg plus metoclopramide 10 mg for all six attacks. Those with grade III or IV received zolmitriptan 2.5 mg.

Step care across attacks. Patients treated the first three attacks with aspirin 800–1000 mg plus metoclopramide 10 mg. Those without adequate relief took zolmitriptan 2.5 mg for the next three attacks.

Step care within attacks. Patients treated all attacks with aspirin 800–1000 mg plus metoclopramide 10 mg first. If adequate relief was not obtained by two hours, they then took zolmitriptan 2.5 mg.

Results

In the three treatments groups, 1062 patients were randomised. Twenty percent of patients withdrew or were lost for various reasons, mostly innocuous. Only 3% withdrew because of an adverse event, and 0.2% because of deteriorating condition. Groups were well balanced.

More patients had a 2-h headache response in the stratified care strategy than for either step care strategy (Figure 3.12.1).

More patients were pain free at 2 h in the stratified care strategy than for either step care strategy (Figure 3.12.2).

Adverse events were equally common in all three groups, and were predominantly mild and transient. Adverse event study withdrawals were evenly distributed across the groups.

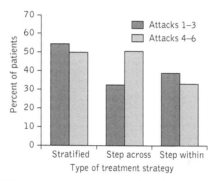

Figure 3.12.1 Two-hour headache response for up to six migraine attacks with different treatment strategies.

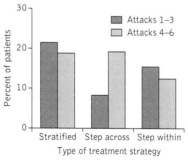

Figure 3.12.2 Two-hour pain free for up to six migraine attacks with different treatment strategies.

Comment

Most guidelines would probably accept a step up approach, similar to that of step up across attacks, but with many more steps. Because of the time involved, and because of repeated failure of treatment, some patients simply become disenchanted and seek other forms of treatment.

Treating the appropriate patient appropriately from the beginning is a better bet. It takes less time, is more effective, and is without the 'hassle factor' for patient and doctor. This is exactly what evidence-based medicine was supposed to be about, and reading the definition of EBM in the context of this trial is rewarding.

References

1. Lipton, R. B. *et al*. (2000). Stratified care vs step care strategies for migraine: The disability in strategies of care (DISC) study: a randomized trial, *JAMA* 284: 2599–605.

3.13 **Prophylaxis for migraine**

People who have frequent migraines will sometimes need other approaches to treatment than just treatment of the acute attacks. This usually means a prophylactic treatment to try and reduce the number of acute attacks. The evidence on the efficacy of migraine prophylaxis is not extensive but is summarised here.

Beta-blockers

Beta-blockers are competitive antagonists of adrenaline and nor-adrenaline at beta-adrenoceptors. Propranolol is the most commonly used of the beta-blockers, although timolol, metoprolol and nadolol are also used in migraine prophylaxis. However, there are a number of important side-effects associated with this class of drugs.

A systematic review of propranolol [1,2] examined headache index (a composite score of frequency, duration and intensity of attacks). Inclusion criteria were adult patients with recurrent migraine and group size of 5 or more. Reviewers looked at propranolol pre-treatment baseline and propranolol versus placebo. Methodological weaknesses were that reviewers may have included non-randomised and non-blinded trials in their review and that reviewers did not attempt to analyse different propranolol doses separately.

When compared with placebo, propranolol was associated with a 34% improvement in patient migraine activity. This percent was derived from weighted trial scores. However, this should be treated with caution given the methodological weaknesses listed above. Reviewers state that most trials looked at propranolol use over a six-month period. One trial continued for 8–16 months, and reported good maintenance. This trial also reported improved migraine ratings when patients were switched to placebo. Comparative figures were not given and adverse effects were not considered.

Anticonvulsants

A systematic review of anticonvulsants in chronic pain [3] identified three randomised trials where prophylactic use of anticonvulsants (carbamazepine, clonazepam or valproate) was compared with placebo in migraine. Two studies had dichotomous outcomes (improve-ment in number of migraine attacks), and 63 of 74 patients benefited with anticonvulsants compared with 17 of 77 given placebo. The relative benefit was 3.9 (2.5–5.9) and the NNT was 1.6 (1.3–2.0). This means that one of two patients suffering from migraine and treated prophylactically with anticonvulsants will have their headache frequency reduced, who would not have done had they been treated with placebo.

Valproate

Bandolier has done its own systematic review on valproate for migraine prevention. The clinical bottom line was that sodium valproate is effective for the prevention of migraine attacks. About half of the patients had a reduction in the number of migraine attacks or days with migraine by about 50%. NNT for at least 50% reduction in migraine frequency for individual studies were 3–4 in three trials, with a pooled result of 3.5 (2.6–5.3) in three trials with 350 patients. The incidence of adverse effects was not insignificant, with nausea, dizziness and drowsiness associated with its use. Women of childbearing age should use the drug with caution due to the possibility of birth defects.

Systematic review

Date review completed: November 2000

Number of trials included: Four randomised controlled trials

Number of patients: 390 patients

Control groups: Placebo

Main outcomes: Migraine frequency (attacks or days), severity and duration, adverse effects

Inclusion criteria were randomised, double-blind trials of sodium valproate for migraine prevention in adults.

Search methods

Comprehensive searches of the following databases were made: MEDLINE (1966–Sept 2000), EMBASE (1980–Sept 2000), Cochrane Library (Issue 3, 2000) and the Oxford Pain Relief Database (1950–1994) and other reviews (Tran *et al.*, 1997). A series of free text searches were undertaken, using generic and trade names for sodium valproate. There was no restriction to language. Retrieved reports were searched for additional trials. Neither individual authors nor pharmaceutical companies were contacted for unpublished data.

Outcomes

The outcome most often quoted was the number of patients with at least 50% reduction in their migraine headache frequency over four weeks at the end of 12 weeks treatment. Adverse effect withdrawal and the number of people having particular adverse effects was also noted.

Findings

Five randomised, double-blind trials were found, all were placebo controlled. Doses of valproate were varied, often were titrated, and often

were titrated against plasma concentration. The lowest starting dose
was 250 mg/day and the highest ending dose was 1500 mg/day.
Patients at baseline had at least two migraine attacks per month, usually for at least six months. The average number of attacks per month
at baseline was six. Migraine was diagnosed using IHS criteria in three
studies, and using very similar criteria in the other.

Trials were of higher methodological quality, with quality scores of
3 and 4 out of 5. Trials were disparate with respect to dosing regimes
and outcome measures but pooling of data for quantitative analysis
was still possible, as all measured at least 50% reduction in migraine
attacks over about 12 weeks. Dichotomous data were used to calculate
NNTs for individual studies.

There were three RCTs with outcomes of at least 50% reduction in
migraine attacks. All three trials used IHS criteria for migraine diagnosis, baseline values of migraine frequency were established during a
4 week run-in period. Twelve week treatment periods were followed
by 4 week washout in the two crossover trials before the second phase
of treatment. All three trials showed that between 44% and 50%
patients achieved at least 50% reduction in the frequency of migraine
days or attacks on sodium valproate compared with 14–21% on placebo
(Figure 3.13.1). The NNTs for individual studies were three to four
(Table 3.13.1).

Combining all three studies, 108/235 patients (46%) had more than
50% reduction in migraine frequency with valproate, compared with

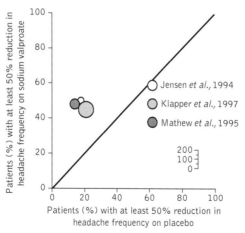

Figure 3.13.1 Reduction in number of migraine attacks or days over
four weeks.

Table 3.13.1 NNT for one patient to achieve at least 50% reduction in migraine frequency over 4 weeks on sodium valproate versus placebo

Study	Sodium valproate dose	Number of patients with at least 50% reduction in migraine frequency		NNT (95% CI)
		Valproate	Placebo	
Jensen et al., 1994	1000–1500 mg/day, plasma concentration around 50 mg/L	17/34	6/34	3.1 (1.9–8.9)
Mathew et al., 1995	give trough Dose titrated to plasma valproate levels 70–120 mg/ L	33/69	5/36	3.0 (2.0–5.7)
Klapper et al., 1997	500–1500 mg/day	58/132	9/44	4.3 (2.6–11)
Combined		108/235	20/114	3.5 (2.6–5.3)

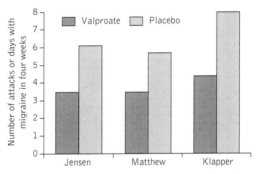

Figure 3.13.2 Mean 4-week migraine attack frequency with sodium valproate or placebo.

20/114 (18%) with placebo. The pooled relative benefit was 2.6 (1.7–4.0) and the pooled NNT was 3.5 (2.6–5.3). Sodium valproate was more effective than placebo in reducing the frequency of migraine attacks by almost 50% (Figure 3.13.2).

Adverse effects

Information on adverse effects was extracted from each trial (Table 3.13.2). There were significantly more withdrawals due to sodium

Table 3.13.2 Adverse effects with sodium valproate and placebo

Adverse effect category	Number of studies	Number with AE with valproate	Number with AE with placebo	Relative risk (95% CI)	NNT (95% CI)
Any adverse effect	3	127/245	44/124	1.4 (0.69–3.0)	nc
Withdrawals due to adverse effects	3	38/245	6/124	3.1 (2.1–4.7)	9.4 (6.0–21)
Particular adverse effects					
Tremor	3	33/220	0/124	47 (10–207)	6.2 (4.7–9.1)
Nausea	3	107/245	14/124	3.3 (2.0–5.4)	3.3 (2.5–4.2)
Dizziness/ vertigo	2	37/175	5/87	2.6 (1.1–6.1)	6.5 (4.3–13)
Drowsiness	3	58/245	9/114	2.6 (1.4–5.2)	6.3 (4.3–12)

valproate than placebo with a number needed to harm (NNH) of 9.4 (6.0–21). Particular adverse effects were nausea, tremor, dizziness and drowsiness with NNHs of 3.1, 6.2, 6.5 and 6.3, respectively. Asthenia, weight gain and hair loss also occurred with sodium valproate but were not significantly more frequent than with placebo.

Comment

We know that anticonvulsants for neuropathic pain are effective so it is no surprise that sodium valproate is so effective at preventing migraines. The adverse effects associated with its use may be a concern for some patients. Newer anticonvulsants coming onto the market with less adverse effects may present better treatment options. So far there are no RCTs to support the use of drugs like gabapentin for migraine prevention, but there are suggestions that migraine prophylaxis is becoming an active research area with a number of new treatments.

References

1. Holroyd, K. A. *et al.* (1991). Propranolol in the management of recurrent migraine: a meta-analytic review, *Headache* 31: 333–340.
2. Tfelt-Hansen, P. (1986). Efficacy of beta blockers in migraine. A critical review, *Cephalalgia* 6(Supp. 5): 15–24.
3. McQuay, H. J. *et al.* (1995). Anticonvulsants for the management of pain – a systematic review, *BMJ* 311: 1047–52.

Section 4
Chronic pain

4.1 **Introduction**

In chronic pain relief, just as in other therapeutic areas, there are often many ways to tackle a particular problem. There may be more or less evidence of benefit for each of the alternatives. The task facing us is to have a way of ranking the relative effectiveness of these interventions, and to couple that with knowledge of any hazards, minor or major. Then we can make informed decisions about which should be offered to patients.

In an ideal world there would be large randomised trials comparing the various interventions. In practice what we have is a relatively small number of small studies. This section is not about how clinical trials are performed in chronic pain, but rather to set a scene in which the available evidence may be placed.

Range of interventions

The range of interventions available for chronic pain management is summarised in Figure 4.1.1.

The same conventional analgesics, from NSAID to opioid, are used in chronic as in acute pain. If analgesics relieve the pain to an adequate extent, and with tolerable or controllable adverse effects, then there is little reason to use other interventions. If analgesics are ineffective other methods have to be considered. If analgesics are effective but cause intolerable or uncontrollable adverse effects then again other methods should be considered.

We know from audits of cancer pain that using analgesics according to the WHO ladder (Figure 4.1.2) can relieve pain for 80% of patients. For most of the 80% the relief will be good, for a minority it will only be moderate. This presumes that the pain is managed optimally, and we know from audit is often not the case. Optimal management requires that the correct drugs are available, and that they are given in the correct dose by the correct route and at the correct time. This needs staff who

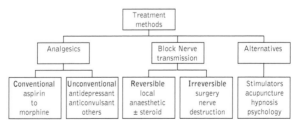

Figure 4.1.1 Treatment methods.

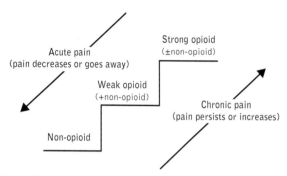

Figure 4.1.2 Schematic WHO 'ladder' for cancer pain management.

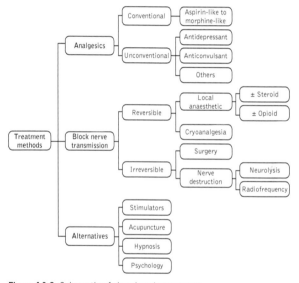

Figure 4.1.3 Schematic of chronic pain treatment.

are well versed in the problems, and who are available to care for the patient. The second problem is the 20% of patients whose pain is not well managed by intelligent use of analgesic guidelines.

The other treatment methods in Figure 4.1.3 are necessary to manage those for whom analgesics fail, and it provides a generalised schematic of how most chronic pain clinics would approach problems.

Non-opioid analgesics

Choosing the best analgesic for long-term use involves the same decisions as in acute pain. Most comparisons are done using single doses, whereas patients with chronic pain take multiple doses. Historically the efficacy of single doses in acute pain has also proved valid in chronic pain. Despite the fact that the drugs in this category are by far the most widely used, there is remarkably little good evidence about their relative efficacy and adverse effects in chronic pain.

No single-dose trial has shown any efficacy advantage of one NSAID over another [1]. The efficacy dose–response curve for NSAIDs is flat compared with the dose response for adverse effects such as gastrointestinal symptoms, dizziness, and drowsiness [2]. Increasing the dose to improve analgesia is therefore more likely to increase adverse effects than to improve analgesia [3–5].

NSAIDs alone produced as good analgesia as single or multiple doses of weak opioids alone or in combination with nonopioid analgesics [6]. Adverse effect incidence and patient dropout rates were the same for multiple doses of NSAIDs or weak opioids in combination with non-opioid analgesics [7,8].

Opioids

In chronic pain there are two particular problems with opioids [9]. The first is that adequate doses are often not available or are not given, primarily because of fears of addiction. The second is that some (rarer) chronic pain states, particularly when the nervous system is damaged, may not respond fully to opiates.

Opioids used for people who are not in pain can induce physical and psychological dependence. This does not happen to patients who receive them for pain relief, for instance after an operation or for severe pain from osteoporotic vertebral collapse. Some governments restrict medical availability on the grounds that if the drugs are available medically this will worsen the street addiction problem. There is no evidence for this. The casualties are patients who are deprived of adequate pain relief.

In chronic pain opioids are usually given by mouth. The dose is worked out by titration over a period of days, and then the drug is given regularly, not waiting for the pain to come back. Initial problems with nausea or dizziness commonly settle. If constipation is likely laxatives are given.

Patients who cannot swallow can try sublingual, transdermal or suppository dosing. Subcutaneous infusion, usually from a small (external) pump is used for terminal patients who cannot manage these other routes. Rarely the epidural route is used for combination infusion of opioid and local anaesthetic.

If patients' pain starts to increase the dose is increased. If sensible dose increases do not produce pain relief, or if increasing the opioid dose provokes intolerable or unmanageable adverse effects, then other methods have to be considered, either as well as the opioid or instead of it. A working rule is that if the pain is in a numb area, which is a marker for a damaged nervous system, we would be less confident that opioids would necessarily produce pain relief [10], and our threshold for using other strategies would be lower.

Unconventional analgesics

Unconventional analgesics [11] are drugs having other indications in other medical settings, and are not normally thought of as analgesics. Treating chronic pain in a tertiary hospital setting we use these drugs for about one third of our patients. The hallmark is pain in a numb area, neuropathic pain.

When the patient has symptoms and signs of nervous system damage in the area of their pain we expect the response to conventional analgesics to be reduced. Conventional analgesics have often failed already, which is why the patient has been referred. If not, we try them, before we embark on empirical testing to see if any of the unconventional analgesics can provide relief.

Antidepressants. Antidepressants work on the nervous system to relieve depression. We use them in much lower dosage (about half) to relieve pain. Classically they were used to relieve pain that was burning rather than shooting in character, and anticonvulsants were used for shooting pains. Now we tend to use antidepressants as first line for both types of pain, because we have greater success and because we believe antidepressants cause fewer adverse effects.

Anticonvulsants. Anticonvulsants have been used for many years to treat the shooting pains of trigeminal neuralgia and of diabetic neuropathy. How they work has never been clear. The catchall explanation was that they stabilised nerve membranes, preventing them carrying spurious messages. The current fashionable explanation is that these drugs acting as antagonists on the N-methyl D-aspartate (NMDA) mechanism. Anticonvulsants can provide good relief in neuropathic pain. Doses required for analgesic effect are close to the anticonvulsant dosing range, and carry a perceived burden of adverse effects.

Others. Clonidine and other alpha-2 adrenergic agonists have analgesic effects, both in conventional pain and in neuropathic pain [12]. They extend the duration of local anaesthetic effect and have a synergistic effect with opioids. Their clinical utility is limited by the adverse effects of sedation and hypotension. In neuropathic pain single doses of clonidine were effective in postherpetic neuralgia [13] and in cancer pain [14]. Baclofen is used by intrathecal pump to treat the painful spasms of cerebral palsy. Ketamine and dextromethorphan, both drugs with NMDA antagonist action, are being used in severe neuropathic pain.

Block nerve transmission

Reversible. Local anaesthetics block nerve conduction reversibly. When the local anaesthetic wears off the pain returns. That is the pharmacologically correct statement, but another old saying, that a series of local anaesthetic blocks can be used to 'break the cycle' of pain and effect a cure, now has some empirical support [15], even if we do not understand the mechanism. Arner and colleagues showed that the duration of pain relief could far outlast the duration of local anaesthetic action, and that prolonged relief could result from a series of blocks [15]. Local anaesthetic blocks can thus be diagnostic and therapeutic. Diagnosis of pain for instance from a 'trapped' lateral cutaneous nerve of thigh can be confirmed by local anaesthetic block. A series of blocks may prevent pain recurring.

Pain clinics use such blocks commonly, for shoulder pain (supra-scapular nerve block [16] or intra-articular [17]), for intercostal neuralgia, for rectus sheath nerve entrapment, postoperative scar pains and other peripheral neuralgias (Table 4.1.1). What is not clear is the extent to which adding steroid to the local anaesthetic makes a difference, either prolonging the duration of effect of a particular procedure or increasing the chance of success of a series of blocks.

Similar injections are done for the trigger points of fibromyalgia, but there do not appear to be any controlled comparisons of injections with other treatments.

Table 4.1.1 Common nerve blocks

Block	Common indications
Trigger point	focal pain (e.g. in muscle)
Peripheral (intercostal, sacral nerves, rectus sheath)	pain in dermatomal distribution
Extradural	Uni or bilateral pain (lumbosacral, cervical, thoracic, etc.) Midline perineal pain
Intrathecal	Unilateral pain (neurolytic injection for pain due to malignancy, limbs, chest, etc.) (Midline perineal pain)
Autonomic Intravenous regional sympathectomy	reflex sympathetic dystrophy
Stellate ganglion	reflex sympathetic dystrophy arm pain brachial plexus nerve compression
Lumbar sympathetic	reflex sympathetic dystrophy lumbosacral plexus nerve compression vascular insufficiency lower limb perineal pain
Coeliac plexus	abdominal pain

Intravenous regional sympathetic blocks (IRSBs) are used widely in patients with reflex sympathetic dystrophy (RSD). A systematic review of randomised trials of IRSBs found them not to be effective (section 4.12).

Two other common (for back pain) pain clinic procedures are epidural steroid injection and facet nerve blocks. Epidural steroids in back pain [18–20] have been studied in two systematic reviews and are covered in section 4.8.

Classically facet joint injection with local anaesthetic and steroid is indicated when pain is worse when sitting, and pain is provoked by lateral rotation and spine extension. Recent studies suggest that whether or not the injection is actually in the facet joint makes little difference [21], and indeed cast some doubt on long-term utility [22]. Short-lived success (less than six weeks) with local anaesthetic and steroid is said to be improved by the use of cryoanalgesia or radiofrequency blocks to the nerves to the joints.

Irreversible. The destructive procedures are aimed at cutting, burning or damaging nerve fibres carrying the pain signals. The flaw in the logic is that the nervous system can all too often rewire, finding a way around the lesion. If that happens, and the pain returns, then it may be even more difficult to manage – severe neuropathic pain can result. In general neurolytic blocks in non-malignant pain are not recommended, because they do not last forever, and recurrent pain may be more difficult to manage, and because of the morbidity. In cancer pain these neurolytic block procedures do have a place, when there is a short (less than three month) prognosis, or where alternatives such as painstaking drug control or long-term epidural infusion are not possible. Similar distinction between cancer and non-cancer pain holds for coeliac plexus block in pancreatic pain. Pain associated with pancreatic cancer responds well to coeliac plexus block [23], and it may also help those with abdominal or perineal pain from tumour in the pelvis. In chronic pancreatitis results are much less convincing.

The limitation is the potential for motor and sphincter damage. This risk is higher with bilateral and repeat procedures, and higher the lower the cord level of the block. Extradural neurolytics have limited efficacy. While claims have been made that the paravertebral approach is preferable, patchy results may be attributed to unpredictable injectate spread. Our results of spinal infusion of a combination of local anaesthetic and opioid are superior to neurolytic blocks, providing good analgesia with minimal irreversible morbidity.

Surgery. The relevant neurosurgical interventions for orthopaedic pain include dorsal column stimulation, rhizotomy, cordotomy and dorsal root entry zone (DREZ) lesions. The indications are usually non-malignant neuropathic pain which has failed to respond to pharmacological measures. The difficulties of trials of uncommon surgical procedures are well known. These procedures are usually documented by glowing case series. Longer term outcomes may not be so good [24].

Alternatives

TENS. The rationale for transcutaneous nerve stimulation (TENS) is the gate theory [25]. If the spinal cord is bombarded with impulses from the TENS machine then it is distracted from transmitting the pathological pain signal. We know that TENS has limited efficacy in acute (and postoperative) pain, and also in labour pain. In chronic pain we have few trials that can really help us (section 4.5).

What we do know is that attention to detail makes considerable difference to TENS efficacy in chronic pain [26]. Patients need to be told that it is useless expecting success unless the machine is connected for at least an hour at a time. They need to be told where to put the electrodes, how to put them on, how to manipulate the stimulus to best advantage, and indeed to turn the machine on.

Physiotherapy and variants. Pain clinics keep a very open mind about other interventions, like acupuncture [27–30; but see section 6]. If patients benefit from alternatives we are only too pleased. The evidence from back pain however suggests that on rigorous outcome measures physiotherapy and other forms of manipulation have but limited success. Such analyses often did not include any measure of quality of life. If they make the patient feel better and they are cheap then it is a decision for the third party payer whether or not these physiotherapy manoeuvres should be offered. There are a number of systematic reviews [31–39], though they are of limited help as there are few good trials.

Behavioural management. Back schools to behavioural management programmes offer a range of help for patients, help to cope with their (usually back) pain problems. Making decisions about the benefits of psychologically-based treatments of medical problems is not easy, and especially difficult to compare with other treatments and to measure relative benefit and cost. Patients whose pain has proved intractable to all reasonable medical and other interventions are chronic consumers of health care – GP or hospital clinic time, analgesic and psychotropic drugs, repeated admissions and sometimes surgery. If rehabilitation treatment enables these patients to carry on more satisfying lives with minimum medical help, how can it be most effectively and economically offered?

Randomised comparison of the St. Thomas' four-week inpatient treatment with eight-week half-day outpatient treatment, with fitness training, planned increases in activity, activity scheduling, drug reduction, relaxation and cognitive therapy as the pain management methods taught by the same staff team [40], showed that for every three patients treated as inpatients rather than outpatients, one patient fewer was taking analgesic or psychotropic drugs. For every four patients treated as inpatients rather than outpatients, one patient fewer sought additional medical advice in the year after treatment. For every five patients treated as inpatients rather than outpatients, one patient more had a 10-min walking distance improved by more than 50%. For every six patients treated as inpatients rather than outpatients, one patient fewer was depressed [42]. Again, there are a number of systematic reviews limited by the quality of trials [43–50].

References

1. Gøtzsche, G. P. (1989). Patients' preference in indomethacin trials: an overview, *Lancet* 1: 88–91.

2. Eisenberg, E. *et al.* (1994). Efficacy and safety of nonsteroidal antiinflammatory drugs for cancer pain: a meta-analysis, *Journal of Clinical Oncology* 12: 2756–65.

3. Henry, D. *et al.* (1996). Variability in risk of gastrointestinal complications with individual non-steroidal anti-inflammatory drugs: results of a collaborative meta-analysis, *BMJ* 312: 1563–6.

4. Silverstein, F. E. *et al.* (1995). Misoprostol reduces serious gastrointestinal complications in patients with rheumatoid arthritis receiving nonsteroidal anti-inflammatory drugs, *Annals of Internal Medicine* 123: 241–9.

5. Shield, M. J. and Morant, S. V. (1996). Misoprostol in patients taking non-steroidal anti-inflammatory drugs, *BMJ* 312: 846.

6. March, L. *et al.* (1994). N of 1 trials comparing a non-steroidal anti-inflammatatory drug with paracetamol in osteoarthritis, *BMJ* 309: 1041–6.

7. Kjærsgaard-Andersen, P. *et al.* (1990). Codeine plus paracetamol versus paracetamol in longer-term treatment of chronic pain due to osteoarthritis of the hip, *Pain* 43: 309–18.

8. Moore, R. A. *et al.* (1998). A systematic review of topically-applied non-steroidal anti-inflammatory drugs, *BMJ* 316: 333–8.

9. McQuay, H. J. (1989). Opioids in chronic pain, *British Journal of Anaesthesia*, 63: 213–26.

10. Jadad, A. R. *et al.* (1992). Morphine responsiveness of chronic pain: double-blind randomised crossover study with patient-controlled analgesia, *Lancet* 339: 1367–71.

11. McQuay, H. J. (1988). Pharmacological treatment of neuralgic and neuro-pathic pain, *Cancer Surveys* 7: 141–59.

12. McQuay, H. J. (1992). Is there a place for alpha2 adrenergic agonists in the control of pain? in: Besson, J. M. and Guilbaud, G. (Eds), *Toward the use of alpha2 adrenergic agonists for the treatment of pain*, Elsevier, Amsterdam, pp. 219–32.

13. Max, M. B. *et al.* (1988). Association of pain relief with drug side effects in postherpetic neuralgia: a single dose study of clonidine, codeine, ibuprofen, and placebo, *Clinical Pharmacology and Therapeutics* 43: 363–71.

14. Eisenach, J. C. *et al.* (1995). Epidural clonidine analgesia for intractable cancer pain. The Epidural Clonidine Study Group, *Pain* 61: 391–9.

15. Arner, A. *et al.* (1990). Prolonged relief of neuralgia after regional anesthetic blocks. A call for further experimental and systematic clinical studies, *Pain* 43: 287–97.

16. Emery, P. *et al.* (1989). Suprascapular nerve block for chronic shoulder pain in rheumatoid arthritis, *BMJ* 299: 1079–80.

17. van der Heijden, C. J. M. *et al.* (1996). Steroid injections for shoulder disorders: a systematic review of randomized clinical trials, *British Journal of General Practice* 46: 309–16.

18. Jadad, A. R. *et al.* (1995). Intravenous regional sympathetic blockade for pain relief in reflex sympathetic dystrophy: a systematic review and a randomized, double-blind crossover study, *Journal of Pain and Symptom Management* 10: 13–20.

19. Watts, R. W. and Silagy, C. A. (1995). A meta-analysis on the efficacy of epidural corticosteroids in the treatment of sciatica, *Anaesthesia and Intensive Care* 23: 564–69.

20. Koes, B. W. *et al.* (1995). Efficacy of epidural steroid injections for low-back pain and sciatica: a systematic review of randomized clinical trials, *Pain* 63: 279–88.

21. Lilius, G. *et al.* (1989). Lumbar facet joint syndrome, *Journal of Bone and Joint Surgery* 71: 681–4.

22. Carette, S. *et al.* (1991). A controlled trial of corticosteroid injections into facet joints for chronic low back pain, *New England Journal of Medicine* 325: 1002–7.

23. Eisenberg, E. *et al.* (1995). Neurolytic celiac plexus block for treatment of cancer pain: a meta-analysis, *Anesthesia & Analgesia* 80: 290–5.

24. Abram, S. E. (1992). Bonica Lecture. Advances in chronic pain management since gate control, *Regional Anesthesia* 18: 66–81.

25. Melzack, R. and Wall, P. D. (1965). *Pain* mechanisms: a new theory, *Science* 150: 971–8.

26. Johnson, M. I. *et al.* (1992). Long term use of transcutaneous electrical nerve stimulation at Newcastle Pain Relief Clinic, *Journal of the Royal Society of Medicine* 85: 267–8.

27. Patel, M. *et al.* (1989). A meta-analysis of acupuncture for chronic pain, *International Journal of Epidemiology* 18: 900–6.

28. ter Riet, G. *et al.* (1990). Acupuncture and chronic pain: a criteria-based meta-analysis, *Journal of Clinical Epidemiology* 43: 1191–9.

29. BhattSanders, D. (1985). Acupuncture for rheumatoid arthritis: an analysis of the literature, *Seminars Arthritis Rheumatology* 14: 225–31.

30. Puett, D. W. and Griffin, M. R. (1994). Published trials of nonmedicinal and noninvasive therapies for hip and knee osteoarthritis, *Annals of Internal Medicine* 121: 133–40.

31. Abenhaim, L. and Bergeron, A. M. (1992). Twenty years of randomized clinical trials of manipulative therapy for back pain: a review, *Clinical Investigative Medicine* 15: 527–35.

32. Anderson, R. *et al.* (1992). A meta-analysis of clinical trials of spinal manipulation, *Journal of Manipulative Physiology and Therapeutics* 15: 181–94.

33. Assendelft, W. J. *et al.* (1992). The efficacy of chiropractic manipulation for back pain: blinded review of relevant randomized clinical trials, *Journal of Manipulative Physiology and Therapeutics* 15: 487–94.

34. Brunarski, D. J. (1984). Clinical trials of spinal manipulation: a critical appraisal and review of the literature, *Journal of Manipulative Physiology and Therapeutics* 7: 243–9.

35. Koes, B. W. *et al.* (1991). Spinal manipulation and mobilisation for back and neck pain: a blinded review, *BMJ* 303: 1298–303.

36. Koes, B. W. *et al.* (1991). Physiotherapy exercises and back pain: a blinded review, *BMJ* 302: 1572–6.

37. Ottenbacher, K. and DiFabio, R. P. (1985). Efficacy of spinal manipulation/mobilization therapy. A meta analysis, *Spine* 10: 833–7.

38. Powell, F. C. *et al.* (1993). A risk/benefit analysis of spinal manipulation therapy for relief of lumbar or cervical pain, *Neurosurgery* 33: 73–8; discussion 78–9.

39. Shekelle, P. G. *et al.* (1992). Spinal manipulation for low-back pain, *Annals Internal Medicine* 117: 590–8.

40. Pither, C. E. and Nicholas, M. K. (1991). Psychological approaches in chronic pain management, *BMJ* 47: 743–61.

41. Bandolier, *More wisdom*, Bandolier 1995.

42. McQuay, H. J. *et al.* (1997). Systematic review of outpatient services for chronic pain control, *Health Technology Assessment* 1(6).

43. Cohen, J. E. *et al.* (1994). Group education interventions for people with low back pain. An overview of the literature, *Spine* 19: 1214–22.

44. Cutler, R. B. *et al.* (1994). Does nonsurgical pain center treatment of chronic pain return patients to work? A review and meta-analysis of the literature, *Spine* 19: 643–52.

45. Fernandez, E. and Turk, D. C. (1989). The utility of cognitive coping strategies for altering pain perception: a meta analysis, *Pain* 38: 123–35.

46. Gebhardt, W. A. (1994). Effectiveness of training to prevent job-related back pain: a meta-analysis, *British Journal of Clinical Psychology* 33: 571–4.

47. Hyman, R. B. *et al.* (1989). The effects of relaxation training on clinical symptoms: a meta analysis, *Nursing Research* 38: 216–20.

48. Malone, M. D. *et al.* (1988). Meta analysis of non medical treatments for chronic pain, *Pain* 34: 231–44.

49. Mullen, P. D. *et al.* (1987). Efficacy of psychoeducational interventions on pain, depression, and disability in people with arthritis: a meta analysis, *Journal of Rheumatology* 14 Supp: 33–9.

50. Suls, J. and Fletcher, B. (1985). The relative efficacy of avoidant and nonavoidant coping strategies: a meta analysis, *Health Psychology* 4: 249–88.

4.2 **Antidepressants for diabetic neuropathy and postherpetic neuralgia**

Clinical bottom line. Antidepressants are effective treatments for diabetic neuropathy (NNT 3.4, 95% confidence interval 2.6–4.7) and postherpetic neuralgia (NNT 2.1, 1.7–3.0) compared with placebo. The NNH for any patient to have a minor adverse effect with antidepressant was 2.7 (2.1–3.9) and for a major adverse effect was 17 (10–43).

For over 30 years the management of neuropathic pain has involved the use of both antidepressants and anticonvulsants, but which drug class should be the first-line choice remains unclear. The dogma that the character of the pain was predictive of the response, burning pain responding to antidepressants and shooting pain to anticonvulsants, was shown to be incorrect in diabetic neuropathy, where patients experiencing both burning and shooting pain responded to tricyclic antidepressants. Most studies on neuropathic pain have involved diabetic neuropathy and postherpetic neuralgia, because these conditions represent the majority of patients with neuropathic pain with discrete diagnoses.

Systematic review

Collins, S. L. *et al.* (2000). Antidepressants and anticonvulsants for diabetic neuropathy and postherpetic neuralgia: a quantitative systematic review, *Journal of Pain and Symptom Management* 20: 449–58.

Date review completed: June 1999

Number of trials included: 19

Number of patients: 358 on antidepressant and 278 on placebo (episodes of treatment)

Control group: Placebo

Main outcomes: Various outcomes equivalent to at least 50% pain relief

Searching involved numerous electronic databases including MEDLINE, EMBASE, CINAHL, Sigle, PubMed and the Cochrane Library, plus in-house databases of randomised controlled trials in pain. The inclusion criteria used were: full journal publication, adult patients, double-blind design, random allocation to treatment groups which included placebo and either an antidepressant or an anticonvulsant for the treatment of chronic pain due to diabetic neuropathy or postherpetic neuralgia. An adequate description of the original authors' method of clinical diagnosis was required to ensure an accurate diagnosis of the two conditions. For postherpetic neuralgia the pain must have been present for more than three months after zoster eruption to limit the chance of spontaneous cessation of symptoms.

A clinically relevant outcome was defined as a measure equivalent to at least 50% pain relief after the longest reported duration of treatment. This was extracted as dichotomous information from the following hierarchy of outcome measures:

- Top two values on a patient reported 5-point global scale of pain relief or effectiveness or improvement.
- Top three values on a patient reported 6-point global scale of pain relief or effectiveness or improvement.
- Top value on a patient reported 3-point global scale of pain relief or effectiveness or improvement.
- The top two values on a patient reported 4-point categorical pain relief scale 50% or more reduction on a visual analogue scale (VAS) of pain intensity.
- A mean score of 6 or less on a 6-item neuropathy scale which included pain and had a maximum possible score of 12.

The majority of studies used a cross-over design and results are presented in terms of patient episodes rather than actual numbers of patients. One patient episode represents the result for one patient completing one part of the cross-over. So for a trial where the patient was crossed-over from placebo to active this would generate two patient episodes.

Adverse effects were classified as minor if reported by a patient who then continued to take the medication and completed the trial. A major adverse effect was one causing the patient to withdraw from the study. Withdrawal due to lack of efficacy was not counted as an adverse effect.

Findings

The studies of antidepressants in diabetic neuropathy and postherpetic neuralgia were small, ranging from 12 to 92 patient episodes in total. Consequently the results of individual trials varied greatly, both in diabetic neuropathy (Figure 4.2.1) and postherpetic neuralgia (Figure 4.2.2).

Pooled results are shown in Table 4.2.1. Over both conditions, 64% of patients had an outcome equivalent to more than 50% pain relief with antidepressant, compared with 30% with placebo. The NNT for at least 50% pain relief compared with placebo was 2.9 (2.4–3.7).

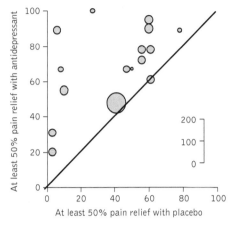

Figure 4.2.1 Trials of antidepressants versus placebo in diabetic neuropathy.

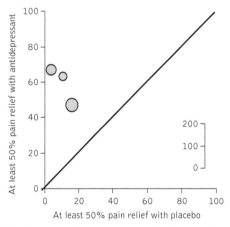

Figure 4.2.2 Trials of antidepressants versus placebo in postherpetic neuralgia.

For every patient who received benefit, one also had a minor adverse effect that did not lead to discontinuation. Nearly 1 patient in 12 discontinued treatment because adverse effects were intolerable, with a NNH of 17 (10–43).

Table 4.2.1 Summary results of efficacy and harm for antidepressants in diabetic neuropathy and postherpetic neuralgia

| | Trials | Patient episodes | Number of patients improved or harmed number/total (%) | | Relative benefit | NNT (95% CI) | NNH (95% CI) |
			Antidepressant	Placebo			
Efficacy							
Diabetic neuropathy	16	491	185/281 (66%)	76/210 (36%)	1.7 (1.4–1.9)	3.4 (2.6–4.7)	
Postherpetic neuralgia	3	145	44/77 (57%)	7/68 (10%)	5.5 (2.7–11)	2.1 (1.7–3.0)	
Both conditions	19	636	229/358 (64%)	83/278 (30%)	1.9 (1.6–2.3)	2.9 (2.4–3.7)	
Harm							
Minor adverse effect	7	281	114/163 (70%)	39/118 (33%)	2.3 (1.8–2.9)		2.7 (2.1–3.9)
Major adverse effect	16	536	27/325 (8%)	5/211 (1%)	2.6 (1.4–5)		17 (10–43)

Comment

This review updated previous reviews and confirmed that antidepressants are effective in patients with diabetic neuropathy and postherpetic neuralgia. The degree of benefit, an outcome equivalent to at least 50% pain relief, was valuable, and with an NNT of 3, efficacy was equivalent to that seen in effective analgesics in acute pain (10 mg intramuscular morphine, for instance). Two thirds of patients given antidepressants benefited. For every patient who benefited, one had a minor adverse effect, but continued with the treatment. There were few differences in the efficacy and harm seen with antidepressants and anticonvulsants.

Other reviews on neuropathic pain

It is an interesting observation that rather a lot of reviews (most systematic) have been done around neuropathic pain. It is impossible to abstract them all, and probably unrewarding, in that they cover virtually the same papers. For those readers with a particular interest, a list of those we have found is given below.

References

Alperand, B. S. and Lewis, P. R. (2002). Treatment of postherpetic neuralgia. A systematic review of the literature, *Journal of Family Practice* 51: 121–8.

Arnold, L. M. *et al.* (2000). Antidepressant treatment of fibromyalgia, *Psychosomatics* 41: 104–13.

Browning, R. *et al.* (2001). Cyclobenzaprine and back pain: a meta-analysis, *Archives of Internal Medicine* 161: 1613–20.

Collins, S. L. *et al.* (2000). Antidepressants and anticonvulsants for diabetic neuropathy and postherpetic neuralgia: a quantitative systematic review, *Journal of Pain and Symptom Management* 20: 449–58.

Denkers, M. R. *et al.* (2002). Dorsal root entry zone lesioning used to treat central neuropathic pain in patients with traumatic spinal cord injury: a systematic review, *Spine* 27: E177–84.

Fishbain, D. A. *et al.* (1998). Do antidepressants have an analgesic effect in psychogenic pain and somatoform pain disorder? A meta-analysis, *Psychosomatic Medicine* 60: 503–9.

Furlanand, A. D. *et al.* (2001). Chemical sympathectomy for neuropathic pain: does it work? Case report and systematic literature review, *Clinical Journal of Pain* 17: 327–36.

Jensen, T. S. *et al.* (2001). The clinical picture of neuropathic pain, *European Journal of Pharmacology* 429: 1–11.

Jung, A. C. *et al.* (1997). The efficacy of selective serotonin reuptake inhibitors for the management of chronic pain, *Journal of General Internal Medicine* 12: 384–90.

Katz, N. (2000). Neuropathic pain in cancer and AIDS, *Clinical Journal of Pain* 16: S41–8.

Koltzenburg, M. (1998). Painful neuropathies, *Current Opinion in Neurology* 11: 515–21.

Ladhaniand, S. and Williams, H. C. (1998). The management of established postherpetic neuralgia: a comparison of the quality and content of traditional vs. systematic reviews, *British Journal of Dermatology* 139: 66–72.

Lancaster, T. *et al.* (1995). Primary care management of acute herpes zoster: systematic review of evidence from randomized controlled trials, *British Journal of General Practice* 45: 39–45.

Lynch, M. E. (2001). Antidepressants as analgesics: a review of randomized controlled trials, *Psychopharmacology of Pain* 26: 30–6.

Martinand, L. A. and Hagen, N. A. (1997). Neuropathic pain in cancer patients: mechanisms syndromes, and clinical controversies, *Journal of Pain and Symptom Management* 14: 99–117.

Martinand, T. J. and Eisenach, J. C. (2001). Pharmacology of opioid and nonopioid analgesics in chronic pain states, *Journal of Pharmacology and Experimental Therapeutics* 299: 811–7.

McQuay, H. *et al.* (1995). Anticonvulsant drugs for management of pain: a systematic review, *BMJ* 311: 1047–52.

McQuay, H. J. (1997). Systematic review of outpatient services for chronic pain control, *Health Technology Assessment* 1.

McQuay, H. J. *et al.* (1996). A systematic review of antidepressants in neuropathic pain, *Pain* 68: 217–27.

Mellegers, M. A. *et al.* (2001). Gabapentin for neuropathic pain: systematic review of controlled and uncontrolled literature, *Clinical Journal of Pain* 17: 284–95.

Nicolucci, A. *et al.* (1996). A meta-analysis of trials on aldose reductase inhibitors in diabetic peripheral neuropathy, *Diabetic Medicine* 13: 1017–26.

Nicolucci, A. *et al.* (1996). The efficacy of tolrestat in the treatment of diabetical peripheral neuropathy. A meta-analysis of individual patient data, *Diabetes Care* 19: 1091–6.

O'Malley, P. G. *et al.* (2000). Treatment of fibromyalgia with antidepressants: a meta-analysis, *Journal of General Internal Medicine* 15: 659–66.

O'Malley, P. G. *et al.* (1999). Antidepressant therapy for unexplained symptoms and symptom syndromes, *Journal of Family Practice* 48: 980–9.

Onghenaand, P. and Van Houdenhove, B. (1992). Antidepressant-induced analgesia in chronic non-malignant pain: a meta-analysis of 39 placebo-controlled studies, *Pain* 49: 205–19.

Padilla, M. *et al.* (2000). Topical medications for orofacial neuropathic pain: a review, *Journal of the American Dental Association* 131: 184–95.

Salerno, S. M. *et al.* (2002). The effect of antidepressant treatment on chronic back pain, *Archives of Internal Medicine* 162: 19–24.

Tomkins, G. E. *et al.* (2001). Treatment of chronic headache with antidepressants: a meta-analysis, *American Journal of Medicine* 111: 54–63.

Volmink, J. *et al.* (1996). Treatments for postherpetic neuralgia: A systematic review of randomized controlled trials, *Family Practice* 13: 84–91.

4.3 Anticonvulsants for diabetic neuropathy and postherpetic neuralgia

Clinical bottom line. Anticonvulsants are effective treatments for diabetic neuropathy (NNT 2.7, 95% confidence interval 2.2–3.8) and postherpetic neuralgia (NNT 3.2, 95% confidence interval 2.4–5.0) compared with placebo, based on four trials. The NNH for any patient to have a minor adverse effect with anticonvulsants was 2.7 (2.2–3.4).

For over 30 years the management of neuropathic pain has involved the use of both antidepressants and anticonvulsants, but which drug class should be first line choice remains unclear. The dogma that the character of the pain was predictive of the response, burning pain responding to antidepressants and shooting pain to anticonvulsants, was shown to be incorrect in diabetic neuropathy, where patients experiencing both burning and shooting pain responded to tricyclic antidepressants. Most studies on neuropathic pain have involved diabetic neuropathy and postherpetic neuralgia, because these conditions represent the majority of patients with neuropathic pain.

Systematic review

Collins, S. L. *et al.* (2000). Antidepressants and anticonvulsants for diabetic neuropathy and postherpetic neuralgia: a quantitative systematic review, *Journal of Pain and Symptom Management* 20: 449–58.

Date review completed: June 1999

Number of trials included: 4 for efficacy, 5 for safety

Number of patients: 270 on anticonvulsant and 276 on placebo (episodes of treatment)

Control group: Placebo

Main outcomes: Various outcomes equivalent to at least 50% pain relief

Searching involved numerous electronic databases including MED-LINE, EMBASE, CINAHL, Sigle, PubMed and the Cochrane Library, plus in-house databases of randomised controlled trials in pain. The inclusion criteria used were: full journal publication, adult patients, double-blind design, random allocation to treatment groups which included placebo and either an antidepressant or an anticonvulsant for the treatment of chronic pain due to diabetic neuropathy or postherpetic neuralgia. An adequate description of the original authors' method of clinical diagnosis was required to ensure an accurate diagnosis of the two conditions. For postherpetic neuralgia the pain

must have been present for more than three months after zoster eruption to limit the chance of spontaneous cessation of symptoms.

A clinically relevant outcome was defined as a measure equivalent
to at least 50% pain relief after the longest reported duration of
treatment. This was extracted as dichotomous information from the
following hierarchy of outcome measures:

- Top two values on a patient reported 5-point global scale of pain
  relief or effectiveness or improvement.
- Top three values on a patient reported 6-point global scale of pain
  relief or effectiveness or improvement.
- Top value on a patient reported 3-point global scale of pain relief or
  effectiveness or improvement.
- The top two values on a patient reported 4-point categorical pain
  relief scale 50% or more reduction on a VAS of pain intensity.
- A mean score of 6 or less on a 6-item neuropathy scale which
  included pain and had a maximum possible score of 12.

The majority of studies used a cross-over design and results are presented
in terms of patient episodes rather than actual numbers of patients. One
patient episode represents the result for one patient completing one
part of the cross-over. So for a trial where the patient was crossed-over
from placebo to active this would generate two patient episodes.

Adverse effects were classified as minor if reported by a patient who
then continued to take the medication and completed the trial.
A major adverse effect was one causing the patient to withdraw from
the study. Withdrawal due to lack of efficacy was not counted as an
adverse effect.

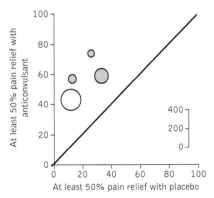

Figure 4.3.1 Trials of anticonvulsants versus placebo in diabetic
neuropathy (filled circles) and postherpetic neuralgia (open circle).

Table 4.3.1 Summary results of efficacy and harm for anticonvulsants in diabetic neuropathy and postherpetic neuralgia

| | Trials | Patient episodes | Number of patients improved or harmed number/total (%) | | Relative benefit | NNT (95% CI) | NNH (95% CI) |
			Anticonvulsant	Placebo			
Efficacy							
Diabetic neuropathy	3	321	100/161 (62%)	41/160 (26%)	2.4 (1.8–3.2)	2.7 (2.2–3.8)	
Postherpetic neuralgia	1	225	47/109 (43%)	14/116 (12%)	3.6 (2.1–6.1)	3.2 (2.4–5.0)	
Both conditions	4	546	147/270 (54%)	55/276 (20%)	2.7 (2.1–3.5)	2.9 (2.4–3.7)	
Harm							
Minor adverse effect	4	492	153/24 (62%)	60/245 (24%)	2.5 (2–3.1)		2.7 (2.2–3.4)
Major adverse effect	5	548	32/276 (12%)	19/272 (7%)	1.6 (0.97–2.7)		N/A

Findings

The studies of anticonvulsants in diabetic neuropathy and postherpetic neuralgia were of medium size, ranging 76–225 patient episodes in total. Consequently the results of individual trials varied greatly (Figure 4.3.1).

Pooled results are shown in Table 4.3.1. Over both conditions, 54% of patients had an outcome equivalent to more than 50% pain relief with anticonvulsant, compared with 20% with placebo. The NNT for at least 50% pain relief compared with placebo was 2.9 (2.4–3.7). For every patient who received benefit, one also had a minor adverse effect that did not lead to discontinuation. Nearly 1 patient in 8 discontinued treatment because adverse effects were intolerable, though this was not significantly different from placebo.

Comment

This review updated previous reviews and confirmed that anticonvulsants are effective in patients with diabetic neuropathy and postherpetic neuralgia. The degree of benefit, an outcome equivalent to at least 50% pain relief, was valuable, and with an NNT of 3, efficacy was equivalent to that seen in effective analgesics in acute pain (10 mg intramuscular morphine, for instance). Over half of patients given anticonvulsants benefited. For every patient who benefited, one had a minor adverse effect, but continued with the treatment. There was no overall difference between results for anticonvulsants and antidepressants.

4.4 **Topical capsaicin for pain relief**

Clinical bottom line. Topically applied capsaicin is useful in alleviating the pain associated with diabetic neuropathy, osteoarthritis and psoriasis. The NNTs for some improvement are 4.2 (2.9–7.5), 3.3 (2.6–4.8) and 3.9 (2.7–7.4) respectively. These may not be the most effective treatments; for example, oral anticonvulsants are more effective in diabetic neuropathy.

It remains to be established whether capsaicin is beneficial in postherpetic neuralgia and post-mastectomy pain. Current evidence, based on very small numbers, suggests no benefit.

Topical capsaicin

Capsaicin is an alkaloid derived from chillies. It first entered European knowledge after Columbus' second voyage to the New World in 1494. There is evidence that capsaicin can deplete substance P in local nerve sensory terminals. Substance P is thought to be associated with initiation and transmission of painful stimuli, as well as a number of diseases including arthritis, psoriasis and inflammatory bowel disease.

Systematic review

Zhang, W. Y., Li and Wan Po, A. (1994). The effectiveness of topically applied capsaicin. A meta-analysis, *Eur J Clin Pharmacol* 46: 517–22.

Date review completed: February 1994

Number of trials included: 13

Number of patients: 991 (480 active/511 control)

Control group: Placebo

Main outcomes: Proportion of patients showing improvement

Inclusion criteria were randomised, double-blind, placebo-controlled trials of topical capsaicin for pain relief; data extractable to show proportion of patients showing improvement. Reviewers calculated odds ratios. We have calculated relative benefits and NNT (with 95% confidence intervals) for some benefit with capsaicin. Reviewers noted that blinding may not be complete owing to the irritant effects of capsaicin when applied to the skin.

Findings

In all the trials for all conditions, topical capsaicin was better than placebo (Figure 4.4.1). The results for individual conditions are shown in Table 4.4.1.

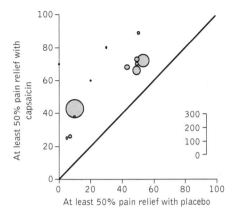

Figure 4.4.1 Efficacy of topical capsaicin for chronic pain in various conditions compared with placebo.

Table 4.4.1 Relative benefit and NNT for topical capsaicin in various conditions

Condition	Number of trials	At least 50% pain relief number/total		Relative benefit (95% CI)	NNT (95% CI)
		Capsaicin	Placebo		
Diabetic neuropathy	4	105/144	81/165	1.5 (1.2–1.8)	4.2 (2.9–7.5)
Osteoarthritis	3	87/192	30/190	2.9 (2.0–4.1)	3.3 (2.6–4.8)
Postherpetic neuralgia	1	4/16	1/16	14 (0.5–32)	NC
Postmastectomy pain	1	5/13	1/10	3.9 (0.5–28)	NC
Psoriasis	4	78/115	55/130	1.6 (1.3–2.0)	3.9 (2.7–7.4)

NC – NNT not calculated (no significant relative benefit).

Diabetic neuropathy. Four trials (144 capsaicin patients, 165 controls) looked at capsaicin 0.075% cream, four times daily for 4–8 weeks. Two of four trials showed significant benefit with capsaicin. When data were pooled for diabetic neuropathy, capsaicin had a NNT of 4.2 (2.9–7.5). For comparison, oral anticonvulsant therapy for diabetic neuropathy in 66 treated patients in two trials had a NNT of 2.5 (1.8–4.0).

Osteoarthritis. Three trials (192 capsaicin patients, 190 controls) looked at capsaicin. Two trials reported on 0.025% and one on

0.075%, four times daily for 4 weeks. The endpoint was articular tenderness or physicians' global assessment of pain relief.

One of three trials showed significant benefit for capsaicin. When the data were pooled for osteoarthritis, capsaicin had a NNT of 2.9 (2.0–4.1).

Postherpetic neuralgia. One trial (16 capsaicin patients, 16 controls) looked at capsaicin 0.075% three or four times daily for 6 weeks. Although this trial reported a significant improvement with capsaicin, the relative benefit of 14 (0.5–3.2) suggested no significant benefit with capsaicin.

Post-mastectomy pain. One trial (13 capsaicin patients, 10 controls) looked at capsaicin 0.075% daily for 6 weeks. Although this trial reported a significant improvement with capsaicin, the relative benefit of 3.9 (0.5–28) suggested no significant benefit with capsaicin.

Psoriasis. Four trials (115 capsaicin patients, 130 controls) looked at capsaicin 0.025% four times daily for 6–8 weeks. The endpoint was much better or better rating of overall appearance. All trials reported improvement on at least one measure. For psoriasis, capsaicin had a NNT of 3.9 (2.7–7.4).

Adverse effects. Reviewers did not include this data, but noted that capsaicin has an irritant effect that may wear off with repeated use.

Comment

There was limited data from this review, now almost a decade since it was completed. An updated review would be useful. Randomised trials published since this review tend to confirm the findings.

4.5 **TENS for chronic pain**

Clinical bottom line. There is no conclusive evidence that TENS is effective for chronic pain.

Systematic review

Carroll, D. *et al.* (2002). Transcutaneous electrical nerve stimulation (TENS) for chronic pain (Cochrane Review), in: The Cochrane Library, Issue 2, 2002, Update Software, Oxford.

Date review completed: June 2000

Number of trials included: 19

Number of patients: 658

Control group: Sham-Tens and other controls

Main outcomes: Various

Inclusion criteria were randomised trials in which the analgesic effect of repeated or continuous use of TENS was studied in patients with chronic pain (defined as pain of at least three months' duration). Various sorts of TENS were included, with sham-TENS, or no treatment controls, or comparisons between different sorts of TENS, with different voltage, frequency or type of machine. Parallel, cross-over, or partial cross-over designs were accepted.

Findings

Trial quality was generally poor because blinding was deemed impossible (active TENS causes tingling sensations). Studies were generally small, with poorly defined treatments and outcomes. Duration of use was variable.

Overall, in 10 of 15 inactive control studies there was a positive analgesic outcome in favour of TENS. The authors considered the results inconclusive.

Comment

TENS is widely used and considered efficacious in chronic pain. Trials did not address the issues properly, especially with respect to duration, as TENS use is generally thought to be required for several months before effects are fully reached. That a review should reach no firm conclusion about its efficacy is disappointing. Another systematic review [1] comes to very similar conclusions.

Reference

1. Brosseau, L. *et al.* (2002). Efficacy of the transcutaneous electrical nerve stimulation for the treatment of chronic low back pain: a meta-analysis, *Spine* 27: 596–603.

4.6 **Fibromyalgia**

Readers who dart to this article in the hope that someone has cracked the problem are going to be disappointed. Those fortified with some Scottish medicine may have the strength to read a little about diagnostic difficulty and therapeutic back-up.

Background

There is a lot of fibromyalgia around. About 10% of the population may have widespread pain, and more in folk in their 60s, and fibromyalgia has a prevalence of 1–2% or so. Diagnosis is difficult and treatments limited. That is getting on for 10,000 and 2000 patients respectively for an average Primary Care Group of 100,000 people.

Diagnosing fibromyalgia

The American College of Rheumatology has produced diagnostic guidelines. The historical feature of fibromyalgia is widespread pain of three months duration or more affecting the axial skeleton and at least two contralateral quadrants of the body. To this definition of widespread pain, for a diagnosis of fibromyalgia patients have to feel pain in 11 of 18 trigger points when they are palpated with the amount of pressure sufficient to blanch a finger nail.

How useful are trigger points? Tricky territory this, because large data sets seem to be lacking. In Cheshire, 250 subjects selected from participants in a chronic pain survey were asked to undergo a trigger point examination [1]. Of the 250, 100 had chronic widespread pain, 100 regional pain and 50 no chronic pain in the survey. On the day of examination, pain state in these patients had shifted. For instance 3/74 with stated chronic widespread pain now had no pain, and 7/39 with no chronic pain now had chronic widespread pain.

According to their status on the day of examination, the criterion of 11 of 18 painful trigger points was found in 40% of patients with chronic widespread pain, 20% of those with regional pain and 5% of those with no pain (Figure 4.6.1). Overall 20 of 132 patients without one of the two criteria of fibromyalgia had at least 11 painful trigger points. By contrast 29% of patients with chronic widespread pain had only 0–4 painful points.

The criterion of 11 painful trigger points looks a poor diagnostic bet. The problems with assessing painful trigger points are several. There is no gold standard against which they can be measured. Experts elicit different numbers [2] in the same patients. Again, perhaps an all or nothing approach to fibromyalgia (with or without trigger points) hides a wider spectrum of disease.

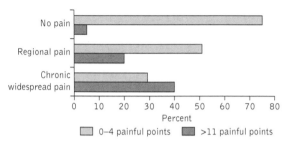

Figure 4.6.1 Trigger points in chronic widespread pain, regional pain and no pain.

Antidepressants for fibromyalgia

Readers should be looking forward to a feast when they hear that three meta-analyses have been published in recent years [3–5]. Unfortunately these only serve up a light snack. Partly that is to do with the raw materials, in that trials have been often small (most with 6–47 patients), some have had poor diagnostic criteria, and many report outcomes in ways that are unhelpful. Partly, though, it is to do with the way that the raw materials have been combined. Only one review [3] tells us about the reporting quality and validity of the trials being combined, making the others somewhat less than useful except as a source of references.

What can be said is that antidepressants have been used for treating fibromyalgia successfully [3]. Trial quality in 13 included trials was good, initial diagnosis predominantly used American College of Rheumatology criteria or its equivalent, and that outcomes were sensibly reported in most.

Results

To improve the symptoms of one patient with fibromyalgia, we have to treat four with antidepressants rather than placebo (95%CI 2.9–6.3). Improvements for fatigue, sleep, overall well-being and pain were significant and moderate using effect sizes. Painful trigger points were not improved.

Comment

There is no neat answer here, only more questions. We use the criterion of 11 painful trigger points to define fibromyalgia, but the most successful treatment does not change the number of trigger points. It helps pain, sleep and other symptoms, and maybe patient and physician assessment of problems, but not the diagnostically defining criterion.

This is food for thought, that meta-analysis of treatment studies can help the understanding of diagnosis. The evidence for the usefulness of trigger points is thin. The evidence that antidepressants help is moderate. But we still do not know what dose of what drug is best for whom, or what we are treating in a disorder that may affect a lot of us.

References

1 Croft, P. *et al.* (1994). Population study of tender points counts and pain as evidence of fibromyalgia, *BMJ* 309: 696–99.

2 Wolfe, F. *et al.* (1992). The fibromyalgia and myofascial pain syndromes: a preliminary study of tender points and trigger points in persons with fibromyalgia, myofascial pain syndrome and no disease, *Journal of Rheumatology* 19: 944–51.

3 O'Malley, P. G. *et al.* (2000). Treatment of fibromyalgia with antidepressants: a meta-analysis, *Journal of General Internal Medicine* 15: 659–66.

4 Arnold, L. M. *et al.* (2000). Antidepressant treatment of fibromyalgia: a meta-analysis and review, *Psychosomatics* 41: 104–13.

5 Rossy, L. A. *et al.* (1999). A meta-analysis of fibromyalgia treatment interventions, *Annals of Behavioural Medicine* 21: 180–91.

4.7   Back pain

This is a complex subject of great importance, and there are some useful publications which are both useful guides into the literature and also provide useful guidance for purchasers and providers. There are few really good reviews of good trials, but there is some terrific good sense. The clinical bottom line is taken from an evidence-based review (2000 references, 800 pages) of back pain and neck pain from the Swedish health technology board [1] which concludes:

* stay active – back pain is common and usually not harmful;
* it is important to identify the rare cases where back pain has a specific cause;
* the consequences of back pain may be more problematic than the pain itself;
* preventative measures are known but not practical;
* the societal costs of back pain are three times higher than the total cost of all types of cancer;
* basic and applied research is urgently needed.

Two other major publications are from the Clinical Standards Advisory Group and are available from HMSO. They are complementary: one examines the epidemiology and cost of back pain [2] while the second develops management guidelines [3].

How big is the problem?

Very big. The sheer amount of information presented for the epidemiology of back pain [1] is staggering, but fascinating. The overall numbers, from population prevalence to those having surgery, are shown in Figure 4.7.1.

The evidence from Britain and elsewhere is that back pain is becoming a bigger problem – not that there is any evidence of changing pathology, but rather due to changed attitudes and expectations. This trend has been particularly noticeable since the mid-1980s. The total number of days in Britain for back incapacity obtained through sickness and invalidity benefit has risen dramatically in recent years (Figure 4.7.2). The British experience is by no means unusual, with other countries seeing an even steeper rise to higher levels.

Contributory factors

* The peak incidence of back pain and sciatica occurs at about age 40–60. Age of onset is spread relatively evenly from 16 years to the early 40s, gradually declines thereafter and is uncommon after

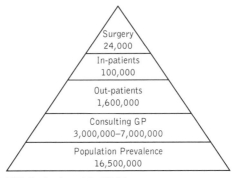

Figure 4.7.1 Back pain and the NHS in one year.

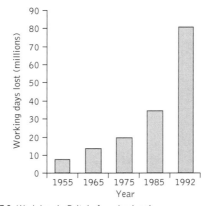

Figure 4.7.2 Work loss in Britain from back pain.

the mid fifties. In those who continue to have back pain it is more likely to be more frequent or constant with increasing age.

• There is little evidence for much difference in back pain in men and women.

• Up to 60% of people with low back pain also have some neck symptoms. Back pain is commonly associated with other complaints.

• There is some, but conflicting, evidence for a relationship between prevalence of low back pain and disability and lower social class. This may largely be related to manual and non-manual occupations.

• There is general though not unanimous agreement that back pain is more common in people in heavy manual occupations and undertaking heavy lifting. People in heavy manual jobs lose significantly more time off work with back pain.

• There is considerable evidence of an increased prevalence of low back pain associated with smoking. This may be due to coincidence with a complex set of demographic social and lifestyle factors.

Disability and work loss

Surveys show that 6% of employed people with back pain report at least one working day lost because of back pain in the previous 4 weeks. This is equivalent to 1.9% of all employed people losing at least one day in four weeks, including 0.3% off for the entire four weeks. The estimate of total working days lost in Britain is 52 million (with 95% confidence intervals of 35–69 million days).

Half the total days lost due to back pain are due to 85% of people who are off work for short periods, most commonly of less than 7 days, and half by the 15% of people who are off work for longer periods of more than one month. The longer a person is off work with back pain, the lower their chances of returning to work. After 6 months there is about a 50% chance of returning to work; this has fallen to about 25% at one year and 10% by two years.

Costs

The estimated cost to the NHS is £481 million a year (min–max range £356–649 million), with non NHS costs (such as private consultations and prescriptions) being an additional £197 million. Cost of DSS benefits is estimated at about £1.4 billion with lost production estimated at £3.8 billion. This breaks down to an annual NHS cost to a purchasing authority of 250,000 people of £2.2 million (range £1.6–£2.9 million). A typical GP practice with five GPs and 10,000 patients would bear costs of about £88,000 (range £65,000–£118,000).

Management guidelines for acute back pain

An overview of the management guidelines for acute back pain is given in the Box. The document from which these are taken [3] develops the background to these ideas and provides two useful algorithms to back this up.

The first algorithm is for diagnostic triage, which includes red flags for possible serious spinal pathology and nerve root problems. The second algorithm is for the primary care management of simple backache, which stresses early activity. Both are easy to follow.

The authors of the CSAG report have done some interesting economic modelling of the effect of the management guidelines and service recommendations on NHS resource use. The analysis is based as much as was possible on the results of controlled trials. It is not a straightforward analysis, because there are implications both for savings and for redistribution of resources to obtain more effective

Table 4.7.1 Effects of guideline implementation on NHS

NHS Resource use	Minimum (%)	Maximum (%)
GP consultation	−7.50	−22.50
X-rays	−12.50	−37.50
Prescribed drugs	−8.00	−25.00
Physical therapy	Reorganisation of NHS physical therapy	

treatment. However, they were able to estimate the maximum and minimum sizes of the effects of guideline implementation on some key resource parameters.

Ongoing research

More studies on back pain treatment are continually being published. One good RCT from Finland recently published in the New England Journal [4] compared bed rest, exercise and ordinary activity in acute low back pain. The conclusion was that continuing ordinary activity within the limits permitted by the pain leads to more rapid recovery than either bed rest or back-mobilising exercises.

References

1. Back pain, neck pain: an evidence-based review. Swedish Council on Technology Assessment in Health Care 2000 (www.sbu.se)
2. Epidemiology Review: The Epidemiology and Cost of Back Pain (1994). Clinical standards Advisory Group. HMSO ISBN 0-11-321889-3.
3. Back Pain (1994). Report of a CSAG Committee on Back Pain. HMSO. ISBN 0-11-321887-7.
4. Malmivaara, A. *et al.* (1995). The treatment of acute low back pain – bed rest, exercises, or ordinary activity? *New England Journal of Medicine* 332: 351–5.

Some systematic reviews on back pain

There are a number of systematic reviews on elements of back pain, usually limited by small numbers of lower quality studies. A flavour of the evidence available can be gained from looking at some of them.

Back schools for low back pain

Clinical bottom line. Back schools appear to be useful in relieving low back pain, but results may not persist beyond 12 months. These findings need to be confirmed with evidence from well-designed trials.

Back schools usually involve information-giving interventions where patients are taught about anatomy and function of the back, mechanical strain and posture. Isometric exercises for abdominal muscles and physical activity programmes are also given. These interventions were originally developed in Sweden, and the content can vary widely.

Systematic review

Koes, B. W., van Tulder, M. W., van der Windt, W. M. and Bouter, L. M. (1994). The efficacy of back schools: a review of randomized clinical trials, *Journal of Clinical Epidemiology* 47: 851–62.

(Also, see the following references.)

Di Fabio, R. P. (1995). Efficacy of comprehensive rehabilitation programs and back school for patients with low back pain: a meta-analysis, *Physical Therapy* 75: 865–78.

Maier-Riehle, H. and Härter, M. (2001). The effects of back schools – a meta-analysis, *International Journal of Rehabilitation Research* 24: 199–206.

Date review completed: 1992

Number of trials included: 16

Number of patients: Not stated

Control group: Active or no treatment

Main outcomes: Various measures of efficacy

Inclusion criteria were randomised controlled trials of back schools for low back pain; back school programme had an education and skills component together with an exercise regimen; intervention given by a trained specialist; full journal publication. Reviewers based their conclusion on the conclusion of original trials, taking quality of trial into account. Measures of efficacy varied between trials.

Findings

Trials varied greatly in quality, very few were blind, and overall quality rating was low. Trials were in a mixture of acute, chronic and recurrent low back pain.

Seven of 16 trials reported better results from back school programme compared with usual care, short-waves, waiting list control, etc. These were generally the higher quality trials, and included the two highest quality trials (score $\geqslant$50 of a possible 100). The four highest quality trials were all positive, and took place in occupational settings. No significant differences were apparent at 12 months, even though some interventions were intensive (e.g. 3–5 weeks of intensive exercise, etc.).

Seven of 16 trials reported no difference or worse outcomes for the back school programme compared with reference treatment (similar to above). In the remaining two trials, authors were unable to draw a conclusion. Both trials were of low quality.

The most recent review comes up with substantially similar conclusions from 18 trials with 1682 patients. Back schools may help in the short term, but not longer than 6 months.

Chiropractic for low back pain

Clinical bottom line. Based on a small, poor quality set of trials, there is no convincing evidence for long-term benefits of chiropractic interventions for acute or chronic low back pain. There may be some short-term pain relief, especially in patients with acute pain. Better quality evidence is required before the question of efficacy can be answered adequately.

Chiropractic is one of the manipulative therapies often used to treat acute and chronic pain. For acute and chronic back pain, chiropractors often use spinal manipulation techniques, although other trained therapists also use this technique.

Systematic review

Assendelft, W. J. J., Koes, B. W., Van der Heijden, G. J. M. G. and Bouter, L. M. (1996). The effectiveness of chiropractic for treatment of low back pain: An update and attempt at statistical pooling, *Journal of Manipulative and Physiological Therapeutics* 19: 499–507.

Date review completed: June 1995

Number of trials included: 8

Number of patients: 1774

Control group: Other treatment or placebo

Main outcomes: Successful treatment, pain rating, functional status

Inclusion criteria were randomised controlled trials of chiropractic treatment for low back pain; treatment included manipulation or mobilisation of the spine; follow-up period greater than one day; English language reports; full journal publication. Chronic pain was defined as duration greater than three weeks, and acute pain was defined as pain $\leqslant 3$ weeks. It was not possible to pool results from trials, so reviewers carried out a vote-counting review based on the main outcome measure for each trial.

Findings

Four trials were in chronic pain, three trials reported on both acute and chronic pain, and one mixed acute and chronic together. Trials were of poor methodological quality, with different patients, interventions, outcomes, follow-up periods.

Acute pain (approximately 300 patients). Three of three trials reported short-term benefit from chiropractic intervention (approximately 3 weeks). Where longer-term data were available, these benefits appear to have been lost.

Chronic pain (approximately 1500 patients). Six trials had relevant data. One trial reported benefit for chronic patients, but reviewers were unable to agree with this finding since there were no statistically significant differences in the original report (6-week outcome). One trial reported some benefit at two but not at 4 weeks. Two trials reported no benefit of chiropractic over control. Of two trials mixing acute and chronic patients, both reported positive overall findings at more than 3 weeks.

Massage for low back pain

Clinical bottom line. There is insufficient evidence to determine whether massage therapy works in the treatment of low back pain. The included trials were methodologically flawed.

Massage relaxes the mind and the muscles and is thought to increase pain threshold. In Europe, it is commonly used in the treatment of low back pain.

Systematic review

Ernst, E. (1999). Massage therapy for low back pain: A systematic review, *Journal of Pain and Symptom Management* 17: 56–69.

Date review completed: July 1997

Number of trials included: Four

Number of patients: (399 total; number per group unknown)

Control groups: Chiropractic/spinal manipulation, electrical stimulation, corset, balneotherapy, traction, no treatment

Main outcomes: Improvement (unspecified); pain; straight leg raising to pain, fingertip floor distance

MEDLINE, Embase and the Cochrane Library were searched (all years to July 1997) for published reports of studies which assessed the effectiveness of massage in the treatment of low back pain. Reference lists of retrieved reports were checked for additional citations and no language restrictions were made. Massage was defined as manual/apparative massage of muscular and soft tissue structure of the back. Trials that assessed massage in combination with other interventions were excluded. Data were extracted in a standardised, predefined manner. Duplicate data were excluded. A descriptive analysis was conducted. Inclusion criteria were: controlled clinical trial, any form of low back pain, one treatment group which had massage therapy as sole form of treatment.

Findings

Four trials were included. The patient population was: non-specific, uncomplicated chronic or subacute LBP (63 patients), uncomplicated chronic or subacute LBP of the lumbosacral region (158), unspecified acute LBP (81), acute or chronic LBP of lumbosacral region (95). Three trials were randomised and single blind, the largest study was neither randomised nor blind. One trial found massage to be significantly inferior to chiropractic manipulation in uncomplicated chronic/subacute LBP. The other studies reported no significant difference between massage and the control treatments, except the non-randomised study which reported massage to be significantly better than no treatment for uncomplicated chronic/subacute LBP at the end of the treatment period.

The studies were small and had major methodological flaws. The lack of randomisation and blinding in one study, and use of single-blinding in the others meant the studies were open to selection and observer bias. Inadequate definitions of massage and improvement were given in the trials and different outcomes and measurement tools were used. The studies were, therefore, of poor quality and validity and unlikely to be capable of providing a true result regarding the effectiveness of massage in low back pain.

NSAIDs for low back pain

Clinical bottom line. The benefit of treating low back pain is unclear. It is unclear from the present review whether these trials have been adequately designed to measure NSAID efficacy compared with placebo and other treatments. There is no convincing evidence to suggest that one particular NSAID is better than another, or that NSAIDs are better than other treatments.

There is no clear consensus regarding optimal management for low back pain, and management varies widely. The rationale for NSAID treatment is based on analgesic and anti-inflammatory properties.

Systematic review

Koes, B. K., Scholten, R. J. P. M., Mens, J. M. A. and Bouter, L. M. (1997). Efficacy of non-steroidal anti-inflammatory drugs for low back pain: a systematic review of randomised clinical trials, *Annals of Rheumatic Disease* 56: 214–23.

Date review completed: 1994

Number of trials included: 26

Control group: Active and placebo

Main outcomes: Pain intensity, pain relief, clinical improvement

Inclusion criteria were randomised, controlled trials of NSAIDs for low back pain; full journal publication; English language. Reviewers assessed trials for quality, and based their conclusions on authors' original conclusions together with data pooling where appropriate. Data were pooled where placebo information was also available, separating out acute and chronic low back pain trials. Peto's odds ratios with 95% confidence intervals were calculated with fixed (heterogeneity present) and random effects models (heterogeneity). Odds ratios were calculated for treatment failures, and therefore a ratio of below one indicates significant benefit of NSAID.

Findings

Trials were of poor to high quality. Unfortunately it was not possible to clearly establish from the review which trials were double-blind, but probably only 10 of 26 were double-blind. This makes understanding review findings difficult. Clearly this information should carry more weight than data from non- or single-blind trials. A brief overview of results is provided, but further work would be required to establish treatment efficacy more accurately. Reviewers did not comment on baseline pain intensity. Clearly trials that did not ensure adequate baseline pain were unlikely to detect an improvement.

Trials differed according to drugs, doses, length of intervention, diagnosis, rescue medication allowed, size and outcomes. Interventions were mainly of 1–2 weeks duration.

NSAID versus placebo. Five of 10 trials reported significant benefit with NSAID. However, looking just at the five trials of highest quality suggests that NSAIDs may not be that effective. Only one of these found a significant benefit of NSAID, and this was only on one day. This trial did not allow rescue medication. A second trial found significant benefit only when it looked at the subgroup of patients with moderate to severe baseline pain. It is unclear whether these trials were adequately designed to measure the effect.

NSAIDs compared with other pharmacological interventions. Nine trials were included. Only one trial had a high quality rating. This trial was very small, but reported that patients with chronic low back pain preferred diflunisal 500 mg twice daily for 4 weeks to paracetamol 1000 mg twice daily (10/16 versus 4/12 rated treatment as good or excellent). Only three of the remaining eight trials reported significant benefit of NSAID compared with a range of other treatments. It is unclear whether any of these trials were adequately designed to measure a difference.

Different NSAID comparisons. Only one low quality trial of the 11 included trials reported a significant difference. It is unclear whether any of these trials were adequately designed to measure a difference.

Adverse effects. Reviewers extracted information on adverse effects where possible. These were usually mild to moderate severity and included abdominal pain and diarrhoea, oedema, dry mouth, rash, dizziness, headache and tiredness.

Physiotherapy exercises for back pain

Clinical bottom line. Trials are of insufficient quality to draw a clear conclusion. It is not clear whether physiotherapy is better than other conservative treatments, or whether it is better than no treatment. It is not possible to establish which types of exercises are the most effective.

About 80% of the population will suffer from back pain during their active lives. This is usually self-limiting, and will disappear within a few months in 90% of patients. However, there is a lack of consensus on which of the many treatments available is the best for chronic back pain. Physiotherapy is widely used for back complaints, usually exercise therapy given alone or in combination with other treatments (e.g. massage, heat, traction, ultrasound or short wave diathermy).

Systematic review

Koes, B. W., Bouter, L. M., Beckerman, H., van der Hiejden, G. J. M. G. and
 Knipschild, P. G. (1991). Physiotherapy exercises and back pain: a blinded
 review, *BMJ* 302: 1572–6.

Date review completed: 1990

Number of trials included: 16

Control group: Active/no intervention/placebo

Main outcomes: Pain, mobility

Inclusion criteria were randomised controlled trials of physiotherapy for back pain; physiotherapy given individually, not in groups; physiotherapy given alone or with additional treatment; back pain present at baseline; full journal publication. Reviewers provided a descriptive summary of trials, methodological assessment together with a 'positive' or 'negative' conclusion for each trial as concluded in the original report.

Findings

Of the 16 trials included, most were of poor methodological quality, and trials were generally not adequately designed to assess the intervention – small group sizes, high rates of loss-to-follow-up, lacked internal sensitivity, poor statistical analysis. Type of exercise, control interventions and length of intervention varied between trials. Ten trials had negative conclusions and six had positive conclusions. Reviewers note that there is a general trend for higher quality trials to have positive results. Blinding status was unclear, but 10 of 16 appeared to be evaluator-blind.

Inactive/placebo comparisons. Four trials compared exercise therapy with no therapy or placebo therapy. One of four trials showed a benefit of exercise therapy for pain and activity at 4 and 12 weeks, but this did not persist to 3 months. The remaining trials showed no benefit for acute pain, sciatic symptoms and chronic low back pain.

Active comparisons. Seven trials compared exercise therapy with other conservative treatments. Two of 7 trials showed significant benefit compared with hot packs and rest and with mini back school (i.e. one session). The second study showed benefit was still present at one year. Five of 7 trials showed no benefit when compared with manual therapy, home care instructions, NSAIDs, manipulation, manipulation and mobilisation or short wave diathermy.

Different exercise therapies compared. Eight trials compared different types of exercise therapy – mainly isometric flexion exercises compared with extension exercises. Four of 8 trials showed no difference (although all were flawed). Four showed some benefit – one favouring 3 months of intensive dynamic back extensor exercises over a less intensive treatment plus massage and heat, one favoured extension over flexion exercises, and two favoured flexion exercises over mobilisation plus other exercises and, in one trial, massage and heat.

Overall comment

The Swedish health technology review concluded that basic and clinical research about back pain was urgently needed. Perhaps because it is so common that we conclude that it is 'only pain', and look on sufferers as unfortunate. We have useful guidelines, but no magic bullets for so common a problem.

4.8 **Epidural corticosteroids for back pain**

Clinical bottom line. Epidural administration of corticosteroids is effective in the management of sciatica, with a NNT of 7.3 (4.7–16) for greater than 75% pain relief in the short-term (1–60 days), and a NNT of 13 (6.6–314) for greater than 50% pain relief in the long-term (12 weeks to one year).

Epidural corticosteroids are commonly used in the treatment of low back pain and sciatica, although steroids are not currently licensed for epidural use in the UK. Steroids have a number of anti-inflammatory properties and an inhibitory effect on C-fibre conduction.

Systematic review

The original review by Watts and Silagy has been updated and presented differently by McQuay and Moore:

McQuay, H. J. and Moore, R. A. (1998). Epidural corticosteroids for sciatica, in: *An evidence-based resource for pain relief*, Oxford University Press, Oxford, Chapter 27.

McQuay, H. J. and Moore, R. A. (1996). Epidural steroids for sciatica, *Anaesthesia and Intensive Care* 24: 284–5.

Watts, R. W. and Silagy, C. A. (1995). A meta-analysis on the efficacy of epidural corticosteroids in the treatment of sciatica, *Anaesthesia and Intensive Care* 23: 564–9.

And see also: Koes, B. W. *et al.* (1995). Efficacy of epidural steroid injections for low-back pain and sciatica: a systematic review of randomized clinical trials, *Pain* 63: 279–88.

Date review completed: 1997

Number of trials included: 12

Number of patients: Short-term relief 664 (319 active/345 control); long-term relief 710 (315 active/395 control)

Control group: Placebo

Main outcomes: At least 75% pain relief for short-term outcomes (1–60 days); at least 50% pain relief for long-term outcomes (12 weeks to 1 year) NNT.

Inclusion criteria were randomised, double-blind trials of steroid treatment of sciatica; caudal or lumbar epidural. Data were extracted from original trials and the number of patients improved on active and control were used to calculate odds ratios, relative benefits and NNT (all with 95% confidence intervals).

Findings

Active treatments included epidural methylprednisolone 80 mg (ten trials), triamcinalone 80 mg (one trial) and hydrocortisone 25 mg (one trial).

Short-term relief

Eleven trials reported on short-term pain relief. Only three of 11 trials showed significant benefit of epidural over placebo. However, when data were pooled, there was an overall significant benefit of 1.5 (1.2–1.9). The NNT for greater than 75% pain relief in the short-term (1–60 days) was 7.3 (4.7–16; Figure 4.8.1).

Long-term relief

Six trials reported on long-term pain relief (Figure 4.8.2). Only one trial showed significant benefit of epidural over placebo. However, when data were pooled, there was an overall significant benefit of 1.3 (1.1–1.5). The NNT for greater than 50% pain relief in the long-term (12 weeks to one year) was 13 (6.6–314).

Adverse effects

Original reports did not compare adverse effects in the active with the placebo groups. Based on seven trials (431 patients), 2.5% suffered dural taps, 2.3% transient headache, 1.9% transient increase in pain, 0.2% irregular menstrual cycle. Long-term effects were not covered in original reports. One reviewer reported evidence from other sources for the risk of neurological sequelae after epidural as 1 in 5000.

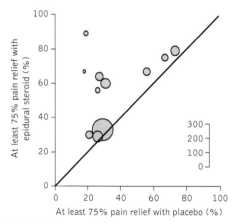

Figure 4.8.1 Epidural steroids for short-term relief (1–60 days).

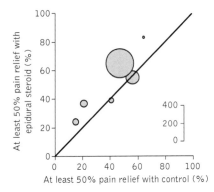

Figure 4.8.2 Epidural steroids for long-term relief (12–52 weeks).

Comment

These NNT values at first sight appear disappointing. Here is an intervention which shows statistically significant improvement compared with control, and yet the clinical benefit, the NNT for one patient to reach the chosen end-point, is 7 for short-term benefit and 13 for long-term. The short-term end-point, however, is quite a high hurdle. Using an easier hurdle of 50% relief rather than 75%, the 'best' NNT achieved by drug treatment of neuropathic pain was just under 3. Patients may choose the epidural if it means they do not have to take medication, particularly if it gives a higher level of relief, even though there is a 1 in 7 chance of this level of response.

The long-term NNT of 13 is perhaps not surprising. Occasional patients in most clinics report a 'cure' as a result of a steroid epidural, but the majority of epidural steroid successes return for repeat epidurals. That one patient has relief lasting between 12 weeks and a year for 12 treated with epidural steroid fits with experience.

The message is that we will have inevitably to expose our practice to the searching type of analysis which Watts and Silagy have used for epidural steroid. This intervention has shown a statistically significant benefit over control. Others will not, and will be discarded. For those interventions which do show statistically significant benefit over control there is then a further stage, which is to define the clinical benefit of the intervention. The NNTs for effectiveness are one possible definition, particularly when coupled with NNTs for minor and major harm (NNT of about 40 for dural tap).

For patients with chronic disease, and in this case chronic painful disease, interventions may be attractive even if their success rate is far lower than would be acceptable in, say, the management of postoperative pain. This means that the interpretation of measures of clinical bene-fit, such as NNTs, has to be context-dependent. For the moment we need the best possible analysis, as Watts and Silagy have demonstrated, of the data available. If the data is poor then that establishes the clin-ical research agenda. If the data is reasonable then we can try to define measures of clinical benefit. The art of clinical practice will then come into play, as patient and doctor juggle the risk and benefit of the alternatives, albeit with better data than we have at present.

4.9 **Steroid injection for shoulder and elbow disorders**

Shoulders

Clinical bottom line. There is currently insufficient evidence to provide a definitive answer on the efficacy of steroid injections. Existing data suggest no compelling evidence. Steroid injections should not be used to alleviate pain associated with shoulder disorders until the effectiveness of this treatment can be demonstrated.

Shoulder disorders are often caused by periarticular soft tissue impairment, with a minority originating from neurological or generalised musculoskeletal conditions, neoplasms or referred pain from the neck or from internal organs. Based on Dutch data, of all newly presented episodes, 23% resolve within one month, 51% within six months and 59% within one year. Steroid injections are used in about 12% of consultations, usually in combination with analgesics, rest or exercise. However, steroid injections are associated with a range of adverse effects including minor and serious ones.

Systematic review

van der Heijden, C. J. M. G., van der Windt, D. A. W. M., Kleijnen, J., Koes, B. W. and Bouter, L. M. (1996). Steroid injections for shoulder disorders: a systematic review of randomized clinical trials, *British Journal of General Practice* 46: 309–16.

Date review completed: November 1995

Number of trials included: 16

Number of patients: 393 (208 active/185 control)

Control group: Active or placebo (only placebo considered here)

Main outcomes: Clinically relevant outcome measures, including treatment success, pain, mobility and functional status. These were used to calculate 'success rates' with 95% confidence intervals.

Inclusion criteria were randomised controlled trials of shoulder pain; pain present at moment of inclusion; treatment by steroid injection; clinically relevant outcome measures. Reviewers calculated 'success rate' of treatments by dividing the number of documented successes at the end of the intervention period by the number of patients randomly allocated to the intervention, with 95% confidence intervals.

Findings

Reviewers noted that methodological quality of most trials was poor. Each trial looked at a variety of time points ranging 2–24 weeks.

Seven trials compared steroid injection with a placebo treatment (usually steroid plus lignocaine versus lignocaine alone or lignocaine with saline). Two of 7 trials reported a significant benefit of steroid injection on at least one key measure, these two trials ranked highest in terms of quality.

We calculated a NNT for success at 4 weeks or later using the three trials comparing steroid injection with saline injection. The NNT was 17 with a confidence interval which included no benefit to any patient. The NNT rose to 33 when the remaining placebo trials were examined.

Elbows

Clinical bottom line. Corticosteroid injections are effective in treating lateral epicondylitis in the short term (2–6 weeks), but there appears to be no longer term benefit. It is unclear whether this form of treatment has benefits over other treatments. Review findings are based on hospitalised patients, and are therefore not generalisable to general practice. Clear recommendations on treatment regime could not be formulated.

Corticosteroid injections are commonly used to alleviate pain in lateral epicondylitis. This condition has an incidence of 4–7 per 1000 per year in general practice, with the average episode lasting between 6 months and 2 years. Dutch data suggest that 10–30% of episodes result in an average of 12 weeks absence from work. Other treatments include analgesic medication, physical therapy and, most radical, surgery.

Systematic review

Assendelft, W. J. J., Hay, E. M., Adshead, R. and Bouter, L. M. (1996).
 Corticosteroid injections for lateral epicondylitis: a systematic overview,
 British Journal of General Practice 46: 209–16.

 Date review completed: 1994

 Number of trials included: 9 (10 comparisons)

 Number of patients: Not stated

 Control group: Placebo or different dose injection

 Main outcomes: Pain outcomes as stated in original reports, success/ failure rates expressed as odds ratios with 95% confidence intervals

Inclusion criteria were randomised controlled trials of corticosteroid injection for lateral epicondylitis. The review aimed to answer questions on optimal treatment regimen and suitability for general practice as well as efficacy. Reviewers used conclusions on efficacy from the original reports, and also extracted data on success rates at follow-up points, with preference given to patient ratings.

Findings

Injection versus placebo. Five trials compared injection plus local anaesthetic with either local anaesthetic alone or with saline. Four of five trials reported significant benefit of injection over placebo.

Injection versus active. One high quality trial compared injection with Cyriax physiotherapy and found significant benefit with injection. Two trials compared injection with naproxen. Naproxen alone was no different to injection, and naproxen with wrist brace was better than injection (although quality of trial lower).

One trial compared injection with elbow band and wrist brace, and found significant benefit with injection. One trial compared injection with ultrasound, phonophoresis and transcutaneous electrical nerve stimulation, and found no differences. One trial compared two injection techniques and found them to be equally effective.

For all included trials, there was a tendency for higher quality trials to show a larger effect, with a pooled odds ratio of 0.15 (0.10–0.23) at 2–6 weeks, indicating a beneficial effect of corticosteroids.

Longer term efficacy. For all included trials there was a general trend that injections were effective in the short term (2–6 weeks), but not after a follow-up of greater than 6 weeks. The odds ratio for more than 6 weeks was 0.73 (0.37–1.44) indicating a lack of long term effect.

Adverse effects

Six trials reported on adverse effects. Three of six stated there were no adverse effects. Three trials reported post-injection pain lasting a few days, but this was not always attributed to corticosteroids. However, the most detailed trial reported that 50% (58/116) of patients injected with corticosteroids and local anaesthetic experienced post-injection pain compared with 31% (9/29) with local anaesthetic alone. Skin atrophy was reported in 27% (31/116) patients compared with 17% (5/29) with local anaesthetic alone.

Comment

The evidence that steroid injections are beneficial is less than compelling. An unresolved issue is this: if steroid is injected together with local anaesthetic, which is giving the long-term benefit? The additional benefit of steroid added to local anaesthetic has yet to be demonstrated.

4.10 **Systemic local anaesthetic-type drugs in chronic pain**

Clinical bottom line. Sodium channel blockers can be used to reduce pain due to nerve damage. Intravenous lignocaine and oral mexiletine both reduce neuropathic pain. Intravenous lignocaine is effective in fibromyalgia (based on small patient numbers), but not in cancer-related pain. Intranasal lignocaine is not effective in myofascial pain (based on small patient numbers).

Lignocaine and related local anaesthetic-type drugs which block sodium channels have been used to relieve clinical pain, as a last resort in cancer-related pain and in other conditions when more traditional treatments fail. It has been demonstrated that the neuroma and the dorsal root ganglion display spontaneous activity and increased sensitivity after peripheral nerve injury. Systemic sodium channel blockers silence the spontaneous activity, and may block glutamate-evoked activity in the dorsal horn of the spinal cord.

Systematic review

Kalso, E., Tramèr, M. R., Moore, R. A. and McQuay, H. J. (1998). Systemic local anaesthetic type drugs in chronic pain: a qualitative systematic review, *European Journal of Pain* 2: 3–14.

Date review completed: September 1996

Number of trials included: 17

Control group: placebo or active control

Main outcomes: findings from original trials

Inclusion criteria were randomised controlled trials of local anaesthetic-type drugs for pain relief; pain outcomes.

Findings

Neuropathic pain

Nine trials were included, with 199 patients and the following pain conditions: peripheral nerve injury, diabetic neuropathy, postherpetic neuralgia, trigeminal neuralgia and dysaesthetic pain following spinal cord injury.

Peripheral nerve injury. Two of two trials showed significantly better pain relief with intravenous lignocaine (intravenous 2 and 5 mg/kg over 45 min) compared with placebo, and a dose response. One of these trials also showed significant reduction of allodynia. One trial showed significantly better pain relief with mexiletine (oral up to 750 mg/day) compared with placebo in patients with peripheral nerve damage of mixed origin.

Diabetic neuropathy. One trial showed a significant effect of lignocaine (intravenous 5 mg/kg over 30 min) up to 8 days compared with placebo, and significant relief of dysaesthesia. One of two trials showed significantly better pain relief with mexiletine (oral 750 mg/day) than placebo. The second trial only showed benefit with post hoc analysis of subgroups.

Postherpetic neuralgia. One trial showed lignocaine (intravenous 2.4–6.0 mg/kg over 1 h) significantly better than placebo, but inferior to intravenous morphine.

Dysaesthetic spinal cord injury. One trial showed no benefit of mexiletine (oral 450 mg/day) compared with placebo in reducing dysaesthetic pain following spinal cord injury.

Trigeminal neuralgia. One trial showed that tocainide (oral 1500 mg/day) was comparable to carbamazepine (oral maximum tolerated dose).

Fibromyalgia
One trial was included. Based on 11 patients, pain relief was significantly better with lignocaine (5 mg/kg over 30 min) at 15 min, and at least 50% pain relief persisted for 4–7 days in three of four responders.

Myofascial facial pain
One trial of 28 patients showed lignocaine (intranasal 30 mg) was not significantly better than placebo.

Cancer-related pain
Three small trials compared lignocaine (intravenous 5 mg/kg) with placebo. In three of three trials lignocaine was no different to placebo (conditions: bony metastases, chemotherapy polyneuropathy, radiotherapy plexopathy and tumour invasion of nerve plexus).

Adverse effects
No arrhythmias were noted in any trial with lignocaine infusion (all but one measured this). Twenty-one of 134 infusions were associated with adverse effects (mainly light-headedness, somnolence, nausea and perioral numbness). Five of these resulted in study withdrawal. One adverse effect was reported in 100 saline infusions. Dose-related adverse effects were reported in 16 of 85 mexiletine patients. These were considered mild, and there were no study withdrawals. Tocainide was associated with three adverse effects in 12 patients

(nausea, apical paraesthesias and skin rash), but is known to cause serious haematological adverse effects including death.

Comment

These results show that sodium channel blockers can reduce pain due to nerve damage. In peripheral nerve injury, diabetic neuropathy or postherpetic neuralgia lignocaine was effective at plasma concentrations of 1.5–5 mg/L. The evidence was strongest in pain due to nerve injury where the decrease in pain intensity was 40–60%. Oral mexiletine 750 mg daily was also effective in these conditions. Allodynia and dysaesthesia were also alleviated. Mexiletine 450 mg had no effect in central pain due to spinal cord injury, perhaps because the effects of these drugs are mainly confined to the peripheral nerves and the dorsal root ganglion. Tocainide has been reported to have caused serious haematological adverse effects including several deaths and should not be used.

Intractable cancer pain is another condition where local anaesthetic type drugs have been advocated. The result of this review is quite unequivocal. Intravenous lignocaine 5 mg/kg, was without effect. Intravenous lignocaine does not give more relief when combined with high doses of opioids and NSAIDs.

The long-term analgesic effects of intravenous lignocaine were not systematically studied. Only two studies reported that pain relief could last for several days. It is not known if subsequent infusions provide longer relief. Long-term systemic administration of lignocaine is not practical, and no controlled studies have been done on either its efficacy or adverse effects in long term use.

The encouraging signal from this review is that a difficult subgroup of neuropathic pains can be helped. Delivering and optimising that benefit will require new approaches. In the meantime the message that all neuropathic pains do not necessarily respond identically is important.

4.11 Cognitive behaviour therapy and behaviour therapy for chronic pain

Clinical bottom line. Diverse studies showed that cognitive behaviour therapy was effective in reducing pain experience, and improving positive behaviour expression, appraisal and coping in individuals with chronic pain.

Systematic review

Morley, S., Eccleston, C. and Williams, A. (1999). Systematic review and meta-analysis of randomised controlled trials of cognitive behaviour therapy and behaviour therapy for chronic pain in adults, excluding headache, *Pain* 80: 1–13.

Date review completed: 1996

Number of trials included: 25

Number of patients: 1672

Control group: Waiting list control, alternative therapy control

Main outcomes: Pain experience, mood/affect depression or other, cognitive coping and appraisal, behaviour expression, behaviour activity, social role functioning

Inclusion criteria were randomised clinical trial which assessed cognitive behaviour therapy or behaviour therapy in the treatment of chronic pain. MEDLINE, PsychLit, Embase and Social Science Citation Index were searched, using a combination of MeSH terms and relevant keywords, for trials which assessed cognitive behaviour therapy or behaviour therapy for the treatment of chronic pain. Bibliographies of retrieved reports and reviews were checked for additional citations. The Oxford Pain Relief Database was also searched. Papers were read by each reviewer. Authors were contacted for additional information if this was lacking from the individual studies. Information was pooled in a meta-analysis and effect size was calculated using Hedge's g. Corrections for small sample size were made. When mean or standard deviations were not presented other available statistics were used to determine the effect size.

Findings

Information from 25 studies (1672 patients) was pooled in a meta-analysis; 19 were randomised and six were not. The average age of

Table 4.11.1 Comparisons of cognitive behavioural therapy with waiting list control

Treatment	Number of comparisons	Mean effect size (95% CI)
Pain experience	28	0.40 (0.22–0.58)
Mood/affect depression	24	0.36 (0.13–0.59)
Mood/affect other	16	0.52 (0.19–0.84)
Cognitive coping & appraisal negative	16	0.50 (0.27–0.73)
Cognitive coping & appraisal positive	11	0.53 (0.28–0.78)
Behaviour expression	12	0.5 (0.22–0.78)
Behaviour activity	14	0.46 (0.25–0.72)
Social role functioning	25	0.60 (0.44–0.76)

patients was 45.3 years and the mean chronicity was 12.3 years. Chronic low back pain, rheumatoid arthritis, osteoarthritis, mixed back pain, fibromyalgia, upper limb pain, and unspecified pain were assessed. Mean treatment duration was 6.7 weeks (range 3–10).

Pain experience (28 comparisons), mood/affect depression (24), mood/affect other (16), cognitive coping and appraisal negative (16), cognitive coping and appraisal positive (11), behaviour expression (12), behaviour activity (14), and social role functioning (25) were assessed in the trials.

Different treatments were grouped into three classes: cognitive behavioural therapy, behavioural therapy and biofeedback.

Waiting list control. Overall treatments were significantly more effective than waiting list control (Table 4.11.1). All three treatments were significantly more effective than waiting list control in changing pain experience, improving social functioning and in reducing negative appraisal and coping. The exception was a single comparison using behavioural therapy in reducing negative appraisal and coping.

Active control. All three cognitive-behavioural treatments were compared with active alternative treatments (e.g. progressive or applied relaxation, routine care, education and occupational therapy). Pooled data showed that cognitive-behavioural treatments were significantly more effective than the alternative treatment controls for pain experience, cognitive coping and appraisal (increasing positive coping), and reducing the expression of pain (Table 4.11.2).

Adverse effects

Adverse effects were not mentioned.

Comment

This systematic review is based on mostly information from randomised controlled trials, though six were not randomised because

Table 4.11.2 Comparisons of cognitive behavioural therapy with active alternative treatments

Treatment	Number of comparisons	Mean effect size (95% CI)
Pain experience	22	0.29 (0.11–0.46)
Mood/affect depression	15	−0.14 (−0.32–0.04)
Mood/affect other	16	0.05 (−0.27–0.37)
Cognitive coping & appraisal negative	14	0.17 (−0.08–0.42)
Cognitive coping & appraisal positive	15	0.40 (0.21–0.62)
Behaviour expression	11	0.27 (0.08–0.47)
Social role functioning	14	0.17 (−0.08–0.34)

they used inappropriate methods to allocate patients to treatment groups. The reviewers' stated that most trials were statistically under powered, information could not be readily dichotomised, and that blinding was rarely possible in these types of studies. Blinding of the observer, but not the patient or therapist, would be possible in active treatment controlled trials. Bias could have occurred in these studies. The appropriateness of waiting list control is also debatable, but probably the best that can be done in most circumstances.

4.12 **Intravenous regional sympathetic blockade for reflex sympathetic dystrophy**

Clinical bottom line. There is no evidence from existing trials that guanethidine used in intravenous regional sympathetic blockade (IRSB) reduces the pain associated with reflex sympathetic dystrophy (RSD). Based on a small number of patients, there is weak evidence that ketanserin and bretylium may provide some relief.

Reflex sympathetic dystrophy describes the constellation of chronic pain conditions associated with hyperactivity of the sympathetic nervous system. Pain is usually constant, severe and unresponsive to conventional analgesics. Intravenous regional sympathetic blockade is an intervention where a drug known to block the sympathetic nervous system is given in high local concentration in the painful limb isolated with a tourniquet.

Systematic review

Jadad, A. R., Carroll, D., Glynn, C. J. and McQuay, H. J. (1995). Intravenous regional sympathetic blockade for pain relief in reflex sympathetic dystrophy: a systematic review and a randomized, double-blind crossover study, *Journal of Pain and Symptom Management* 10: 13–20.

Date review completed: May 1993

Number of trials included: 8

Number of patients: Not stated, but group size ranged 6–21

Control group:

Main outcomes: Original trial findings (reviewers do not state which outcomes were used)

Inclusion criteria were trials of patients with chronic pain associated with RSD; randomised and/or double-blind; administration of an IRSB to at least one of the treatment groups. Data pooling was not possible. Original trial findings were used as outcomes.

Findings

Eight trials were included. Most used guanethidine as the active substance, but reserpine, bretylium, droperidol and ketanserin were used as alternatives. Two of 8 trials (17 patients in total) showed some advantage of IRSB over control. These trials used ketanserin and bretylium.

Adverse effects

In at least one trial a number of patients suffered from hypotension. Results from other trials were not reported.

Comment

Persistent pain due to RSD use is usually difficult to control, and can be very frustrating for patients and carers. IRSB has been the mainstay of management, but the results of randomised trials is disappointing.

4.13 **Treatments for intermittent claudication**

Intermittent claudication is an early symptom of peripheral arterial disease. Its incidence increases with age. Between the ages of 45 and 65 years there are 7–19 cases per 10,000, but 54–61 cases per 10,000 between the ages of 65 and 74 years. This section reviews the evidence on treatments.

Exercise

Clinical bottom line. Walking exercises are useful in improving walking distance and pain-free walking distance in patients with intermittent claudication. Percentage improvement in walking time or distance ranged from 28% to 210% with exercise interventions. Data from this review and other sources suggest that patients should be encouraged to exercise for at least 30 min, three times a week for 6 months.

Systematic review

Brandsma, J. W., Robeer, B. G., van den Heuvel, S. *et al.* (1998). The effect of exercises on walking distance of patients with intermittent claudication: a study of randomized clinical trials, *Physical Therapy* 78: 278–88.

Date review completed: 1998

Number of trials included: 10

Number of patients: 291

Control group: Untreated, placebo medication or active control

Main outcomes: Improvement in pain-free walking distance or time, maximum walking distance or time

Inclusion criteria were randomised controlled trials of exercise for intermittent claudication due to peripheral arterial occlusive disease in the lower extremities; walking distance as an outcome; use of treadmill for evaluations. Reviewers extracted data on pain-free or maximum walking times or distances, and used pre- and postintervention scores to calculate a percent change from baseline.

Findings

All of the included trials were small, with group sizes ranging from seven to 25, and exercise interventions varied in intensity, duration and content. Five of 10 trials had an untreated control group (no intervention or placebo drug), and the remaining trials had an active intervention, either pharmacological, surgical or strength training of lower extremities only. Nine of 10 trials included walking as part of

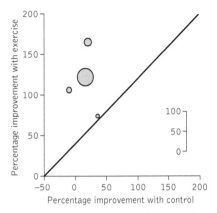

Figure 4.13.1 Effects of exercise on walking distance or time compared with placebo in patients with intermittent claudication.

the exercise intervention. All the studies were small, the largest involving 75 patients.

Ten of ten trials found improvement on walking time or distance with the exercise intervention. This ranged from 28% to 210% (unweighted mean 105%; Figure 4.13.1). This compared with a range of −10 to 36% improvement in patients receiving no treatment or placebo. The two trials with the smallest improvements in patients receiving exercise interventions were either of short duration or low intensity.

Although little data is provided on the exact nature of the exercise interventions, this review together with a second review suggest that patients should be encouraged to exercise for at least 30 min, three times a week for 6 months. No adverse events were reported.

Ginkgo biloba

Clinical bottom line. Ginkgo biloba extracts at doses of 120–160 mg over 12–24 weeks increased mean pain free walking distance by an average of 33 metres (95% confidence interval 22–43 m) compared with placebo in high quality randomised trials.

Systematic review

Pittler, M. H. and Ernst, E. (2000). Ginkgo biloba extract for the treatment of intermittent claudication: a meta-analysis of randomized trials, *American Journal of Medicine*, 108: 276–81.

Date review completed: 1998

Number of trials included: 8

Number of patients: 385 total

Control groups: Placebo

Main outcomes: Pain free walking distance an maximal walking distance

Inclusion criteria were randomised double blind comparisons of ginkgo versus placebo. Authors sought data from original trials to be able to obtain it in a form suitable for pooling, and to verify important study details. Studies using ginkgo in combination with other therapies were not included, nor those not assessing walking distance.

MEDLINE, Embase, Biosis, Amed and CISCOM were searched to June 1998 for published reports. Bibliographies of retrieved reports were checked for additional citations and no language restrictions were made. Manufacturers of ginkgo preparations were contacted for published and unpublished information. Data were extracted in a standardised, predefined manner by the two reviewers.

Findings

There were eight studies with pain free walking distance, defined using devices that forced patients to walk at a set speed. Intermittent claudication was according to predefined criteria. The quality scores were 3 (out of 5) or better for all trials, ensuring that bias was minimised.

Ginkgo biloba extracts at doses of 120–160 mg over 12–24 weeks increased mean pain free walking distance by an average of 33 m (95% confidence interval 22–43 m) compared with placebo in high quality randomised trials (Figure 4.13.2).

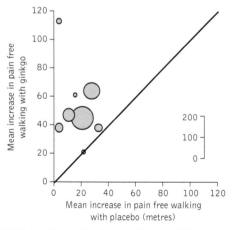

Figure 4.13.2 Pain free walking distance with ginkgo biloba and placebo.

Some trials reported no adverse events, but when they were reported they comprised abdominal complaints, nausea and dyspepsia.

Smoking cessation and nafronyl

Clinical bottom line. Nafronyl improves pain-free walking distance and total walking distance in patients with stage II intermittent claudication by approximately 60 and 70 m, respectively. No high quality data is available to assess the effects of smoking cessation. Studies have produced conflicting results, and there is therefore currently a lack of evidence for the effectiveness of this information.

Systematic review

Girolami, B., Bernadi, E., Prins, M. H. *et al.* (1999). Treatment of intermittent claudication with physical training, smoking cessation, pentoxifylline, or nafronyl, *Archives of Internal Medicine* 159: 337–45.

Date review completed: December 1996

Number of trials included: 6 nafronyl/4 smoking cessation

Number of patients: 629/866 smoking cessation

Control group: Placebo/no intervention

Main outcomes: Pain-free and total walking distance/time, ankle-brachial index, ankle pressure and peak blood flow

Inclusion criteria were controlled trials of smoking cessation or nafronyl for intermittent claudication at stage II of the disease; randomised and non-randomised trials; trials not in selected population groups; placebo or inactive comparison; English language reports. Reviewers pooled data from randomised trials only. This was calculated by combining the mean difference from each trial with 95% confidence interval. Descriptive summaries of studies and results were otherwise provided.

Findings

Smoking cessation. Four non-randomised cohort studies of 866 patients were included. These compared patients who stopped smoking with those who continued. It is difficult to interpret these findings owing to the lack of randomisation and therefore potential differences between groups. One small trial showed no difference on a number of measures. One trial showed that after 7 years 8.6% of smoking patients (26/304) had developed Fontaine stage III illness severity compared with none (0/39) of the stopped-smokers (95% CI 5.4–11.6%). A further trial of 415 patients failed to show any difference between groups. The fourth study did not provide extractable data.

Nafronyl. Six randomised, double-blind trials compared nafronyl with placebo over three to six months. Doses ranged from 400 to 800 mg/day.

Data for pain-free walking distance was available for four trials, three of which showed significant improvement. Pooled mean difference was 59 m (95% CI, 30–87). There was also a significant improvement in total walking distance based on information from two trials (pooled mean difference 71 m, 95% CI 13–129).

Reviewers did not consider adverse effects.

Pentoxifylline and smoking cessation

Clinical bottom line. Although pentoxifylline is associated with significant benefit in pain-free and maximum walking distances, based on small numbers of patients, this is unlikely to be of clinical relevance.

There is insufficient data to assess whether smoking cessation is of benefit for intermittent claudication.

Systematic review

Radack, K. and Wyderski, R. J. (1990). Conservative management of intermittent claudication, *Annals of Internal Medicine* 113: 135–46.

Date review completed: April 1989

Number of trials included: 12 (pentoxifylline) + 2 (smoking cessation)

Number of patients: 529 pentoxifylline/smoking cessation not stated

Control group: Placebo or active

Main outcomes: Improvement in pain-free or maximum walking distance

Inclusion criteria were randomised, double-blind trials of pentoxifylline or controlled trials of smoking cessation for intermittent claudication; English language. For pentoxifylline trials reviewers calculated effect sizes with 95% confidence intervals, from means and standard deviations or standard errors. Effect sizes were regarded as showing a significant difference when the confidence intervals did not cross one. An improvement of at least 100% was regarded as a clinically relevant outcome measure. A change of at least 25% from baseline was regarded as an acceptable alternative where it was not possible to extract precise data. Reviewers also assessed the relationship between trial quality and outcome.

Findings

Pentoxifylline. Twelve trials were included in 529 patients. Ten were placebo-controlled, and two compared pentoxifylline with either flunarizine or nylidrin. Trials varied in terms of inclusion criteria, baseline measures, etc. Doses ranged 600–1200 mg/day, and treatment duration ranged 8–1 year.

Effectiveness of pentoxifylline varied considerably across trials, as did placebo response rates, and reviewers did not feel that data pooling was therefore appropriate. Of the 10 placebo-controlled trials, five trials had significant effect sizes, suggesting that pentoxifylline was significantly better than placebo. Efficacy did not seem to be a reflection of dose or treatment duration. Of the active trials, one showed pentoxifylline 1200 mg/day to be significantly better than nylidrin 6 mg/day, and the other showed no difference between pentoxifylline 1200 mg/day and flunarizine 15 mg/day. There was no relationship between trial outcome and quality.

To answer the question of clinical relevance, numbers of patients experiencing at least 25% improvement and 100% improvement on walking were calculated, based on five trials where these data were extractable.

At least 25% improvement from baseline. The pooled benefit for at least 25% improvement in pain-free walking distance in 141 patients was 0.16 (0.01 to 0.31, 95% confidence interval) when compared with placebo. This suggests a very small gain attributable to pentoxifylline, and that this is of no clinical significance.

At least 100% improvement from baseline. The pooled benefit for at least 100% improvement in pain-free walking distance in 137 patients was 0.16 (0.03–0.29, 95% confidence interval) when compared with placebo. The pooled benefit for at least 100% improvement in maximum walking distance in 153 patients was 0.27 (0.13–0.41, 95% confidence interval) when compared with placebo. These findings suggest that only a modest gain is attributable to pentoxifylline, and that this is of limited clinical significance.

Smoking cessation. Two trials were found. One non-randomised, non-blinded trial compared 15 patients who chose to give up smoking with 46 patients who did not over approximately 10 months. They found significant improvement in maximum walking distance (approximately 60 m), although it is unclear whether this is of clinical significance or not. The second trial concluded that there was no benefit of smoking cessation on treadmill walking distance.

Adverse effects were not covered in this review.

Beta-blockers

Clinical bottom line. For short-term beta-blocker interventions (up to eight weeks), compared with placebo there appear to be no significant differences in walking capacity. However, this is based on trials with very small group sizes, and longer-term trials are needed to answer the question of whether it is advisable to prescribe beta-blockers for long-term use in patients with peripheral arterial disease.

Beta-adrenergic blockers have been contraindicated in peripheral arterial disease because of the perceived risk that these drugs could worsen intermittent claudication. The concern is that interventions which might lower systemic arterial blood pressure could potentially adversely affect limbs with impaired blood flow. Standard anti-hypertensive therapy is therefore sometimes not recommended, and beta-blockers in particular, which diminish cardiac output and block skeletal muscle vasodilation, have been avoided.

Systematic review

Radack, K. and Deck, C. (1991). Beta-adrenergic blocker therapy does not worsen intermittent claudication in subjects with peripheral arterial disease. A meta-analysis of randomized controlled trials, *Archives of Internal Medicine* 151: 1769–76.

Date review completed: 1990

Number of trials included: 11

Number of patients: 284 (crossover patients included twice)

Control group: Placebo or other inactive control

Main outcomes: Changes in pain-free walking distance

Inclusion criteria were randomised controlled trials comparing beta-blockers with placebo or other inactive control; patients with symptomatic peripheral arterial disease of the lower extremities; English language reports; walking capacity outcomes. Differences between the mean change in walking capacity during treatment and control periods were extracted from trials together with standard deviations. Standard errors were converted to standard deviations. These data were used to calculate an effect size with 95% confidence intervals. In most cases, the data were extracted for pain-free walking distances. Individual effect sizes were weighted by trial size and pooled for overall effect size. Effect sizes were regarded as significantly different to placebo when confidence intervals overlapped zero.

Findings

Trials were generally in middle-aged male patients with mild to moderate stable intermittent claudication that had usually persisted for at least six months. Trials varied in terms of treatment protocols, doses, duration (10 days to 8 weeks), clinical end points and trial quality. Included drugs were non-selective beta-adrenergic antagonists (propranolol hydrochloride), or $beta_1$-selective antagonists (metoprolol tartrate, atenolol and labetalol hydrochloride) or beta-blockers with intrinsic sympathomimetic activity (pindolol and acebutolol).

Of the eleven included trials, four had group sizes of less than ten, and the largest group was 23. Eight trials were double-blind, and a further two were blinded for outcomes. In 11 of 11 trials there were no significant differences in effect size between beta-blockers and placebo for either pain-free or maximum walking distance.

Walking capacity. Seven comparisons were included in the analysis of pain-free walking distance. Effect sizes were small, with 5 of 7 comparisons having negative values suggesting reduced, but not significantly reduced, pain-free walking distance with beta-blockers when compared with placebo. The overall treatment effect size was −0.24 (−0.62 to 0.14), and was not significant.

Six comparisons were included in the analysis of maximum walking distance. Effect sizes were small, with 4 of 6 comparisons having negative values suggesting reduced, but not significantly reduced, maximum walking distance with beta-blockers when compared with placebo. The overall treatment effect size was −0.29 (−0.71 to 0.12), and was not significant.

Other measures. These included pain-free and maximum exercise times and peak calf blood flow. Although methods of measuring these varied, there were no significant differences on any of the exercise outcomes. In one of three trials there was a significant improvement in peak calf blood flow, although the clinical relevance of this is unclear.

Adverse effects were not covered in this review.

Comment

Intermittent claudication is a topic that has been the subject of several systematic reviews, of varying quality. The individual trials have been of differing quality, but no large, randomised high quality studies exist. So whatever conclusions the reviews come to has to be regarded with some misgivings about whether we can trust the results we find. In a large review looking at pharmacological management, a good Canadian team [1] concluded that with medical therapy patients walked 60 m further with therapy than with placebo, but that only half of that was pain free, and suggested that pentoxifylline was better than naftidrofuryl. Antithrombotic medication gave only a small, if statistically significant, increase in pain free walking distance [2]. There is also a review [3] of the results of aortic bifurcation graft surgery over time. All reviewers agree that better studies need to be performed, with more attention to outcomes, and much more attention to adverse effects of treatments.

References

1. Moher, D. *et al.* (2000). Pharmacological management of intermittent claudication: a meta-analysis of randomised trials, *Drugs* 59: 1057–70.

2. Girolami, B. *et al.* (1999). Antithrombotic drugs in the primary medical management of intermittent claudication: a meta-analysis, *Thrombosis and Haemostasis* 81: 715–22.

3. de Vries, S. O. and Hunink, M. G. (1997). Results of aortic bifurcation grafts for aortoiliac occlusive disease: a meta-analysis, *Journal of Vascular Surgery* 26: 558–69.

4.14 **Cannabis for pain relief and for spasticity**

Pain relief

Clinical bottom line. Cannabinoid derivatives tested in cancer, chronic non-malignant or acute pain proved no better than the least effective analgesics, but with many adverse events, including psychotropic adverse events.

Systematic review

Campbell, F. A., Tramèr, M. R., Carroll, D., Reynolds, D. J. M., Moore, R. A. and McQuay, H. J. (2001). Are cannabinoids an effective and safe treatment option in the management of pain? A qualitative systematic review, *BMJ* 323: 13–16.

The search used a number of electronic databases to look for trials of cannabis or cannabinoids given by any route of administration with analgesic or placebo for acute, chronic, or chronic non-malignant, or cancer pain.

Findings

There were nine full publications of randomised trials where pain was measured. Two were in acute postoperative pain, two in chronic non-malignant pain, and five in cancer pain.

Acute pain. Two trials (72 patients) showed intramuscular levo-mantradol to be more effective than placebo. Adverse effects were common though mild.

Chronic non-malignant pain. Two trials in two patients (both N of 1 trials with one patient in each) tetrahydrocannabinol 5 or 10 mg was better than placebo and about equivalent to codeine 50 mg.

Cancer pain. Five trials with 128 patients. Tetrahydrocannabinol was roughly equivalent to codeine 60 mg in one trial. An analogue was also found to be equivalent to codeine 60 mg. Higher doses of tetrahydrocannabinol produced many adverse effects. At lower doses adverse effects were still more frequent than with standard analgesics.

Comment

These trials were not exceptionally large, nor particularly well designed. They showed some analgesic efficacy for cannabinoids, but equivalent to analgesics which perform poorly. Codeine 60 mg, for instance, can barely be distinguished from placebo even in meta-analysis, where the NNT is about 16. Other analgesics have NNTs of 2. Given that this comes with higher rates of adverse effects, and that higher doses are ruled out by adverse effects, cannabinoids are unlikely to have any useful place in analgesia in their present formulations.

Cannabis for spasticity

Clinical bottom line. There is only limited evidence mainly from anecdotal reports that cannabis (smoked or oral) benefits spasticity from multiple sclerosis or spinal cord injury. Some randomised N of 1 studies support this. The weight of evidence is not great, and more recent, though small, randomised trials show absolutely no effect, with some adverse effects.

Cannabis is commonly thought to be beneficial to patients with multiple sclerosis, especially those with spasticity. There are no modern randomised double-blind trials of any size, though there is one currently ongoing, whose design and objectives can be seen on the Internet. It will be some time before that trial is completed and reports.

Bandolier therefore set out to examine what evidence does exist, and searched for papers on cannabis (plus its other names) using PubMed and the Cochrane Library, and reviews, reference lists, and official reports. What we found is given in Table 4.14.1, together with the reference for each and a brief summary of what the paper was and found. Reviews and peripherally interesting papers are also included.

Results

Most of the results were anecdotal and impossible to interpret. Where test, abstinence and retest had been conducted, sometimes with blinded observations, results were reproducible. This was true also of two N of 1 designs, one of which was randomised, and double-blind, and with identical looking preparations of cannabinoid, codeine and placebo. There are several studies that were randomised and double-blind, but not always examining useful clinical outcomes. Because studies were often very small, and with self-selecting patients who were usually (though not always) previous cannabis users, the small benefits seen must be regarded as disappointing. They could easily be wrong just by the random play of chance.

Oral preparations of cannabinoids helped most, but not all patients, and some seemed only to respond to the smoked version. In the last few years some scientific basis has been adduced to support cannabinoid involvement in the control of spasticity, perhaps with endogenous cannabinoids being involved with maintaining spastic tone. The most recent randomised trial was negative, though small. Significant adverse events were reported.

Comment

There are few conclusions to be drawn from this. With case reports we are unlikely to know how many people who have tried cannabinoids and failed, so the bias we find from publication of positive results will be massive. Even the N of 1 trials were done in known responders. There may be patients who respond to cannabinoids and whose spasticity or other symptoms may be allieviated. They may be common, or rare as hen's teeth. We will have to wait for the results of the ongoing large randomised trial underway in the UK for the bigger picture.

What we do see is that newer studies, or those with better and designs less open to bias, are being more negative. The hope must be (and hope it has to be now) that something in the method of delivery of drug will confer unexpected benefits.

Table 4.14.1 Studies in cannabis and spasticity

Reference	Summary
O'Shaughnessy, W. B. (1842). On the preparation of Indian hemp or gunjah, *Transactions of the Medical and Physical Society of Bombay* 8: 421–461.	Paper available in full on-line. A terrific historical narrative coupled with a series of cases where cannabis was used. Spasm of tetanus was particularly well controlled.
Reynolds, J. R. (1890). Therapeutic use and toxic effects of Cannabis indica, *Lancet* 1: 637–8.	An interesting discourse on use of ethanolic extracts of cannabis. Regarded cannabis as useful in chronic painful conditions and spasm (but not epilepsy). Descriptive, but acutely observed by Fellow of the Royal Society and Physician to Queen Victoria.
Dunn, M. and Davis, R. (1974). The perceived effects of cannabis on spinal cord injured males, *Paraplegia* 12: 175.	Informal survey on 10 patients with spinal cord injury and spasm and pain who already took cannabis. Decreases spasticity in 5/8, decreased phantom pain in 4/9 with smoked cannabis.
Cunha et al. (1980). Chronic administration of cannabidiol to healthy volunteers and epileptic patients, *Pharmacology* 21: 175–85.	Randomised, double blind study of 200–300 mg cannabidiol daily or placebo in 15 patients with epilepsy with frequent convulsions Absence of convulsive crisis over 3–18 weeks in 4/8 on cannabidiol and 1/8 on placebo (sic).
Petro, D. J. (1980). Marihuana as a therapeutic agent for muscle spasm or spasticity, *Psychosomatics* 21: 81–5.	This is a case report of two cases, one of whom had MS. Nocturnal leg spasms were relieved by smoking cannabis within five minutes. Abstention led to increased spasticity and pain, again relieved by use of cannabis.
Petro and Ellenberger (1980). Treatment of human spasticity with delta 9-tetrahydrocannabinol, *Journal of Clinical Pharmacology* 21: (Suppl. 8–9): 413S–16S.	Nine patients with spasticity related to MS were examined by a blinded observer before an 90 min intervals after oral capsules with 10 mg, 5 mg or no synthetic THC. THC, but not placebo, was associated with a reduced spasticity score lasting for about 4 h. Big improvements with 4/9 with THC and 1/9 with placebo. Subjective highs were experienced by one patient after THC and one after placebo.
Malec et al. (1982). Cannabis effect on spasticity in spinal cord injury, *Arch Phys Med rehabil* 63: 116–18.	Questionnaire to spinal cord injury patients. 9/24 users reported no spasticity while using cannabis, 11/24 reported some benefit.

Clifford, D. B. (1983). Tetrahydrocannabinol for the treatment of tremor in multiple sclerosis, *Ann Neurol* 13: 669–71.	Eight patients with MS, disabling tremors and ataxia were given THC or single-blind placebo (?oral) and effect on tremor investigated. Two patients had some subjective and objective improvement with THC but not placebo.
Snider, R. R. and Consroe, P. (1984). Treatment of Meige syndrome with cannabidiol, *Neurology* 34 (Suppl 1): 147.	Case report of use of cannabidiol in patient with severe cranial dystonia (Meige Syndrome) with severe untreatable spasms. 400 mg cannabidiol daily reduced spasm frequency by 50%, and withdrawal led to return of spasms to previous level.
Consroe *et al.* (1986). Open label evaluation of cannabinoid in dystonic movement disorders, *Int. J. Neurosci.* 30: 277–82.	Five patients with dystonia in open-label study with oral cannabidiol (100–600 mg/day). Improvement in dystonia scores in all five (20–50%). Some adverse events\ (lightheadedness, hypotension) and two patients had exacerbation of resting tremor.
Ungerleider *et al.* (1987). Delta-9-THC in the treatment of spasticity associated with multiple sclerosis, *Adv Alcohol Subst Abuse 7*: 39–50.	13 patients with MS and spasticity unable to take other drugs. Random assignment to double-blind crossover between THC and placebo (five days) with two day washout. Decreased spasticity with increasing THC dose. Significant benefit by patient, but not physician, scoring of spasticity.
Meinck *et al.* (1989). Effect of cannabinoids on spasticity and ataxia in multiple sclerosis, *J Neurol* 263: 120–2.	Chronic motor handicaps of one MS patient improved acutely while smoking cannabis cigarette.
Maurer *et al.* (1990). Delta-9-tetrahydrocannabinol shows antispastic and analgesic effects in a single case double-blind trial, *Eur Arch Psychiatry Clin Neurosci* 240: 1–4.	N of 1 randomised comparison of oral THC 5mg, codeine 50 mg and placebo in patient with spasticity due to spinal cord injury. Three treatments used 18 times each. THC significantly better than placebo for sleep pain spasticity, micturition, concentration and mood. THC better than codeine for spasticity.
Greenberg *et al.* (1994). Short-term effects of smoking marijuana on balance in patients with multiple sclerosis and normal volunteers, *Clin Pharm Ther* 55: 324–8.	Randomised, double blind study of inhaled cannabis on postural (balance) responses in normal subjects and MS patients Technical paper that says that cannabis gives patients and MS sufferers worse balance control.
Martyn *et al.* (1995). Nabilone in the treatment of multiple sclerosis, *Lancet* 345: 579.	N of 1 trial of nabilone 1 mg every second day or placebo for four successive periods of four weeks in man with severe spasticity and MS. Nabilone reduced frequency of nocturia and severity of muscle spasm and improved well being.
Voth and Schwartz. (1997). Medicinal applications of delta-9-tetrahydrocannabinol and marijuana, *Ann Intern Med* 126: 791–8.	Systematic review of medicinal applications of cannabis, to 1996. No additional information on spasticity or MS.

Table 4.14.1 continued

Reference	Summary
Consroe et al. (1997). The perceived effects of smoked cannabis on patients with multiple sclerosis, Eur Neurol 38: 44–8.	Questionnaire findings of 112 US and UK patients with MS and who used cannabis. Signs or symptoms reported to be much better in over 60% of patients were spasticity at sleep onset, pain in muscles, spasticity at night, pain in legs at night, tremor, depression, anxiety, spasticity on waking or walking.
Taylor, H. G. (1998). Analysis of the medical use of marijuana and its societal implications, J Am Pharm Assoc (Wash) 38(2): 220–7. (Systematic Review).	Systematic review of medicinal applications of cannabis, to 1997. No additional information on spasticity or MS.
Schon, F. et al. (1999). Suppression of pendular nystagmus by smoking cannabis in a patient with multiple sclerosis, Neurology 53: 2209.	Report of a patient with MS whose nystagmus improved with smoked, not oral cannabis, and was partly related to serum cannabinoids.
Dell'Osso, L. F. (2000). Suppression of pendular nystagmus by smoking cannabis in a patient with multiple sclerosis, Neurology 54: 2190–1.	Letter. Another case report, but with no data.
Schon, F. et al. (2000). Suppression of pendular nystagmus by smoking cannabis in a patient with multiple sclerosis, Neurology 54: 2190–1.	Response to letter. Reports original patient's nystagmus also responded to drinking red wine.
Williamson and Evans. (2000). Cannabinoids in clinical practice, Drugs 60: 1303–14.	A review that does not add much. It incorrectly identifies a questionnaire study as a trial, appearing to add more weight of evidence than there is.
Baker et al. (2000). Cannabinoids control spasticity and tremor in a multiple sclerosis model, Nature 404: 84–87.	Use of cannabinoid receptor agonism with THC and other agents ameliorated tremor and spasticity in mice with relapsing experimental allergic encephalomyelitis, an autoimmune model of MS.

Carter and Rosen. (2001). Marijuana in the management of amyotropic lateral sclerosis, *Am J Hosp Palliat Care* 18: 264–70.

Useful pharmacological review, but no clinical data, so speculative.

Baker *et al.* (2001). Endocannabinoids control spasticity in a multiple sclerosis model, *FASEB J* 15(2): 300–2.

Experimental work in mice suggesting that natural cannabinoids help control spastic tone.

Robson, P. (2001). Therapeutic effects of cannabis and cannabinoids, *British Journal of Psychiatry* 178: 107–115.

Review. No additional studies.

Fox, S. H. *et al.* (2002). Randomised, double-blind, placebo-controlled trial to assess the potential of cannabinoid receptor stimulation in the treatment of dystonia, *Movement Disorder* 17: 145–9.

Nabilone was ineffective in patients with generalised and segmental primary dystonia.

Killestein, J. *et al.* (2002). Safety, tolerability and efficacy of orally administered cannabinoids in MS, *Neurology* 58: 1404–7.

This was a randomised crossover trial of placebo, THC and plan extract given orally in 16 patients with progressive MS and spasticity. Four weeks of treatment with placebo, 2.5–5 mg THC, or plant extract with equivalent THC (identical appearance) was followed by four weeks of washout before the next treatment. A lower dose was used for two weeks, and doubled, if well tolerated, for the second two weeks of treatment. Active treatments conferred no benefit. Plant extract, but not THC, had significantly more adverse events. Five patients on plant extract reported subjective increased spasticity and one had an episode of acute psychosis.

Martin, B. R. (2002). Identification of the endogenous cannabinoid system through integrative pharmacological approaches, *J Pharm Exp Ther* 301: 790–6.

A really interesting bit of basic pharmacology, which for most of us will be a bit academic. But a useful read if one wants to try to get a grip on what may be going on.

Section 5
Arthritis

5.1 **Arthritis and joints**

Introduction

There has been a major change in the conduct of clinical trials in arthritis with the advent of COX-2 selective inhibitors (called, for convenience, coxibs). Previously, trials were characterised by being small, short, and having uncertain outcomes. Subsequently they have become large, of long duration, and often have many outcomes measured, though few reported.

A view of outcomes reported in trials before the late 1980s can be gained from a study of reporting outcomes up to 1998 [1]. A search was made for all randomised double-blind trials that compared two of the 22 NSAIDs available in Denmark published up to August 1998. The final sample was 144 trial reports.

These were examined for a number of outcomes commonly used in arthritis research that are measured on ordinal or interval scales, and therefore potentially useful for meta-analysis (global evaluation, pain, number of tender joints and grip strength). The reports were examined to see if the information was useable in meta-analysis. The definitions were optimal and usable. Optimal was information on the original ordered categories (number in each category), and usable required information on patients in two or more ordered categories. The main results are shown in Table 5.1.1 for the 144 reports.

The median sample size was 60 patients, increasing in time to 110 patients per trial. The most common problem was the lack of standard deviations, or confidence intervals, or other useful statistical outcomes.

Gøtzsche comments that many of the studies are full of misleading statements unsupported by data, comments that are biases in themselves. Similar comments about 'non-significantly greater than' effects, or similar, are to be found in many trials of conventional and unconventional treatments. Moreover, the size of these trials is so small that even large differences might be missed. He calculated that for one drug to be half as effective as another and this not to be overlooked,

Table 5.1.1 Arthritis outcomes reported in clinical trials

	Global evaluation	Pain	Joint count	Grip strength
Number of trials	127	98	123	124
Percent optimal	41	28	33	27
Percent usable	69	48	40	3

a trial would need nearly 300 patients. For a difference of 25%, it would need nearly 1200 patients.

We have to be vigilant. Even meta-analysis can be useless if trials themselves are useless. Gathering small piles of junk together gives one large pile of junk. Systematic review and meta-analysis should be about picking the nuggets of gold from the dross.

Outcomes

One of the most difficult problems in arthritis trials is the very large number of different outcomes that are used. Global evaluation (by the patient), or pain, may seem to be sensible outcomes, but there are others. Grip strength, the number of painful joints, pain walking on a flat surface, pain at rest, pain at night, morning stiffness and many others have been and are being used. They are probably all relevant to a greater or lesser extent, and to different extents to different patients.

In rheumatoid arthritis the most commonly used (though perhaps difficult to explain and use) measure is the American College of Rheumatology (ACR) response criteria, a composite measure of seven indices:

- tender joint count,
- swollen joint count,
- global disease activity assessed by observer,
- global disease activity assessed by patient,
- patient assessment of pain,
- physical disability score (like health assessment questionnaire),
- acute phase response (CRP measurement, or ESR).

The ACR 20 response is defined as a 20% improvement in the first two of these, plus a 20% improvement in any three of the remaining five items. This is not an easy outcome to reach, though also being used now are ACR 50 and ACR 70, which are similar to the ACR 20 but at 50% and 70% improvements. These are very high hurdles of treatment efficacy and represent very significant clinical improvement. Despite the obvious relevance of these composite outcomes, they are not always easy to use or to explain to patients.

In rheumatoid and osteoarthritis, another commonly-used outcome is the WOMAC scale, where patients measure their pain using a 100-mm scale after walking on a flat surface. Typically in these trials patients initially on NSAID or other analgesic will have the analgesic stopped. Pain then gets much worse (called a 'flare'), and then they begin taking the treatment to which they have been randomised for periods of up to one year or more.

The mean value on the VAS pain scales usually begins at about 35 mm on the original NSAID, rises to about 75 mm without treatment, and then returns to 35 mm on treatment again (Figure 5.1.1).

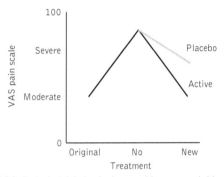

Figure 5.1.1 Typical trial design in rheumatoid or osteoarthritis.

Over 30 mm on the VAS scale equates with moderate pain, and over 60 mm severe pain [2]. So even on treatment the average arthritis patient has pain sufficiently severe to fulfil an entry criterion for clinical trials in acute pain. Disappointing is that the trials never define what is adequate control of pain, or tell us how many patients have a specified level of pain relief.

Placebo can be used as well as active drugs, and often there appears to be some analgesic action from placebo (Figure 5.1.1). Some people take this as being the effect of placebo, forgetting that these trials will almost always have an escape analgesic, which can be paracetamol, or paracetamol plus opioid combination.

Who to treat, and with what?

Another difficulty that trials almost never help with is the vexed question of who to treat, and with what. Common experience is that some patients do not do well on paracetamol, and move on to NSAIDs. But not all do well on NSAIDS, and move to other treatments or back to paracetamol. There is almost no information on this, though analysis of discontinuation rates in clinical trials would probably help, though it has not been done. The best we have is a large questionnaire study about what patients with rheumatoid arthritis, osteoarthritis and fibromyalgia think [3].

As part of a long-term prospective study going on since 1974, 2085 participants were mailed a six-monthly questionnaire. All had clinically defined rheumatoid arthritis, osteoarthritis or fibromyalgia. In July 1998 four additional questions were asked about the use of paracetamol. These addressed use of paracetamol, effectiveness, effectiveness compared with NSAIDs and satisfaction compared with NSAIDs considering both effectiveness and adverse effects.

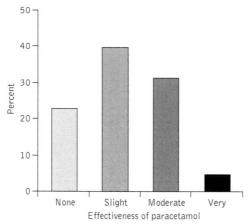

Figure 5.1.2 How 1187 patients rated the effectiveness of paracetamol.

The questionnaire was returned by 1799 patients (86%), of whom 1187 had taken paracetamol. There were 825 responders with rheumatoid arthritis, 668 with osteoarthritis and 286 with fibromyalgia.

Of those who had taken paracetamol, 37% had found it moderately or very effective and 63% found it slight or not effective (Figure 5.1.2).

Responses on questions of efficacy and satisfaction compared with NSAIDs were similar. About 60% found paracetamol less satisfactory than NSAIDs, 25% found it about the same, and 13% found it more satisfactory (Figure 5.1.3), with a similar result for comparison of effectiveness and adverse effects.

There were minor differences between responders and non-responders in the survey, and minor differences between disease states and with age, but none of any obvious importance. Obviously this is much less satisfactory than a properly conducted, large, long-term randomised trial. It demonstrates that for a significant minority of patients paracetamol can be effective, and given the cost and safety issues, it is reasonable as a first choice, or as an addition to NSAIDs. It also shows that for many patients it simply is not good enough, and that patients may not be best served by persevering with an ineffective medicine.

Comment

The quality of trials in arthritis and joint disorders is improving, but we still do not have the best type of information – that about individual patients and information about which patient is most likely to

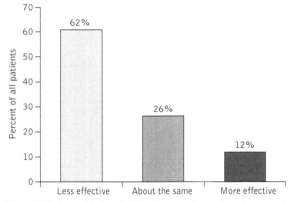

Figure 5.1.3 How patients rated effectiveness of paracetamol compared with NSAIDs.

benefit from what treatment. The next few years may see some developments.

And finally, it is not stated anywhere else, but is worth saying here, that for many patients with diseased joints, replacement operation is probably the most effective option. The fact that treatment is often delayed, by months or even years (in the UK in particular) does not make analgesic management a better option.

References

1. Gøtzsche, P. C. (2001). Reporting of outcomes in arthritis trials measured on ordinal and interval scales is inadequate in relation to meta-analysis, *Annals of Rheumatic Disease* 60: 349–52.
2. Collins, S. L., Moore, R. A. and McQuay, H. J. (1997). The visual analogue pain intensity scale: what is moderate pain in millimetres? *Pain* 72: 95–8.
3. Wolfe, F., Zhao, S. and Lane, N. (2000). Preference for nonsteroidal antiinflammatory drugs over acetaminophen by rheumatic disease patients, *Arthritis & Rheumatism* 43: 378–85.

5.2 **Lifestyle and exercise**

With many bone and joint problems, exercise or other lifestyle interventions are recommended. This is not a bad thing. There is abundant evidence that taking moderate exercise, like walking, improves well-being and reduces the risk of cardiovascular problems. A reasonably brisk walk of a mile a day is sufficient. Again, diet, including a reasonable amount of fruit and vegetables, whole grain bread or rice, and regular fish, protects both against cardiovascular disease, but also cancer. People who adopt a healthy lifestyle live longer and better. The Bandolier 10 tips for healthy living summarise the recommendations from the evidence, and are reproduced in section 9.3.

What about lifestyle affecting arthritis, either by exercise or diet? There are systematic reviews, but usually of a small number of relatively small and poor trials. Because exercise and lifestyle are so often regarded as being important, this section will briefly review the reviews.

Diet

Fasting and vegetarian diet in rheumatoid arthritis

Few trials likely to be bias free (randomised, blind), and valid (longer duration) exist. The results are mixed, but a cautious interpretation may be that there is no evidence of lack of effect, while what evidence we have suggests some benefit.

Clinical observation has been that diet may improve the symptoms of rheumatoid arthritis. The biology underlying any dietary influences is not exact. Some food additives are taken by patients with rheumatoid arthritis (RA). It has also become traditional in some centres for patients to fast, followed by a vegan or vegetarian diet with add-back of foods not associated with symptom worsening. This may be accompanied by holistic approaches involving physiotherapy, exercise and psychotherapy.

A systematic review [1] has examined the evidence-base for fasting and vegetarian diet. Only MEDLINE was searched (up to 1997), and reference lists checked. Criteria for inclusion were trials with follow-up information for at least three months, and full journal publication.

The review found 31 reports. Only one was randomised. A further randomised report with just under three months duration was also included. The other reports were observational studies, or controlled studies. Most were very small, with few having more than 30 patients in total, or 30 patients per group. The main findings in each study are reported, including clinical and biochemical or immunological findings. Pooling of clinical finding data was done for two randomised and two non-randomised studies separately and together, showing an overall effect size of about 0.8. This is quite a large effect.

Exercise

Because most of the reviews on exercise examine rather poor trials, the first example is a recent well conducted randomised trial showing that exercise can prevent disability.

Exercise prevents disability in older adults

As the population ages, the proportion of people having difficulty performing essential everyday activities is on the increase. This type of disability affects people's quality of life, limits their independence and increases the requirements for both formal and informal care. Clearly, there is a need to develop strategies to increase older adults' active years of life. This study [2] examines whether an exercise programme can prevent this type of disability, known as activities of daily living (or ADL) disability.

Study

Participants were 250 adults, initially free of ADL disability, from the Fitness Arthritis and Seniors Trial, a randomised controlled trial of aerobic or resistance exercise among older adults with knee osteoarthritis. Participants were recruited from the community through local advertisements and mailings. Eligibility criteria were: aged 60 years or older; pain in the knee/s on most days; difficulty with at least one activity, for example, climbing stairs; and radiographic evidence of knee osteoarthritis. Exclusion criteria were: a medical condition that prevented safe participation in an exercise programme; inflammatory arthritis; exercising regularly; and an inability to walk 128 m in 6 min.

Participants were randomly assigned to one of three groups: 80 in the attention control group; 88 in the aerobic exercise programme; and 82 in the resistance exercise programme. Both programmes were supervised by exercise therapists.

Attention control group. Participants attended monthly group sessions on arthritis management (months 1–3); and were telephoned to update health status and provide support (months 4–18).

Aerobic exercise programme. Participants attended an indoor track three times a week for 1 h, consisting of 10 min warm-up/cool-down and 40 min walking (months 1–3); and were visited and telephoned to offer assistance and support in developing a walking programme at home (months 4–18).

Resistance exercise programme. Participants attended three 1-h sessions a week, consisting of 10 min warm-up/cool-down and 40 min of 2 sets of 12 repetitions of 9 exercises, for example, biceps curl, leg curl (months 1–3); and continued these exercises at home (months 4–18).

Demographics and clinical conditions were assessed at baseline, including hypertension, chronic co-morbid conditions (e.g. coronary heart disease) and intensity of knee pain. Self-reported disability was assessed with a 30-item questionnaire every three months during the 18-month follow-up period. ADL disability was defined as experiencing difficulty in bathing, eating, dressing, transferring from a bed to a chair or using the toilet.

Results

The average age of participants, free of disability at baseline, was 69 years and 68% were women. Demographics, co-morbidity, intensity of knee pain, walking speed and disability scores did not differ across the three groups. Adherence to the exercise programmes declined over time, with 56% completing the aerobic exercise programme and 61% completing the resistance programme.

The incidence of ADL disability was lower in the exercise groups (37%) than in the attention group (53%).

Participation in an exercise programme was associated with a 43% reduced risk of ADL disability (relative risk 0.57, 95% confidence interval 0.38–0.85). Those participating in the aerobic exercise programme had a 47% reduced risk and those in the resistance programme had a 40% reduced risk, compared with those in the attention group (relative risks and 95% confidence intervals: 0.53, 0.33–0.85; and 0.60, 0.38 to 0.97). These results were adjusted for several variables including age, body mass index, walking speed, disability and knee pain scores.

Participants who attended the most exercise sessions had the lowest risk of ADL disability. For the 28 participants who completed 78% or more of the aerobic exercise sessions, the relative risk was 0.38 (95% confidence interval 0.17–0.82) compared with those in the attention group. The results were similar for the 26 participants who completed 81% or more of the resistance exercise programme (0.43, 0.19–0.97).

Comment

This study was relatively small so the relative risks should not be taken too literally. Nevertheless, it showed that exercise can reduce the incidence of ADL disability in older adults with knee osteoarthritis and in the short term. Further research is needed to investigate the incidence rate in the long-term (which would include looking at whether older adults can maintain regular exercise for longer than 18 months). Participants were a selected group of patients with knee osteoarthritis (chosen because they are at high risk for ADL disability), so the results may not entirely generalise to the average population.

The preventive effect of exercise appeared to be similar for the aerobic and resistance programmes. However, further analyses examined the incidence of disability in four specific activities. Aerobic exercise was associated with a reduced risk of disability in three of the activities (bathing, dressing and transferring from a bed to a chair), whereas resistance exercise was associated with a reduced risk of disability in one activity (bathing). The lack of significance could be due to the small numbers in the analysis or it could be that aerobic exercise is more beneficial. Nevertheless, it is probable that most people, particularly older people, would choose walking as a form of exercise rather than resistance training. In any case, activities such as walking combine both aerobic exercise and a certain amount of resistance training. Swimming is another ideal activity, especially for those who suffer from joint or bone conditions.

Exercise therapy for OA of the hip or knee

There is limited evidence that exercise provides modest reductions in pain and disability in patients with mild or moderate osteoarthritis of the hip or knee. The majority of trials were small, of low validity and had insufficient power.

Systematic review

Van Baar, M. E., Assendelft, W. J. J., Dekker, J., Oostendorp, R. A. B. and
  Bulsma, J. W. J. (1999). Effectiveness of exercise therapy in patients with
  osteoarthritis of the hip or knee, *Arthritis and Rheumatism* 42: 1361–9.

  Date review completed: September 1997

  Number of trials included: 11

  *Number of patients: (mean number of patients per group in the two
  studies of high quality and sufficient power was 100–146)*

  Control groups: Placebo, no treatment

  *Main outcomes: Pain; self-reported disability; observed disability;
  patient's global assessment of treatment effect*

Inclusion criteria were randomised controlled trial which assessed exercise therapy in patients with osteoarthritis (OA) of the hip or knee and used the outcomes listed above. MEDLINE (1966–1997), EMBASE (1988–1997), CINAHL (1982–1997) and the Cochrane Controlled Trials Register were searched. Bibliographies of retrieved reports were checked for additional citations. No language restrictions were made. The validity of the trials and their power to detect a difference between treatments were assessed. Effect sizes, with 95% confidence intervals, were calculated.

Findings

Eleven studies were included. Only one study assessed OA of the hip. Two trials were described as being of adequate validity and sufficient power and are discussed here. These assessed the effect of aerobic or resistance exercises in patients with mild-to-moderate OA of the hip or knee over 12 weeks. There were between 100–146 patients per treatment group.

In one study aerobic exercise was more effective than resistance exercise; the effect sizes were 0.31 (0.28–0.34) and 0.47 (0.44–0.5) respectively. The second trial assessed a combination of strengthening and range-of-motion exercises and functional training; the effect size for pain was higher, 0.58 (0.54–0.62).

Modest improvements were reported in the two high quality studies. The effect sizes were highest for patients randomised to aerobic exercise for both self-reported disability, 0.41 (0.38–0.44), and for observed disability in walking, 0.89 (0.85–0.93).

The reviewers' stated that adverse effects of exercise therapy were not often mentioned in the trials. No further information was provided.

Comment

The reviewers stated that different outcome measurement tools were used in the trials, most were small and no information about the long-term, beneficial or adverse effects, of exercise were provided. The reviewers concluded that there is some evidence for small to modest beneficial effects of exercise in the treatment of OA of the hip or knee. These conclusions are based mainly on the results of the two trials of adequate validity and power. The studies of lower validity and inadequate power showed variable results and reported on few of the outcomes of interest.

Dynamic exercise therapy for rheumatoid arthritis

Dynamic exercise therapy (aerobic exercise) appears to be effective in improving physical capacity (aerobic capacity, muscle strength and joint mobility) but less effective in improving functional ability when compared with other forms of exercise or no exercise. Based on small patient numbers, dynamic exercise therapy does not increase pain. It does not appear to exacerbate disease activity or radiological progression, but there is currently insufficient evidence to draw a firm conclusion.

Exercise therapy has traditionally been used for patients with rheumatoid arthritis to preserve joint mobility and maintain muscle strength. Interventions have often been designed to put limited stress on joints, with non-weight-bearing, isometric exercise. One rationale for this has been that a more intense intervention might cause pain and damage joints or cause increased disease activity.

Systematic review

Van den Ende, C. H. M. *et al.* (1998). Dynamic exercise therapy in rheumatoid arthritis: a systematic review, *British Journal of Rheumatology* 37: 677–87.

Date review completed: October 1996

Number of trials included: 6

Number of patients: 277

Control group: Other exercise or no exercise

Main outcomes: Joint mobility, muscle strength, aerobic capacity, daily functioning

Inclusion criteria were randomised controlled trials of dynamic exercise therapy for rheumatoid arthritis; other exercise or no exercise control groups; full length articles including unpublished; intervention sufficient to improve aerobic function; outcome measures standardised or accepted in measuring symptom changes in rheumatoid arthritis; English, Dutch, French or German language articles.

Appropriate exercise interventions were defined as exercise frequency at least twice a week with each session of at least 20 min, exercises likely to increase heart rate to exceed 60% of maximal heart rate, and duration of exercise programme at least 6 weeks.

Mean data with standard deviations were extracted, together with (where possible) mean changes from baseline with standard deviations. Data pooling was not possible because trials were not similar enough, so conclusions from original reports were summarised.

Findings

Disease duration was for a minimum of seven years, and patients were predominantly on stable medication with non-active to moderately active disease and mildly restricted daily functioning. Mean ages ranged from 48 to 67. Length of exercise intervention ranged from eight weeks to two years.

The results from the six trials suggest that dynamic exercise therapy is effective in improving physical capacity (aerobic capacity, muscle strength and joint mobility) but less effective in improving functional ability. Details of findings are given in the review.

This review specifically set out to answer the question of whether dynamic exercise therapy had any deleterious effects. This was assessed by measuring pain, disease activity and radiological progression.

Pain worse?

Changes in pain were used to assess whether pain was exacerbated by exercise. In three of three trials there was no significant difference between dynamic exercise and control group on measures of pain. No detrimental effects of exercise were observed for disease activity or radiological progression, but reviewers point out that this is based on very limited data.

Comment

Good lifestyle, including exercise, is obviously a good thing in and of itself. It may also benefit arthritis.

References

1. Müller, H. *et al*. (2001). Fasting followed by vegetarian diet in patients with rheumatoid arthritis: a systematic review, *Scandinavian Journal of Rheumatology* 30: 1–10.
2. Penninx, B. W. J. H. *et al*. (2001). Physical exercise and the prevention of disability in activities of daily living in older persons with osteoarthritis, *Archives of Internal Medicine* 161: 2309–16.

5.3 **NSAIDs for treating osteoarthritis**

Clinical bottom line. NSAIDs effectively relieve pain by about half and increase mobility in about 60% of people with osteoarthritis. There is insufficient information to rank their effectiveness, but what information we have suggests that daily doses of diclofenac (100–150 mg) and naproxen (500–750 mg) are more effective than low doses of ibuprofen, and more effective than paracetamol.

Non-steroidal anti-inflammatory drugs (NSAIDs) have become the common choice for treating rheumatological conditions like osteoarthritis, rheumatoid arthritis and gout. About 25 million prescriptions are written in the UK every year and most general practitioners will write a number of prescriptions every day because these are common conditions. About 4% of all prescriptions in the UK are for NSAIDs, and 70% of GP prescriptions for analgesics are for NSAIDs.

Osteoarthritis is the most common form of arthritis and is associated with significant disability and impaired quality of life because of increasing pain, loss of mobility, and consequently loss of independence as people get older or the disease worsens. Osteoarthritis is the main reason why people have hip and knee replacement operations.

Systematic reviews

Two Cochrane reviews on NSAIDs in OA of the hip and knee have been combined because there is no prior reason to suspect that they should be different in response to NSAIDs. In order to try to tease out more information in a very difficult area, the papers included in the original reviews have been obtained and re-analysed.

Towheed, T., Shea, B., Wells, G. and Hochberg, M. (1999). Analgesia and non-aspirin, non-steroidal anti-inflammatory drugs for osteoarthritis of the hip. Cochrane Library, May 21 1999.

Watson, M. C., Brookes, S. T., Kirwan, J. R. and Faulkner, A. (1999). Non-aspirin, non-steroidal anti-inflammatory drugs (NSAIDS) for osteoarthritis of the knee. Cochrane Library (May 21 1999).

Note: Four papers originally included have been omitted because they dealt with opioids, combination of NSAID with other compounds, suppositories (all others being oral), and naproxen/paracetamol combinations.

Date reviews completed: Nov 1996, August 1997

Number of trials: 29

Number of patients: 3014

Control groups: Most studies compared two NSAIDs. Only a very few included a placebo

Main outcomes: Studies used a variety of outcomes, and many gave only mean results without dispersion. For this summary, information has been taken from patient global evaluations available in dichotomous form and equivalent to at least 50% improvement or relief of pain. No statistical calculations were possible.

Inclusion criteria were randomised controlled trials of NSAIDs in patients with osteoarthritis of the hip and/or knee, compared with placebo, or other NSAID, or analgesic.

Findings

Despite extensive searching, only 29 trials were found which fulfilled these inclusion criteria; over 1100 trials were originally identified by one of the reviews. The trials were small, with 67 as the median number of patients in the trials. Only five studies had more than 200 patients. The trials were short, with 6 weeks as the median duration, either of the trial if parallel group or one treatment period if cross-over design. Only three trials lasted more than 10 weeks.

Because the design of trials of NSAIDs in OA left much to be desired – they were small, short, and had poor reporting of results – the information on efficacy and harm that follows should be taken as indicative only.

Effectiveness of NSAIDs

A large number of different outcomes were used in the trials, but few were reported in detail. Pain at rest, pain on movement and patient and physician global evaluations were the most commonly used outcomes. Mobility was occasionally judged by walking times, and joint flexion and/or tenderness were sometimes assessed.

Where results were reported, they were frequently given as mean values without dispersion. Many trials described 'improvement', but not one defined what improvement actually meant – though it was implied that this would be any improvement from baseline rather than a prior definition of what constituted sufficient quality of life or pain reduction for the patient.

Almost all trials put patients on simple analgesics like paracetamol for one or two weeks before treatment, and some allowed paracetamol during treatment as additional analgesia. In these cases it was universally stated that paracetamol had to be discontinued before assessments were made.

The most commonly reported outcome with dichotomous information was the patient global evaluation of treatment, shown graphically in Figure 5.3.1 where the results of global evaluations as good or better (equivalent to at least half pain relief) are given.

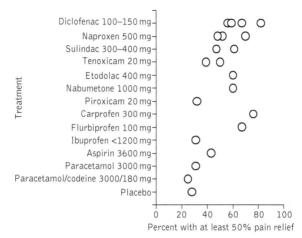

Figure 5.3.1 Global outcome equating to at least 50% pain relief in individual trials.

Placebo, paracetamol and paracetamol/codeine, low dose ibuprofen (< 1200 mg/day) and piroxicam were the least effective treatments with 20–40% of patients with at least 50% pain relief. Diclofenac 100–150 mg was the NSAID for which there was most data (four trials) and this showed consistently good responses of between 59% and 82% of patients with at least 50% pain relief.

Harm with NSAIDs

Most of the trials give information on harm at various levels. Table 5.3.1 contains the information collected from the trials for adverse effect discontinuations, which were essentially the same at below 10% across all treatments, including placebo. It is worth noting that very high adverse effect discontinuation rates were seen in the study comparing paracetamol and paracetamol plus codeine.

Upper gastrointestinal problems, including dyspepsia, abdominal pain, nausea, vomiting etc., were higher at about 20% with NSAIDs than the 9% recorded with placebo. For dyspepsia alone the distinction was less clear. Bleeding episodes, including positive faecal occult bloods, melaena, ulcers and GI bleeding were reported in 21 patients. This is 0.7% of all patients in the 29 trials, including placebo, paracetamol, and non-NSAID treatments.

Comment

The amount of information is not large for such commonly-used drugs. Much of the research on NSAIDs and arthritis has concentrated

Table 5.3.1 Overall reporting of measures of harm in RCTs of NSAIDs in OA

Drug	Number of trials	Number of patients	Percent affected
Adverse effect discontinuations			
Etodolac 400–800 mg	11	642	9
Diclofenac 100–150 mg	10	435	9
Naproxen 500–1000 mg	8	415	8
Piroxicam 20 mg	5	330	9
Nabumetone 1000–1500 mg	2	124	8
Flurbiprofen 100–150 mg	2	110	5
Placebo	3	185	10
Upper gastrointestinal problems			
Etodolac 400–800 mg	12	746	18
Diclofenac 100–150 mg	8	367	20
Naproxen 500–1000 mg	8	415	17
Piroxicam 20 mg	4	311	23
Placebo	4	291	9
Dyspepsia			
Etodolac 400–800 mg	10	630	9
Piroxicam 20 mg	4	285	16
Naproxen 500–1000 mg	3	250	19
Placebo	3	185	11

Data calculated when at least 100 treated patients or two studies available. Upper GI problems includes dyspepsia, abdominal pain, nausea, vomiting, etc.

on small head-to-head comparisons performed mainly for registration or marketing purposes, rather than to illuminate the treatment of arthritis or chronic pain.

5.4 **Topically applied non-steroidal anti-inflammatory drugs for chronic pain**

Clinical bottom line. Topical NSAIDs provide effective pain relief. This relief seems comparable to that offered by oral NSAIDs. Topical NSAIDs had a combined number-needed-to-treat (NNT) of 3.1 (2.7–3.8) for at least 50% pain relief at two weeks after beginning treatment. Importantly, topical application of NSAIDs is not associated with serious side effects, and therefore provides an effective method of pain relief without the gastrointestinal effects seen with the same drugs taken orally.

Oral NSAIDs are associated with increased risk of adverse effects such as gastrointestinal problems. The question arises therefore whether topical NSAIDs, which are widely available without prescription, are more suitable for a number of conditions. However, it has also been argued that topical NSAIDs have no action other than as rubefacients.

Systematic review

Moore, R. A., Carroll, D., Wiffen, P. J., Tramer, M. and McQuay, H. J. (1998). Quantitive systematic review of topically-applied non-steroidal anti-inflammatory drugs, *BMJ* 316: 333–8.

Date review completed: September 1996

Number of trials included: 13 placebo controlled/12 active controlled

Number of patients: 1161 in placebo-controlled trials plus 1272 in active-controlled trials

Control group: Topically applied placebo, other topical NSAIDs, other formulations or route of administration

Main outcomes: Successful treatment defined as at least 50% pain relief using standard pain scales at approximately two weeks after start of treatment. Number-needed-to-treat, relative risk and relative benefit (with 95% confidence intervals).

Inclusion criteria were randomised controlled trials of NSAIDs with pain outcomes; chronic pain conditions (arthritic and rheumatic); full journal publication and unpublished drug company trials. Trials in vaginitis, oral and buccal conditions, thrombophlebitis and experimental pain were excluded. Dichotomous data on pain outcomes were extracted from trials for analysis. At least 50% pain relief was regarded as a clinically relevant outcome. From the dichotomous data, information on the proportion, and then the number of patients who achieved at least 50% pain relief were calculated. A NNT for at least 50% pain relief and the relative risk and benefit of the treatment were then calculated. The review also included a meta-analysis of topical NSAID use in acute pain.

Findings

Topical NSAID versus placebo

Most trials were in single joint arthritis and rheumatological disorders. Twelve trials reported dichotomous outcomes (Figure 5.4.1). Seven of 12 trials showed significant benefit of topical NSAID over placebo. The trial with no dichotomous outcomes also reported significant benefit of topical NSAID over placebo. When the data were combined, the pooled relative benefit was 2.0 (1.5–2.7), with a NNT of 3.1 (2.7–3.8) for successful treatment. Results for studies with higher quality scores, and larger numbers, were similar to the overall result (Table 5.4.1).

Topical NSAID versus oral NSAID

Two trials compared topical with oral NSAIDs. Neither showed significant benefit of oral over topical.

Adverse effects

There were no significant differences in the frequency of local or systemic adverse effects or drug-related withdrawals (Table 5.4.1).

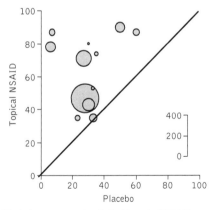

Figure 5.4.1 At least 50% pain relief with topical NSAID versus placebo.

Table 5.4.1 Results for chronic painful conditions (combined data for efficacy/adverse events)

	Trials	Patients	Average number of treated patients	Response with placebo (%)	Response with active (%)	Relative benefit (95% CI)	NNT (95% CI)
Combined efficacy data	12	1097		30	65	2.0 (1.5–2.7)	3.1 (2.7–3.8)
Trials of quality score 3–5 only	9	987	55	27	62	2.2 (1.5–3.1)	3.1 (2.6–3.8)
Trials with treatment groups >40 patients	6	836	70	29	61	2.0 (1.7–2.4)	3.3 (2.8–4.3)
Trials with treatment groups <40 patients	6	261	22	31	69	2.2 (1.5–3.1)	2.6 (2.0–3.6)
Local adverse effects				5.3	5.9	0.9 (0.4–1.7)	
Systemic adverse effects				1.3	1.1	1.1 (0.5–2.3)	
Withdrawal due to adverse effects				0.7	0.7	1.0 (0.4–2.4)	

Response is either proportion of patients achieving at least 50% pain relief or percent of patients having an adverse effect.

Comment

Topical NSAIDs were effective in short-term (two week) clinical trials compared with placebo. It was not just the rubbing. What is not known is their efficacy over longer periods, nor is it known whether any one NSAID is better than another for this indication.

5.5 **Coxibs for treating rheumatoid and osteoarthritis**

Coxibs are drug that selectively inhibit the cyclooxygenase-2 enzyme without inhibiting cyclooxygenase-1. This, of course, is at normal (licensed) doses, and as doses increase some inhibition of cyclooxygenase-1 is likely. The importance of the difference between coxibs and standard NSAIDs, is that NSAIDs inhibit both enzymes. There are many different ways of measuring cyclooxygenase activity and inhibition, and much is made about how different drugs inhibit different enzymes in different systems, little of which is relevant to the properties of the drugs in clinical practice.

The key issue is this. Cyclooxygenase-1 is largely constitutive and responsible for, among other functions, protecting the stomach and duodenum from acid attack. Inhibition leads to poorer protection, and the development of erosions and ulcers, bleeding, and even death from a bleeding ulcer (see section 5.6). Cyclooxygenase-2 is largely inducible and responsible for actions that lead to pain. Inhibition should reduce pain. Cyclooxygenase-2 is constitutive in brain and kidney.

What we should expect from coxibs, therefore, is what we get from NSAIDs, but with better gastrointestinal safety. This supposes that there are no other issues that have yet to be revealed. Certainly, there should be no expectation for better efficacy, other than from longer duration of action.

Efficacy of coxibs

What we do have for the coxibs is a large body of evidence from large trials that are often also of long duration. The available evidence for rofecoxib is shown in Table 5.5.1, for celecoxib in Table 5.5.2 and for etoricoxib in Table 5.5.3. They show the coxibs to be more effective than placebo, and as effective as maximum daily doses of standard NSAIDs (ibuprofen 2400 mg, diclofenac 150 mg, naproxen 1000 mg daily).

Discontinuations

Much attention has been given to the gastrointestinal adverse effects of coxibs compared with NSAIDs. In clinical practice this is just one of the reasons why patients discontinue treatment. For instance, we know that over about 6 weeks, 5–10% of patients discontinue with NSAID or placebo because of adverse events (section 5.4). Knowing the rate of total discontinuation, adverse event discontinuations and discontinuations because of lack of effect is useful, and the results for placebo, paracetamol, NSAID and rofecoxib and celecoxib are shown in Table 5.5.4 and total discontinuations in Figure 5.5.1.

Table 5.5.1 Clinical trials of rofecoxib in rheumatoid and osteoarthritis

Reference	Design	Patients	Treatments	Outcomes	Results	Discontinuations
Rheumatoid arthritis						
Schnitzer et al. Clin Therap 1999 21: 1688–1702.	Randomised, double blind, placebo controlled over 8 weeks	RA with VAS pain score of >40 mm, >8 tender joints and >5 swollen joints	Rofecoxib 5 mg (n = 158) Rofecoxib 25 mg (n = 171) Rofecoxib 50 mg (n = 161) Placebo (n = 168) (7800 mg paracetamol allowed/2 weeks)	ACR 20 response, patient assessment of pain and disease activity. Adverse events	Higher doses of rofecoxib significantly better than placebo for all efficacy outcomes. Maximum effect after 2–4 weeks	Total discontinuations similar to placebo (15–20%). Smaller number through lack of efficacy.
Bombardier et al. NEJM 2000 343: 1520–28.	Randomised, double blind, comparison with naproxen for median of 9 months	RA at least 50 years old, or 40 on steroids.	Rofecoxib 50 mg (n = 4047) Naproxen 1000 mg (n = 4029)	Global assessment of disease activity	No difference between rofecoxib 50 mg and naproxen 1000 mg	Total discontinuations similar in both groups (about 29%). Significant reduction in perforations, ulcers, and bleeds with rofecoxib.
Osteoarthritis						
Laine et al. Gastroenterol	Randomised comparison of	Randomised comparison of	Rofecoxib 25 mg (n = 195)	No efficacy measures	No efficacy results	Total discontinuations were 30–34% for

Reference	Design	Treatment	Efficacy measures	Results
1999 117: 776–83.	rofecoxib with ibuprofen and placebo for 12 weeks	Rofecoxib 50 mg (n = 186) Ibuprofen 2400 mg (n = 184) Placebo (n = 177) (paracetamol allowed daily)	No efficacy results	placebo and rofecoxib, 61% with ibuprofen, but these included endoscopic ulcers and erosions
Hawkey et al. Arth Rheum 2000 43: 370–7	Randomised comparison of rofecoxib with ibuprofen and placebo for 12 weeks	Rofecoxib 25 mg (n = 195) Rofecoxib 50 mg (n = 186) Ibuprofen 2400 mg (n = 184) Placebo (n = 177) (paracetamol allowed daily)	No efficacy measures	Total discontinuations were 29–34% for placebo and rofecoxib, 59% with ibuprofen, but these included endoscopic ulcers and erosions
Cannon et al. Arth Rheum 2000 43: 978–987	Randomised, double blind comparison of doses of rofecoxib with diclofenac over 1 year. Patients at least 40 years old with OA of hip two or knee and at least 40 mm on VAS pain scale.	Rofecoxib 12.5 mg (n = 259) Rofecoxib 25 mg (n = 257) Diclofenac 150 mg (n = 268)	WOMAC pain on walking, patients assessment of response and physician assessment of disease status	All three treatments were comparable on all three outcomes. Maximum effect after 2–4 weeks. Total discontinuations similar in all groups (38–46%)

Table 5.5.1 continued

Reference	Design	Patients	Treatments	Outcomes	Results	Discontinuations
Day et al. Arch Intern Med 2000 160: 1781–7.	Randomised, double blind comparison of two doses of rofecoxib with ibuprofen and placebo over 6 weeks	Patients at least 40 years old with OA of hip or knee and at least 40 mm on VAS pain scale	Rofecoxib 12.5 mg ($n = 244$) Rofecoxib 25 mg ($n = 242$) Ibuprofen 2400 mg ($n = 249$) Placebo ($n = 74$) (2,600 mg paracetamol allowed daily)	WOMAC pain on walking, patients assessment of response and physician assessment of disease status	All three treatments were comparable on all three outcomes and better than placebo. Maximum effect after 2–4 weeks	Total discontinuations ranged from 6–14%, with more lack of efficacy discontinuations with placebo and more adverse event discontinuations with ibuprofen
Saag et al. Arch Fam Med 2000 9: 1124–34. Study 1	Randomised, double blind comparison of two doses of rofecoxib with ibuprofen and placebo over 6 weeks	Patients at least 40 years old with OA of hip or knee and at least 40 mm on VAS pain scale	Rofecoxib 12.5 mg ($n = 219$) Rofecoxib 25 mg ($n = 227$) Ibuprofen 2400 mg ($n = 221$) Placebo ($n = 69$) (paracetamol allowed daily)	WOMAC pain on walking, physical functioning and morning stiffness	All three treatments were comparable on all three outcomes and better than placebo. Maximum effect after 2–4 weeks	Total discontinuations ranged from 11–28%, with more lack of efficacy discontinuations with placebo

Study	Design	Patients	Treatments	Outcomes	Results	Discontinuations
Saag et al. Arch Fam Med 2000 9: 1124–34. Study 2	Randomised, double blind comparison of two doses of rofecoxib with diclofenac over 1 year	Patients at least 40 years old with OA of hip or knee and at least 40 mm on VAS pain scale	Rofecoxib 12.5 mg (n = 231) Rofecoxib 25 mg (n = 232) Diclofenac 150 mg (n = 230)	WOMAC pain on walking, physical functioning and morning stiffness	All three treatments were of comparable efficacy	Total discontinuations similar in all groups (32–36%)
Geba et al. JAMA 2002 287: 64–71.	Randomised double blind comparison of two doses of rofecoxib with celecoxib and paracetamol for 6 weeks	Patients at least 40 years old with OA of hip or knee and at least 40 mm on VAS pain scale	Rofecoxib 12.5 mg (n = 96) Rofecoxib 25 mg (n = 95) Celecoxib 200 mg (n = 97) Paracetamol 2400 mg (n = 94)	WOMAC pain on walking, at night and at rest, and patient global evaluation	Rofecoxib 25 mg was generally superior to other treatments	Total discontinuations were 17–30%
Lisse et al. (ADVANTAGE) 2002	Randomised, double blind, comparison with naproxen for 12 weeks	Patients at least 40 years old with OA of hip or knee for at least 6 months	Rofecoxib 25 mg (n = 2785) Naproxen 1000 mg (n = 2772)	Patient global assessment, SF-36 and others	No difference between treatments	Lack of efficacy discontinuations 6.4% in both groups

Table 5.5.2 Clinical trials of celecoxib in rheumatoid and osteoarthritis

Reference	Design	Patients	Treatments	Outcomes	Results	Discontinuations
Rheumatoid arthritis						
Simon et al. Arth Rheum 1998 41: 1591–1602.	Randomised double blind comparison of celecoxib with placebo over 4 weeks	Patients with RA in a flare state with at least six tender and three swollen joints	Celecoxib 80 mg (n = 81) Celecoxib 400 mg (n = 82) Celecoxib 800 mg (n = 82) Placebo (n = 85)	Physician and patient global assessment, pain, swelling, tenderness and others	Higher doses of celecoxib better than placebo	Lack of efficacy discontinuations were 4–18%
Emery et al. Lancet 1999 354: 2106–2011	Randomised double blind comparison of celecoxib and diclofenac over 6 months	Patients with RA of at least six months duration	Celecoxib 400 mg (n = 326) Diclofenac 150 mg (n = 329)	Patient and physician assessments and ACR 20 plus pain plus others	Treatments same efficacy for almost all outcomes	Total discontinuations were 20% for celecoxib and 28% for diclofenac
Simon et al. JAMA 1999 282: 1921–1928	Randomised double blind comparison of celecoxib and naproxen and placebo over 3 months	Patients with RA of at least three months duration and at least six tender and three swollen joints	Celecoxib 200 mg (n = 240) Celecoxib 400 mg (n = 235) Celecoxib 800 mg (n = 218) Naproxen 1000 mg (n = 225) Placebo (n = 231)	Number of tender and swollen joints, patients assessment, ACR-20	All active treatments similar and superior to placebo	Total discontinuations were 33–56%, predominantly lack of efficacy
Osteoarthritis						
Simon et al. Arth Rheum 1998 41: 1591–1602.	Randomised double blind comparison of celecoxib with placebo over 2 weeks	Patients with OA of the knee in a flare state	Celecoxib 80 mg (n = 73) Celecoxib 200 mg (n = 76) Celecoxib 400 mg (n = 73) Placebo (n = 71)	Physician and patient global assessment, pain, and others	Higher doses of celecoxib better than placebo	Lack of efficacy discontinuations were 1–14%

Reference	Study design	Patients	Treatments	Outcomes	Results	Overall
Bensen et al. Mayo Clin Proc 1999 74: 1095–105.	Randomised double blind comparison of celecoxib with naproxen and placebo over 6 months	Patients with OA with worsening on treatment discontinuation	Celecoxib 100 mg (n = 203) Celecoxib 200 mg (n = 197) Celecoxib 400 mg (n = 202) Naproxen 1000 mg (n = 198) Placebo (n = 203)	Physician and patient global assessment, WOMAC and others	Active treatments better than placebo, with maximum effect at 2–4 weeks.	Overall discontinuation was 43%, mainly due to lack of effect, but numbers in tables do not add up.
Williams et al. J Clin Rheumatol 2000 6: 65–74.	Randomised double blind comparison of celecoxib with placebo over 6 weeks	Patients with OA of the knee with worsening on treatment discontinuation	Celecoxib 200 mg (n = 231) Celecoxib 200 mg (n = 223) Placebo (n = 232)	Physician and patient global assessment, functional capacity, and Lequesne index	Active treatments similar and superior to placebo	Overall discontinuation was 16–37%, with lack of effect predominating for placebo
Silverstein et al. JAMA 2000 284: 1247–55.	Randomised double blind comparison of celecoxib with ibuprofen and diclofenac for up to 13 months (6 months reported)	Patients over 18 years with RA or OA for at least 3 months	Celecoxib 800 mg (n = 3987) Ibuprofen 2,400 mg or diclofenac 150 mg (n = 3981)	No efficacy assessment	No efficacy result	Total withdrawals were 29% with celecoxib and 45% with NSAID (57% of patients had 6 months treatment)

Table 5.5.3 Clinical trials of etoricoxib in rheumatoid arthritis

Reference	Design	Patients	Treatments	Outcomes	Results	Discontinuations
Rheumatoid arthritis						
Collantes et al. BMC Family Practice 2002 3:10	Randomised double blind comparison of etoricoxib with placebo or naproxen over 12 weeks	Patients with RA in a flare state with at least six tender and three swollen joints, and have RA for at least 6 months	Etoricoxib 90 mg (*n* = 353) Naproxen 1000 mg (*n* = 181) Placebo (*n* = 357)	Many different clinical and laboratory findings	Etoricoxib and naproxen were equally efficacious, and both better than placebo	Lack of efficacy discontinuations were 25% with placebo, 13% with etoricoxib and 11% with naproxen

Table 5.5.4 Discontinuations in clinical trials of coxibs

Drug	2–6 weeks		8–12 weeks		24–26 weeks		36–52 weeks	
	Percent	Number	Percent	Number	Percent	Number	Percent	Number
Total discontinuation								
Placebo	28	531	31	973				
Paracetamol	31	94						
NSAID	13	470	29	423	43	4640	30	4527
Rofecoxib	12	1123	16	332	24	769	31	5026
Celecoxib	14	864	27	1295	39	4269		
Adverse event discontinuation								
Placebo	6.0	531	4.6	973				
Paracetamol	6.4	94						
NSAID	6.4	470	4.7	423	20	4311	16	4527
Rofecoxib	5.3	1123	5.4	332	9.8	769	16	5026
Celecoxib	4.4	864	5.9	1295	19	3943		
Lack of efficacy discontinuation								
Placebo	19.0	531	20.0	973				
Paracetamol	17.0	94						
NSAID	6.0	470	8.3	3195	14	4311	7.1	4527
Rofecoxib	5.1	1123	6.4	3117	16	769	8.0	5026
Celecoxib	6.9	864	19.0	1295	13	3943		

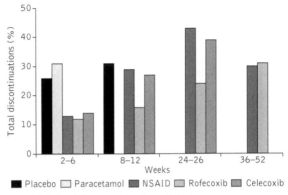

Figure 5.5.1 Total discontinuations in coxib trials.

Total discontinuations with placebo are high early, mainly because of lack of effect (though paracetamol is usually given as escape analgesic). Paracetamol has much the same discontinuation rate. NSAIDs and coxibs have more discontinuations later. The message, though, is that even with the potentially greater safety of coxibs, 30–40% of patients will need their medicine changed for some reason within six months to one year. With paracetamol it may be higher.

Comment

Efficacy is not an issue, in the sense that the coxibs work as effectively as NSAIDs. What we do not have is any analysis to tell us which patients do well on what drugs, and why. We are still left with patients with arthritis whose average pain is moderate while on treatment. Even more relevant, but what we don't have, is some sensible care pathway, based on good evidence.

5.6 **Adverse effects of NSAIDs and coxibs**

NSAID gastrointesinal adverse effects

Epidemiological studies associating NSAID use and upper GI problems and published in the 1990s have been reviewed and the data pooled [1] to give a much clearer picture of risks. To be included studies had to:

+ be case control or cohort studies on non-aspirin NSAIDs;

+ include data on bleeding, perforation, or other serious upper gastrointestinal tract event resulting in hospital admission or referral to a specialist;

+ have data to calculate relative risk.

Eighteen such studies were found. All had specific definitions of exposure and outcome and similar ascertainment for comparison groups. All but two attempted to control for potential confounding factors, like age, sex, history of ulcer or concomitant medicines.

The main results are summarised in Figures 5.6.1 and 5.6.2. Compared with nonusers, NSAID users had a higher risk of upper GI bleed (UGIB) when they were current NSAID users and used a higher dose. The duration of use was unimportant, but different NSAIDs had different risks, with ibuprofen (especially doses below 2400 mg a day) being least harmful.

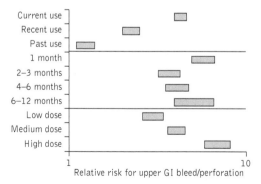

Figure 5.6.1 Risk of UGIB for NSAID users compared with non-users.

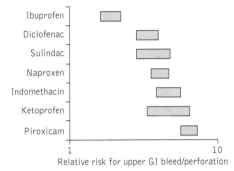

Figure 5.6.2 Risk of UGIB for particular NSAIDs, users compared with non-users.

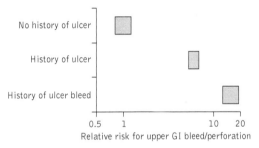

Figure 5.6.3 Effect of history of ulcer in users of NSAIDs.

The effect of ulcer history and age is shown in Figures 5.6.3 and 5.6.4. People with a history of ulcer or with a previous bleed who took NSAIDs were at much greater risk than those with no history of ulcer who took NSAIDs. Older folk who took NSAIDs were at greater risk than under 50s who took NSAIDs.

In this set of high quality studies, there was a clear effect of size on the estimate of relative risk of upper gastrointestinal bleed with NSAID. The pooled estimate was 3.8 (3.6–4.1).

The risk to the individual

Relative risks are useful, but not always transferable to risks for individuals. A large systematic review looked at all studies of NSAID or aspirin use for more than two months to try to estimate the absolute risk of NSAID use [2]. It concluded that bleeding or perforation occurred in about 0.7% of patients in randomised trials taking an

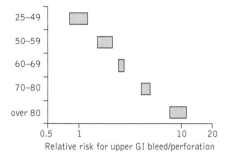

Figure 5.6.4 Effect of age in users of NSAIDs.

NSAID, and that bleeding or perforation carried a mortality risk of about 10%. Taking an NSAID for two months or more carried an absolute risk of:

1 in 5 for presence of an endoscopic ulcer,

1 in 70 of a symptomatic ulcer,

1 in 150 of a bleeding ulcer,

1 in 1200 of dying from a bleeding ulcer.

For comparison, the chance of dying on the roads in the UK in any one year is a (crude) 1 in 17,000.

The burden of NSAID adverse effects in the UK

There are three large-scale surveys, each looking at about 1% of the population, which can inform the arguments about the burden of NSAID adverse events in the UK [3–5].

Blower *et al.*

A retrospective case-control survey of emergency admissions for upper gastrointestinal disease in two English general hospitals covering 1% of the UK population (in Rotherham and Stockport) gives some good estimates [3]. Records of all community deaths attributed to upper gastrointestinal disease were also surveyed. Matched controls were identified from emergency admissions for other causes.

There were 620 emergency admissions over one year in 1990/91, with controls for 460 cases. Controls were matched for GP practice, sex, age and date of admission. Unmatched cases were retained in the analysis.

Results

Cases and controls were well matched, except for musculoskeletal disease (24% versus 3%). Cases were more likely to be using NSAIDs

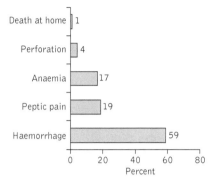

Figure 5.6.5 Presentation of cases by number and percent of total.

(31% versus 16%), H2-receptor antagonists (20% versus 5%), ferrous sulphate (9% versus 2%) and prednisolone (7% versus 3%).

Cases presented largely (59%) as haemorrhage (Figure 5.6.5), with a small proportion presenting as perforation, and 1% dying at home. Blood transfusion was required in 36% of all cases, and in 50% of those taking NSAIDs. NSAID users needed significantly more blood transfused than non-users. NSAID users also required a significantly longer stay (24% had a hospital stay of more than 14 days). NSAID users were more likely to die: overall mortality was 20% in NSAID users compared with 14% in non-users.

Extrapolation to the UK
These results suggest an overall incidence of upper gastrointestinal emergencies in the UK of 147 per 100,000 of the adult population, with an incidence of gastrointestinal haemorrhage of 87/100,000. This would indicate about 65,000 such crises a year in the UK. The study estimated that 1.9% of NSAID users in the Rotherham and Stockport area were admitted to hospital each year with upper gastrointestinal emergencies. The NSAID-attributable number of NSAID-associated emergency admissions in the UK would be about 12,000, with about 2500 deaths.

The data from this study also gave age-related NSAID-specific incidence figures which have been used [6] to calculate the burden of hospital admissions for an average Primary Care Group of 100,000 people (Table 5.6.1). It shows that there would be 24 emergency admissions, and about five deaths, in any one year.

Based on these figures for hospital admission, plus information on the likely cost of co-prescribing with acid-suppressing medicines, the

Table 5.6.1 Calculations of NSAID-related admissions for an average Primary Care Group of 100,000 people

Age range (years)	Percent of total population	Number	Percent prescribed NSAIDs	Number prescribed NSAIDs	Annual incidence of upper GI crisis (%)	Annual number admitted to hospital from an average PCG	Annual UK total admissions
16–45	42	42,000	5	2100	0.07	1	802
45–64	19	19,000	17	3230	0.146	5	2641
65–74	12	12,000	19	2280	0.187	4	2224
≥75	7	7000	22	1540	0.904	14	6514
						24	12,181

cost to the UK of NSAID gastrointestinal adverse events is about £250 million a year [6]. This is equivalent to an adverse event cost of about £50 a year for every patient prescribed an NSAID.

Hawkey *et al.*

Another study in Nottingham [4] prospectively interviewed 500 patients over 60 years admitted to the city's two hospitals with peptic ulcer bleeding over a 5-year period. A structured questionnaire was used to determine NSAID use. General practice prescribing was also examined for patients admitted, looking at 103 general practices responsible for half a million people.

Results

Overall NSAID prescribing varied greatly, by about 6-fold from lowest to highest prescribing practices, even when patient mix was taken into account. NSAID prescribing was the main determinant of emergency GI admissions from practices. Raw prescribing rates were between 137 items per 1000 population and 833 items per 1000. The average admission rate for bleeding peptic ulcer was 15 per 100,000 per year. Analysis indicated a 0.23% (95% confidence interval 0.08–0.31%) increase in the rate of ulcer bleeding of all causes in the elderly for each increase of 1 NSAID prescription per 1000 patients. This is equivalent to one episode of ulcer bleeding in the elderly per 2,823 (95% confidence interval 2095–8116) prescriptions.

MacDonald *et al.*

This cohort study from Scotland [5] looked at the relative risk of hospital admission for 52,000 people over 50 who received at least one NSAID prescription and 74,000 controls who did not. About 2% of the NSAID cohort were admitted to hospital with a gastrointestinal event over three years, compared with 1.4% of controls – suggesting that about 0.2% of the over 50s population can be admitted in any one year because of NSAID-related gastrointestinal events. The risk of gastrointestinal bleeding or perforation was similar at all times after first day of NSAID exposure.

Renal failure

People who work in renal units will tell you about the association between NSAIDs and acute renal failure. The problem has been to get a reliable estimate of the risk. There have been some small studies, but a new, large study from Tennessee gives us a better picture [7].

The study was conducted among all members of the Tennessee Medicaid programme aged 65 years or more in 1987–91 and enrolled for at least one year. Those with first admission to hospital for acute renal failure (admission creatinine level of 180 μmol/L or more at admission) were the cases of community acquired acute renal failure. Controls were randomly selected for all persons in the study population. Exclusions were people with end stage renal disease and those with hospital acquired acute renal failure. NSAID exposure was ascertained from prescriptions filled in the year before the index date.

Results

There were 1799 cases with an annual incidence of community acquired acute renal failure of 4.5 admissions per 1000. The median hospital stay was eight days. Thirty-six percent died within 30 days. Forty-two percent were classified as having new renal disease. The remainder were classified as having chronic renal failure with acute exacerbation based on a prior creatinine level above 122 μmol/L, a documented history of chronic renal failure or imaging studies compatible with chronic renal disease. There were 9899 controls. Controls were less likely to be nursing home residents or be 85 years or older.

NSAID use was higher (18%) in cases than in controls (11%). For current NSAID use the odds ratio was 1.6 (95% confidence interval 1.3–1.9). Those who had stopped using NSAIDs within the past 30 days had no increased risk of renal failure. For certain NSAIDs where there was sufficient information, ibuprofen and indomethacin, there was a dose response for risk. For individual NSAIDs, ibuprofen, piroxicam, fenoprofen and indomethacin had the greatest increased risk, with odds ratios of about 2.

A previous detailed study [8], though on smaller numbers, indicated that previous renal disease, or gout, but particularly a combined history of gout plus previous renal disease were major risks for renal failure with NSAIDs. Patients using NSAIDs with half-lives of 12 h or more in the previous week had particularly increased risk of renal failure.

Congestive heart failure

It seems as if we also have to begin to worry about NSAIDs being related to congestive heart failure (CHF) in older people [9].

This study at two hospitals in New South Wales (population about 450,000) enrolled as cases consecutive patients between 1993 and 1995 where the medical officer admitting the case and the attending physician agreed that the primary reason for admission was CHF. Patients admitted for other reasons with incidental CHF were not included. Study nurses ensured that all included cases met Framingham criteria for CHF. Controls (target two per case) were patients of the same sex and within five years of age admitted to the same hospital, but with no clinical or radiological signs of CHF.

Results

There were 365 cases and 658 controls, with a mean age of 76 years. Most cases had moderate or severe CHF. Use of non-aspirin NSAIDs was 17% in the cases in the week before admission, compared with

12% in controls. The adjusted odds ratio was 2.1 (5% confidence interval 1.2–3.3) for all cases, and 2.8 (1.5–5.1) for the 272 cases with first admission for CHF.

CHF was far more likely in those patients with a prior history of heart disease, in which the odds ratio was 26 (5.8–119). Complicated statistical analysis confirmed the effect of pre-existing heart disease, and also suggested that NSAIDs with longer half lives (naproxen, piroxicam and tenoxicam) had much higher risk than those with short half lives (ibuprofen, diclofenac, for instance), though on small numbers in a sub group analysis.

Comment

Table 5.6.2 puts all this into the perspective of an average PCG of 100,000 for the over-65s. In this group there would be 18 hospital admissions every year for upper gastrointestinal bleeding, 10 for acute renal failure and 22 for congestive heart failure. These latter seem high, but in both cases the bulk of the events would be in those aged 75 and over. Age is certainly the issue.

Also important is that for renal failure and CHF the mechanism seems to be uncovering incipient disease. For renal failure there are several, if smaller, studies. For CHF there is at least one other confirmatory study [10]. For both there appears to be plausible mechanisms, dose-response relationships, and particular association with NSAIDs with longer half-lives. Renal failure has a high mortality, and CHF is also serious, as treatment is unlikely to restore patient's functioning to previous levels.

The good news is that, for most older patients, sensible assessment and pertinent guidance should mean that many of these events could be avoided. While the new coxibs are not associated with elevated risks of gastrointestinal bleeding, there is no evidence, or indeed likelihood, that they will not precipitate renal failure or CHF.

Put in a humanitarian and economic context, these 50 first hospital admissions a year per PCG of 100,000 population is equivalent to 30,000 admissions a year in the UK. Most are avoidable. The information we have suggests the average stay to be about a week, costing about £1400 each. That is something like £40–50 million a year for the NHS.

Table 5.6.2 Impact of NSAID adverse effects on a typical population of 100,000

Event	Cases per year
Upper GI bleed	18
Acute renal failure	10
Congestive heart failure	22

Information based on average PCG of 100,000 patients where 3800 over-65s take NSAIDs

Coxib gastrointestinal adverse events

The evidence that coxibs reduce gastrointestinal adverse events comes principally from two sources. First is the demonstration that coxibs cause less gastric or duodenal damage than NSAIDs by looking through an endoscope, where the target is (usually) erosion or small ulcers 3–5 mm across. More relevant is the demonstration of a reduced incidence of serious gastrointestinal adverse events, usually called perforations, ulcer, or bleeds (PUBs).

An example of the former comes from two randomised double blind studies [11,12] that examined endoscopic gastroduodenal ulcers in 1427 patients with osteoarthritis. Patients were randomised to placebo, 25 or 50 mg rofecoxib daily, or 2400 ibuprofen daily for up to 6 months with active treatment and three months with placebo. The combined results (Figure 5.6.6) showed that the cumulative incidence of ulcers of ≥3 mm was no different for placebo or rofecoxib up to three months. At six months the incidence was much higher with ibuprofen (46%) than with rofecoxib (12%), with a number needed to treat of 2.9 (95% confidence interval 2.5–3.4) for rofecoxib. This means that for every three patients treated with rofecoxib 25/50 mg daily rather than ibuprofen 2400 mg daily for 6 months, one endoscopically detected ulcer ≥3 mm would be prevented.

Evidence supporting reduced incidence of PUBs is summarised in Table 5.6.3. Two pre-planned meta-analyses and at least one large, prospective randomised trial confirm that coxibs result in lower rates of PUBs. One of the trials has been severely criticised, though, and while the reference and details are given, the results are not because it is not clear that they can be trusted. One excellent feature of these studies was that the gastrointestinal events were judged on predefined grounds, and the judgement made by an independent adjudication committee blinded to the treatment.

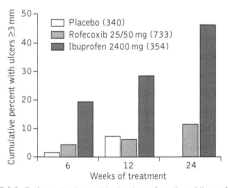

Figure 5.6.6 Endoscopic ulcers with placebo, rofecoxib and ibuprofen.

Table 5.6.3 Evidence of reduced PUBs with coxibs

Reference	Design	Included patients	Major exclusions	Treatments	Outcome	Results
Langman et al. JAMA 1999 282: 1929–23.	Prespecified meta-analysis of 8 randomised, double-blind trials of rofecoxib in osteoarthritis. Total 5435 patients with mean follow up of about 5 months for active treatments	Typically patients were aged 40 years or older, with clinical and radiological evidence of OA of knee or hip, and with pain at least 40 mm (moderate) when not treated. Mean age was 63 years, range 38–94, 75% women, 44% smokers	Premenopausal women, patients with renal impairment, clinically significant abnormalities, positive faecal occult blood, moderate-severe angina, uncontrolled congestive heart failure, stroke or TIA with last two years, recent cancer, allergy to paracetamol or NSAID. Use of aspirin, corticosteroid, warfarin or ticlopidine	Rofecoxib 12.5, 25, 50 mg Ibuprofen 2400 mg, diclofenac 150 mg, nabumetone 1500 mg Placebo	Predefined perforation, active ulcer, clinically significant haemorrhage, adjudicated by independent, external blind committee	Significant reduction in PUB rate with rofecoxib compared with NSAID with 49 PUBs. Cumulative incidence after 12 months was 1.3% versus 1.8% and relative risk over 12 months 0.5 (0.3–1). No difference between rofecoxib and placebo over 4 months
Bombardier et al. NEJM 2000 343: 1520–28.	Randomised, double blind comparison of rofecoxib and naproxen in 8076 patients with RA for mean follow up of 9 months	Age at least 50 years, or 40 with glucocorticoid therapy, with RA. Mean age 58 years, 79% women.	History of other inflammatory arthritis, upper gastrointestinal surgery, inflammatory bowel disease, renal impairment, positive faecal occult blood test, unstable medical condition, recent cancer, or alcohol or drug abuse, or stroke within 2 years, or MI or	Rofecoxib 50 mg naproxen 1000 mg	Predefined perforation, active ulcer, clinically significant haemorrhage, adjudicated by independent,	Significant reduction in PUB rate with rofecoxib compared with naproxen with events in 177 patients. The relative risk was 0.5 (0.3–0.6). For complicated events the

Reference	Design	Inclusion criteria	Exclusion criteria	Drugs	Outcome definition	Results/Comments
Silverstein et al. JAMA 2000 284:1247–55.	Randomised, double blind comparison of celecoxib and ibuprofen or diclofenac in 8059 patients with OA and RA and mean follow up of 6 months	Patients 18 or older with RA or OA for at least 3 months. Mean age 60 years, range 20–90, 69% women, 16% smokers	Active gastrointestinal, renal or hepatic disease, or coagulation disorder, cancer bypass surgery within 1 year. use of aspirin, corticosteroid, warfarin or ticlopidine, acid suppressants and cyclosporin	Celecoxib 800 mg Ibuprofen 2400 mg Diclofenac 150 mg	Predefined perforation, active ulcer, clinically significant haemorrhage, adjudicated by independent, blind external adjudication committee blind external adjudication committee	relative risk was 0.4 (0.2–0.8) This study and its conduct and reporting have been heavily criticised (BMJ, 2002). It is not possible to say what the true result of this trial is
Goldstein et al. Am J Gastroenterol 2000 95:1681–90.	Pooled analysis of 14 randomised, double blind trials of celecoxib and NSAIDs for arthritis. Total 11,008 patients over 2–24 weeks	Not specifically described, but similar to other inclusion criteria	Not specifically described, but similar to other exclusion criteria	Celecoxib 50–800 mg Ibuprofen 2400 mg Diclofenac 100–150 mg Naproxen 1000 mg Placebo	Predefined for criteria outcomes with adjudication by independent, blind external committee	There were 11 ulcer complications, 2 on celecoxib and 9 on NSAID, with annualised incidences of 0.2% and 1.7% respectively. Statistically significant

Coxib renal adverse events

There is no expectation that renal adverse events of coxibs should be any different from those of standard NSAIDs. A pooled analysis of nine OA studies with rofecoxib appears to confirm that [13]. In over 5000 patients the incidence of lower extremity oedema was about 1% with placebo, and 3.4–4.3% with rofecoxib at various doses, or NSAIDs. Hypertension incidence was again about 1% with placebo and 2–4% with rofecoxib and NSAIDs.

Coxibs and cardiovascular events

A potential problem with coxibs was raised when a large randomised gastrointestinal safety study [14] noted that, while overall mortality was similar in patients given rofecoxib and naproxen (0.5% and 0.4%, respectively), myocardial infarction occurred more frequently with rofecoxib (0.4% versus 0.1%), and was statistically significant. Because aspirin use was not allowed in the trial, the question was whether rofecoxib caused myocardial infarction, or whether naproxen prevented it.

A review of 5435 patients in eight early studies showed similar event rates for the composite end point of cardiovascular, haemorrhagic and unknown death, myocardial infarction and cerebrovascular accident when rofecoxib was compared with conventional NSAID or placebo [15]. An even larger analysis of 23 trials with more than 28,000 patients suggested that naproxen was protective [16]. Again, using the same combined end point, it showed no difference between patients taking rofecoxib and those taking placebo, nor between rofecoxib and conventional NSAIDs. What it did show was a reduced rate of events with naproxen, and particularly for nonfatal myocardial infarction (myocardial infarction plus resuscitated cardiac arrest (Figure 5.6.7).

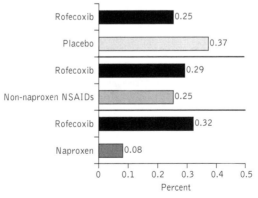

Figure 5.6.7 Pairwise comparison of non-fatal myocardial infarction for rofecoxib with placebo, non-naproxen NSAIDs and naproxen.

Comment

One of the most important features of the advent of coxibs has been the subsequent concentration on all adverse events from NSAIDs, and not just those associated with the gastrointestinal tract. For example, we now have much more light cast on the potential inhibition of NSAIDs on aspirin effects on platelets. Concomitant administration of ibuprofen, but not paracetamol, diclofenac or rofecoxib, antagonises the irreversible platelet aggregation from aspirin [17]. This potential for interactions between NSAIDs, coxibs and aspirin is important, because many patients with arthritis will have co-morbid conditions, some of which may require the use of low-dose aspirin.

Choosing the right balance of care for predominantly elderly people with the deleterious affects of ageing, and arthritis and other disorders, is becoming more complex. This is a good thing, because it is a topic that needs attention, but at the time of writing (June 2002), clear answers are not forthcoming. Adverse event information will be an important driver, though.

References

1. Hernández-Diaz, S. and García Rodriguez, L. A. (2000). Association between nonsteroidal anti-inflammatory drugs and upper gastrointestinal tract bleeding and perforation: an overview of epidemiological studies published in the 1990s, *Archives of Internal Medicine* 160: 2093–9.

2. Tramèr, M. R. *et al.* (2000). Quantitative estimation of rare adverse effects which follow a biological progression – a new model applied to chronic NSAID use, *Pain* 85: 169–82.

3. Blower, A. L. *et al.* (1997). Emergency admissions for upper gastrointestinal disease and their relation to NSAID use, *Alimentary Pharmacology and Therapeutics* 11: 283–91.

4. Hawkey, C. J. *et al.* (1997). Prescribing of nonsteroidal anti-inflammatory drugs in general practice: determinants and consequences, *Alimentary Pharmacology and Therapeutics* 11: 293–8.

5. MacDonald, T. M. *et al.* (1997). Association of upper gastrointestinal toxicity of non-steroidal anti-inflammatory drugs with continued exposure: cohort study. *BMJ* 315: 1333–7.

6. Moore, R. A. and Phillips, C. J. (1997). Cost of NSAID adverse effects to the UK National Health Service, *Journal of Medical Economics* 2: 45–55.

7. Griffin, M. R. *et al.* (2000). Nonsteroidal antiinflammattory drugs and acute renal failure in elderly persons, *American Journal of Epidemiology* 151: 488–96.

8. Henry, D. *et al.* (1997). Consumption of non-steroidal anti-inflammatory drugs and the development of functional renal impairment in elderly subjects. Results of a case-control study, *British Journal of Clinical Pharmacology* 44: 85–90.

9. Page, J. and Henry, D. (2000). Consumption of NSAIDs and the development of congestive heart failure in elderly patients: An underrecognized public health problem, *Archives of Internal Medicine* 160: 777–84.

10. Heerdink, E. R. *et al.* (1998). NSAIDs associated with increased risk of congestive heart failure in elderly patients taking diuretics, *Archives of Internal Medicine* 158: 1108–12.

11. Laine, L. *et al.* (1999). A randomized trial comparing the effect of rofecoxib, a cyclooxygenase 2-specific inhibitor, with that of ibuprofen on the gastroduodenal mucosa of patients with osteoarthritis, *Gastroenterology* 117: 776–83.

12. Hawkey, C. *et al.* (2000). Comparison of the effect of rofecoxib (a cyclooxygenase 2 inhibitor), ibuprofen, and placebo on the gastroduodenal mucosa of patients with osteoarthritis, *Arthritis & Rheumatism* 43: 370–77.

13. Gertz, B. J. *et al.* (2002). A comparison of adverse renovascular experiences among osteoarthritis patients treated with rofecoxib and comparator non-selective non-steroidal anti-inflammatory agents, *Current Medical Research & Opinion* 18: 82–91.

14. Bombardier, C. *et al.* (2000). Comparison of upper gastrointestinal toxicity of rofecoxib and naproxen in patients with rheumatoid arthritis. VIGOR Study Group, *NEJM* 343: 1520–28.

15. Reicin, A. S. *et al.* (2002). Comparison of cardiovascular thrombotic events in patients with osteoarthritis treated with rofecoxib versus nonselective nonsteroidal anti-inflammatory drugs (ibuprofen, diclofenac, and nabumetone). *Am J Cardiol* 89: 204–9.

16. Konstam, M. A. *et al.* (2001). Cardiovascular thrombotic events in controlled, clinical trials of rofecoxib, *Circulation* 104: 2280–8.

17. Catella-Lawson, F. *et al.* (2001). Cyclooxygenase inhibitors and the antiplatelet effects of aspirin, *NEJM* 345: 1809–17.

5.7 **Paracetamol (acetaminophen) for osteoarthritis**

Clinical bottom line. Four trials confirm clinical judgement, that paracetamol 4000 mg daily is better than placebo but probably inferior to top daily doses of NSAIDs. About a quarter of patients will discontinue over 4–6 weeks.

Systematic review

This Bandolier review was concluded in June 2002.

Date review completed: June 2002

Number of trials included: 4

Number of patients: 951

Control group: Placebo and active controls

Main outcomes: Improvement on a number of measures, and discontinuations

The main inclusion criteria were that trials had to be randomised and double blind, to have paracetamol (acetaminophen) at sensible doses of 3000 or 4000 mg a day (without any other added active agent), have a duration of at least four weeks, have at least 50 patients in the trial, and be in osteoarthritis.

Findings

There were only four trials that fulfilled these inclusion criteria, and the main results are outlined in Table 5.7.1. Paracetamol 4000 mg daily was better than placebo in one trial, about the same as ibuprofen, but inferior to diclofenac and rofecoxib at usual daily doses. Total discontinuations in 345 patients over 4–6 weeks were 27%, 8% because of adverse events and 9% because of lack of efficacy.

Comment

Based on this paucity of information it is hard to draw any sensible conclusions, other than such trials as we have broadly confirm clinical judgement, that paracetamol 4000 mg daily is effective for some patients, but will generally be inferior to top doses of NSAIDs.

Table 5.7.1 Trials of paracetamol in osteoarthritis

Reference	Design	Included patients	Major exclusions	Treatments	Outcome	Results	Total discontinuations
Geba et al. JAMA 2002 287: 64–71	Randomised, double-blind parallel group comparison with rofecoxib and celecoxib for 6 weeks	Symptomatic OA knee for six months, minimum VAS of 40 mm while off drug	Concurrent medical or arthritic disease with potential to confound or interfere, hypersensitivity	Paracetamol 4000 mg ($n = 94$) Rofecoxib 12.5 mg ($n = 96$) Rofecoxib 25 mg ($n = 95$) Celecoxib 200 mg ($n = 97$)	Pain on walking, pain at rest, at night, morning stiffness, global response	Both rofecoxib doses Significantly better than paracetamol (good, excellent response on patient global assessment)	Paracetamol 4000 mg (29/94) Rofecoxib 12.5 mg (17/96) Rofecoxib 25 mg (18/95) Celecoxib 200 mg (17/97)
Pincus et al. Arth Rheum 2001 44: 1587–98	Randomised, double-blind cross-over comparison with diclofenac + misoprostol for 6 weeks each period	Symptomatic OA of hip or knee, age over 40 years, VAS score of 30 mm or more	Severe comorbidity, hypersensitivity	Paracetamol 4000 mg ($n = 115$) Diclofenac 150 mg plus misoprostol 400 μg ($n = 112$)	Pain on walking, pain at rest, at night, morning stiffness, and others	Diclofenac had more efficacy, but more adverse effects than paracetamol	Paracetamol 4000 mg (33/115) Diclofenac 150 mg (40/112)

Study	Design	Population	Exclusion criteria	Treatments	Outcomes	Results	Adverse events
Bradley et al. NEJM 1991 325: 87–91	Randomised, double-blind parallel group comparison with ibuprofen for 4 weeks	OA knee with pain for at least three months, over 30 years	History of surgery, intraarticular corticosteroids, RA	Paracetamol 4000 mg ($n = 60$) Ibuprofen 1200 mg ($n = 61$) Ibuprofen 2400 mg ($n = 61$)	Tenderness, swelling, time for 50 foot walk	No difference between treatments	Paracetamol 4000 mg (16/61) Ibuprofen 1200 mg (12/62) Ibuprofen 2400 mg (12/61)
Kjaersgaard-Andersen et al. Pain 1990 43: 309–18	Randomised double-blind comparison of paracetamol with paracetamol and codeine over 4 weeks	Clinical and radiographic evidence of OA hip with chronic pain	Significant impairment of lungs, liver or kidneys, or peptic ulcer history	Paracetamol 3000 mg ($n = 75$) Paracetamol 3000 mg plus codeine 60 mg ($n = 83$)	Pain and adverse events	Trial discontinued early because of adverse events	Paracetamol 3000 mg (17/75) Paracetamol 3000 mg plus codeine 60 mg (43/83)

5.8 **TNF antibodies and rheumatoid arthritis**

Clinical bottom line. Anti-TNF treatments for rheumatoid arthritis are effective. The NNT for the ACR 20 outcome is about 2–3; for ACR 50 is about 4, and for ACR 70 is 7–11.

A real difficulty with original treatments is that evidence emerges slowly. This is particularly the case for chronic diseases where treatments may have to be assessed over long periods. This slow emergence means that initially there can be some difficulty in assessing whether the treatment works, how well it works, in whom it works, and what the economics are if it does work.

There comes a point, though, when there is sufficient evidence on which to pass a judgement, which is one reason the UK government set up its National Institute for Clinical Excellence (NICE). As part of its work, NICE now publishes on its Internet site the evidence on which its judgements are based. The way in which it assessed the evidence on anti-TNF treatments for rheumatoid arthritis [1] demonstrates a growing quality and maturity in its processes.

NICE evidence

The 138-page report from Birmingham is a good background read on rheumatoid arthritis and its treatment. It examines the background, diagnosis, pathology, current service provision, the interventions, its search strategy, the results in the form of a meta-analysis of major outcomes, detailed summaries of the trials involved including adverse events, and the health economic arguments, as well as the implications for the NHS.

Technology

Infliximab and etenercept are partially humanised monoclonal antibodies aiming to reduce the actions of circulating tumour necrosis factor (TNF).

Efficacy

With rheumatoid arthritis there are many possible outcomes, starting with the number of painful or swollen joints, through to health assessment questionnaires and quality of life. The most commonly used (though perhaps difficult to explain and use) measure is the ACR response criteria, a composite measure of seven indices:

* tender joint count,
* swollen joint count,

* global disease activity assessed by observer,
* global disease activity assessed by patient,
* patient assessment of pain,
* physical disability score (like health assessment questionnaire),
* acute phase response (CRP measurement, or ESR).

The ACR 20 response is defined as a 20% improvement in the first two of these, plus a 20% improvement in any three of the remaining five items. This is not an easy outcome to reach, though also being used now are ACR 50 and ACR 70, which are similar to the ACR 20 but at 50% and 70% improvements. These are very high hurdles of treatment efficacy and represent very significant clinical improvement.

Results

To at least give a flavour of the results obtained with these two monoclonal antibodies, the results for ACR 20, 50 and 70 are looked at here. There are issues about dose, and about duration. The NICE evidence combines different doses and duration, but shows that, in the main, this is a reasonable thing to do, at least for now.

Results were consistent between trials comparing the new treatments with placebo. Those for the ACR 20 for infliximab are shown in Figure 5.8.1, and for etenercept in Figure 5.8.2. The results for ACR 20, 50 and 70 outcomes are in Table 5.8.1. NNTs were about 2–3 for ACR 20, about 4 for ACR 50, and about 8 for ACR 70.

The analysis also shows that what happens with placebo depends on the difficulty of the outcome. With placebo about 14% of rheumatoid

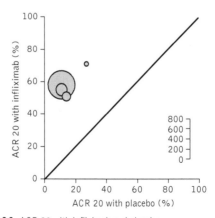

Figure 5.8.1 ACR 20 with infliximab and placebo.

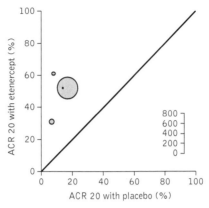

Figure 5.8.2 ACR 20 with etenercept and placebo.

arthritis patients achieved ACR 20. As the hurdle was raised to ACR 50 and 70, the percentage of patients achieving the outcome fell to about 6% and 1% respectively (Table 5.8.1).

Good information about adverse events is also given in the report, though not recounted here.

Comment

Given the evidence outlined in the report, it is clear why the British Society for Rheumatology recommended that infliximab and etenercept should be used if the following criteria were met:

• patients satisfy ACR classification for RA;

• patients have highly active RA;

• patients should have failed treatment on methotrexate and at least one other disease modifying agent;

• treated patients should be entered on a central register, with drugs, does, outcomes and toxicity reported on a quarterly basis.

Early referral

An essential accompaniment to the NICE evidence is an evidence-based early referral recommendation for newly diagnosed rheumatoid arthritis [2]. Based on a wide literature search by an international group of influential group of rheumatologists, this review provides clear support for the observations that permanent structural damage occurs early in the course of active rheumatoid arthritis and that early disease modifying drug intervention slows the progression of structural joint damage and improves long term outcomes, as well as overall quality of life.

Table 5.8.1 NNTs for infliximab and etenercept versus placebo at longest duration, and pooling all doses

Treatment	Outcome	Trials	Outcome [number/total (%)] with		Relative benefit (95% CI)	NNT (95% CI)
			Treatment	Placebo		
Infliximab	ACR 20	4	458/803 (57)	35/259 (14)	4.3 (3.1–5.9)	2.3 (2.0–2.6)
	ACR 50	4	232/803 (29)	14/259 (5)	5.5 (3.3–9.2)	4.3 (3.6–5.2)
	ACR 70	3	68/667 (10)	2/215 (1)	12 (3–47)	11 (8–15)
Etenercept	ACR 20	4	245/497 (49)	19/133 (14)	3.6 (2.3–5.4)	2.9 (2.4–3.6)
	ACR 50	4	161/497 (32)	10/133 (8)	4.5 (2.4–8.3)	4.0 (3.2–5.3)
	ACR 70	1	60/340 (18)	2/88 (2)	8 (2–31)	6.5 (4.9–9.7)

It provides an early referral algorithm for newly diagnosed rheumatoid arthritis. It is advised in the event of clinical suspicion of RA, supported by the presence of any of the following:

1. at least three swollen joints;
2. a positive 'squeeze' test (composite compression test) that clinically evaluates a group of small adjacent joints such as metacarpophalangeal and metatarsalophalyngeal;
3. morning stiffness of at least 30 min.

Important points were:

• patients with RA have been shown to have an improved long term outcome, when treated by a rheumatologist;
• there is evidence that delay of more than 12 weeks in treatment results in a missed opportunity to improve long term outcome;
• RF positivity, a raised acute phase response, and erosions on X-ray are associated with poor outcome, but absence at presentation should not preclude diagnosis or referral;
• NSAIDs can mask signs and symptoms at presentation;
• corticosteroids should not be prescribed without an accurate diagnosis.

Overall comment

There is much new in the field of rheumatoid arthritis, and probably much more to come, backed by good evidence, especially new evidence. Given that RA is the most common form of inflammatory arthritis affecting 0.5–1% of the population, and with a large economic impact because about 90% of patients have some form of disability with two decades, this is of increasing importance. Some or all of this could be incorporated into the delivery of a quality service.

References

1. Jobanputra, P. *et al.* (2002). The clinical effectiveness and cost-effectiveness of new drug treatments for rheumatoid arthritis: etenercept and infliximab. NICE 2002 (http://www.nice.org.uk/Docref.asp?d=29675)
2. Emery, P. *et al.* (2002). Early referral recommendation for newly diagnosed rheumatoid arthritis: evidence based development of a clinical guide, *Annals of Rheumatic Disease* 61: 290–7.

5.9 **Fish oil for rheumatoid arthritis**

Clinical bottom line. Fish oil supplementation in adequate doses improves outcomes for patients with rheumatoid arthritis.

Systematic review

Fortin, P. R. *et al.* (1995). Validation of a meta-analysis: the effects of fish oil in rheumatoid arthritis, *Journal of Clinical Epidemiology* 48: 1379–90.

Date review completed: 1994

Number of trials included: 10

Number of patients: 408

Control group: Placebo

Main outcomes: Improvement on a number of measures (tender and swollen joints, morning stiffness, grip strength and global assessments

The main inclusion criteria were that trials had to be randomised and double blind, to have a placebo control with results reported at baseline and follow up, and with a parallel or cross-over design. One quasi-randomised study was included.

This study used a search of MEDLINE from 1991, supplemented with additional searches and contacts to manufacturers. The review also obtained individual patient results and looked at results from an analysis of mean results of published material, and from an individual patient basis.

Findings

At three months, fish oil use resulted in a significant reduction in tender joint count by 3 joints, and reduced morning stiffness by 26 min.

Comment

This interesting methodological paper showed that the analysis of results on an individual basis largely confirmed those based on mean results reported in individual publications. Fish oil is helpful in rheumatoid arthritis. A subsequent randomised trial [1] compared fish oil (40 mg/kg/day) in 50 patients with rheumatoid arthritis, and reached similar conclusions.

Reference

1. Volker, D. *et al.* (2000). Efficacy of fish oil concentrate in the treatment of rheumatoid arthritis, *Journal of Rheumatology* 27: 2343–6.

5.10 **Sulfasalazine for rheumatoid arthritis**

Clinical bottom line. Sulfasalazine was better than placebo on a number of outcomes important in rheumatoid arthritis, including swollen and painful joints, morning stiffness and pain.

Systematic review

Winblatt, M. E. *et al.* (1999). Sulfasalazine treatment for rheumatoid arthritis: a metaanalysis of 15 randomized trials, *Journal of Rheumatology* 26: 2123–30.

Date review completed: 1998

Number of trials included: 8

Number of patients: 8551 on sulfasalazine, 315 on placebo

Control group: Placebo

Main outcomes: Improvement on a number of measures (tender and swollen joints, morning stiffness, grip strength and global assessments)

The main inclusion criteria were that trials had to be randomised and double blind, to have a placebo control and sulfasalazine treatment. Three databases were searched, and only full publications in peer-reviewed journals were included.

Findings

The review provides a descriptive reporting system. Sulfasalazine was significantly better than placebo on a number of outcomes

Table 5.10.1 Outcomes in studies of sulfasalazine and placebo

Outcome	Sulfasalazine	Placebo
Number randomised	552	351
Adverse event withdrawals (%)	24	7
Lack of efficacy withdrawals (%)	11	28
ESR (%reduction)	37	14
Morning stiffness duration (%reduction)	61	33
Pain VAS (%reduction)	42	15
Articular index (%reduction)	46	20
Number of swollen joints (%reduction)	51	26
Number of painful joints (%reduction)	59	33
Patient global assessment (%reduction)	26	14

(Table 5.10.1), though not all outcomes were reported in all studies. More patients on sulfasalazine discontinued because of adverse effects (rash, abnormal liver function tests) than on placebo, but lack of efficacy discontinuations were many fewer than with placebo. Morning stiffness, pain, the number of tender and swollen joints and patient global assessment were all significantly better with sulfasalazine.

Comment

The majority of the studies used 2 g of sulfasalazine a day, and results are also given for 3 g a day in two studies. There are also comparisons with other treatments for rheumatoid arthritis (hydroxychloroquinine, penicillamine, and gold), but in few studies with limited numbers of patients.

Section 6
Complementary and alternative therapies

6.1 **Complementary and alternative therapies**

Introduction

This is a difficult topic for all sorts of reasons. Most importantly, it is different things to different people. For some, it is the one thing that seems to bring some relief in incredibly difficult situations. For others it is a sort of health fashion accessory. Most frustrating is the continual shifting of goal posts, as evidence for or against one variant of a therapy is talked down because of some slight difference in therapy delivery – different acupuncture points, or homeopathy dilution, or ways of doing massage. Most obviously is the blindingly obvious – that for most complementary or alternative therapies (CAT for convenience), or diagnostic procedures, there is absolutely no evidence whatsoever.

One argument is that even if CATs do not work, then at least they are safe. Not so. Acupuncture does go wrong, and can cause serious harm, or even death. More important, perhaps, and certainly more difficult to measure, is the harm done by CAT practitioners delaying or stopping conventional diagnosis or therapy, often with catastrophic consequences.

There has to be a balance. CAT practitioners take billions of pounds, dollars, and euros each year from the public, often without any objective evidence of benefit. In other circumstances (doctors and diet pills, bogus saving schemes) this would be scandal of immense proportions. Our societies are prepared to allow this, though.

The one thing that we must do in consequence is to try and ensure that we know as much as we can about CAT therapies for pain. In evaluating CAT, the standards have to be the same as those for pharmacological or surgical interventions. That means that trials should be randomised, double-blind, large, and valid, as well as reporting useful outcomes over a sensible timescale. Looking at what happens when we do nothing (use a placebo) can be very instructive.

Systematic review of CAT

Systematic reviews of CAT also have to have the same rigor as those of conventional therapies. If they do not, they will be wrong. Some examples of the need for quality are instructive.

Acupuncture and dental pain

For instance, a review of acupuncture in dental pain [1] concluded that it worked. A more detailed examination [2] concluded that this was something of an overestimate.

Of the 16 trials included in the review, five were not randomised, two made no attempt at blinding and three were simply too small to provide meaningful data. Of the remaining six trials, two were on experimental dental pain and one trial an inadequate placebo condition. We are then left with three trials, with a total of 110 patients, from which we may draw conclusions. And none of these trials is particularly instructive, because none looks at everyday clinical situations, but were rather contrived.

Yet the results of this review are held up as 'proving' that acupuncture should be used for dental pain. We think that overstates the case massively, and that the correct conclusion is that there is no evidence that acupuncture is effective for dental pain.

Acupuncture trials and quality

Another systematic review across all of chronic pain draws attention to the fact that the number of clinical trials of high quality that showed acupuncture to be effective is visibly small [3]. There are only three, at best.

Trials were defined as positive if acupuncture was found to be significantly better than control, neutral if there was no significant difference between acupuncture and control, and negative when acupuncture was significantly worse than control. A 'p' value of 0.05 was used to define statistical significance.

There were 50 trials with 2394 patients. Thirty-four trials (68%) had a quality score of 2 or less on a five-point scale. Controls included waiting lists, inert controls, sham acupuncture and active controls, usually transcutaneous electrical nerve stimulation.

The main results are shown in Table 6.1.1. Most high quality studies (quality score 2 or more) either showed no benefit or that acupuncture

Table 6.1.1 Effect of quality of trial reporting on whether trials of acupuncture in chronic pain are better, the same, or worse than control

	Trials		Patients	
	Number	Percent	Number	Percent
Quality score 3 or more				
Acupuncture better than control	3	19	111	12
Acupuncture same as control	12	75	715	79
Acupuncture worse than control	1	6	77	9
	16	100	903	100
Quality score 2 or less				
Acupuncture better than control	16	47	643	43
Acupuncture same as control	16	47	736	49
Acupuncture worse than control	2	6	112	8
	34	100	1491	100

was worse than control. Forty to 50% of the trials or patients showed acupuncture to be better than control. Studies of low methodological quality showed significantly higher treatment effect than those of high quality.

Without labouring the point about poor quality studies overestimating effects of treatment, or that evidence for acupuncture is thin on the ground, this study demonstrates both with some clarity. It is worth commenting that for chronic pain where acupuncture is much used, the absence of significant effect is all too apparent. Only three studies showed a benefit, and they contained only 12% of the total patients studied in high quality trials. As a balance, one trial with 9% of the total patients studied in high quality trials showed less effect than an active treatment. The remainder of the high quality studies showed no difference at all between acupuncture and control.

Many of the studies were small. Of the 19 positive studies, 14 enrolled fewer than 50 patients, and the smallest number was 12. Overall, positive studies were smaller than neutral studies, which were smaller than negative studies. We might conclude that there is some residual bias in this, which would result in an even more negative conclusion.

Geographical bias in complementary therapy

Bandolier was a guest at a discussion on alternative medicine. One comment made was that: 'The Chinese have been doing this sort of thing for thousands of years: surely it can't be wrong?' The immediate reaction was that the Chinese suffered to the same extent as everyone else to the great plagues of the 6th and 14th centuries, and Chinese historians record many, many major depredations over the centuries. Perhaps it all comes down to how you look at things, standards set, and societal values. A systematic review [4] set out to answer the question whether some countries produce only positive results.

There were two searches. The first used MEDLINE to retrieve papers on acupuncture with abstracts available over 30 years. Papers had to have patients receiving acupuncture who were compared with patients receiving placebo, no treatment or a no acupuncture control. The second search looked for randomised or controlled clinical trials published in China, Taiwan, Japan or Russia/USSR between 1991 and 1995. In addition, 330 most recent randomised or controlled trials published in England were sought. These studies had to have patients receiving a treatment other than acupuncture compared with patients receiving a control intervention.

Reviewers blinded to the country of origin then retrieved and examined the abstracts. The outcome was a superiority of treatment over control based on an author statement, at least one statement of statistical superiority, or at least one outcome described as superior to control.

For acupuncture, there was a wide discrepancy between countries of origin and the proportion of trials showing superiority of acupuncture. Countries in North America, Western Europe and Australasia were positive for acupuncture about half the time, or less. Those from Eastern Europe and especially East Asia were positive nearly all the time (Figure 6.1.1).

The four countries which had 100% positive rates for acupuncture were compared with England for positive rates for randomised or controlled trials where acupuncture was not being tested. They also had very high rates of positive trials here as well (Table 6.1.2), as high as 97% for Russia/USSR and 99% for China. Rates for England were consistently lower.

The authors of this review did a terrific job in trying to eradicate bias from their analysis. They acknowledge that because they included controlled trials, and looked only at abstracts, they will have included

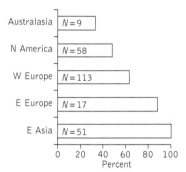

Figure 6.6.1 Percentage of controlled trials of acupuncture showing superiority of acupuncture from five regions, with number of studies.

Table 6.1.2 Proportion of trials with treatment better than control for randomised or controlled non-acupuncture studies, and from acupuncture studies, from five countries

Country	Randomised or controlled trials		Acupuncture trials	
	Number	Positive (%)	Number	Positive (%)
England	107	75	20	60
China	109	99	36	100
Japan	120	89	5	100
Russia/USSR	29	97	11	91
Taiwan	40	95	6	100

studies with known methodological bias. They also acknowledge that authors can and do make misleading or mistaken comments about trial results in abstracts.

That having been said, there remains a gulf between studies reported from different parts of the world. Bias may be institutionalised in some places, or may just be harder to detect in others.

The inference is obvious. Quality is much more important than quantity. No matter how many trials of inadequate or biased design we have, they do not match up to one trial of adequate size and methodological rigor. Quality is first, and everything else is nowhere.

'All was wrong because not all was right' is a quotation from George Crabbe that might usefully govern the interpretation of evidence. It applies to all therapies.

Why bogus therapies seem to work

Context is as important as quality. There is a great website (www.quackwatch.com) worth visiting if you are concerned about the benefits or otherwise of alternative therapies. One page is devoted to why 'bogus' therapies seem to work. The points are well made and some apply just as much to conventional as alternative therapies. Most of the points are where non-scientific belief can be nullified by proper scientific method.

Many diseases are self-limiting

The old saying is that a cold will go away in a week or in seven days if you treat it. Determining whether an intervention has made a difference is therefore difficult. Unless rigorous study methods are applied, an apparent benefit cannot be ascribed to the intervention or the natural course of the disease.

Many diseases are cyclical

Allergies, multiple sclerosis, arthritis and gastrointestinal problems like irritable bowel syndrome all have their ups and downs. Sufferers may seek therapy on a down, so that when an up comes that has to be due to the therapy, doesn't it. Again, only rigorous study design combats this.

Placebo effect

Both the above contribute to what is called a placebo effect. It can be seen as the natural course of things. For instance, some people need no pain relief after surgery [5], making a pre-emptive intervention which claims to reduce pain after surgery a sure win, especially without a placebo. There will always be some people publicly to declaim its value. Natural 'placebo' rates depend on what the problem is and what the benefit is. There will always be some people who benefit without an intervention.

Bets are 'hedged'

'My auntie was under the doctor for six months, but it was only when she started on homeopathy that she got better'. The fact that the poor infantry slaved away for six months is forgotten in the glamour of magic.

Original diagnosis may be wrong

Bandolier has highlighted the difficulty of diagnosis. If the diagnosis is wrong, then miraculous cures are less miraculous.

Mood improvement or cure

Alternative healers often have much more time to spend with their patient than a harassed GP loaded down with kilograms of guidelines and tight prescribing budgets, and in the UK limited to about 7 min per patient, if that. Is it any wonder that alternative healers who spend half an hour with a patient can make them feel better? That mood change is sometimes seen as the cure.

Psychological investment in alternatives

Alternative healing can be as simple as some herbal remedy bought from a shop. Sometimes it can involve huge amounts of time, massive involvement of the family, and an intense psychological investment in believing that something (anything) will work. It is not surprising, then, that many people find some redeeming value in the treatment.

Comment

The issue with CAT is not personal choice, but who should pay, and who should take responsibility when things go wrong. In health services that are over-stretched and under-funded, there can be no place for therapies with no proof of efficacy or effectiveness. When effective therapies for cancer and severe chronic disease are being withheld because of concerns over cost, not of effectiveness, it is well to remember that the most expensive medicine is the one that does not work.

Bandolier's law of inverse claims

A quick screening test to determine whether or not to read about a new product or service is offered by this law. It states that the more benefits claimed for a product, the less likely any of them are to be true. Take, as an example, an E-mail received for Ericson's Alkali-Mine Coral Calcium from Okinawa. The E-blurb states that 'over 150 diseases are linked to ionic calcium deficiency', and that 'reports from users' show 'total or partial relief from symptoms of . . .'. The list starts with arthritis and goes on to include athlete's foot and most other ailments.

Debunking the absurd

Imagine for a moment that *Bandolier*'s editor comes up to you (or, worse, a sick patient) and says that he can see that your aura is disturbed. He then says that for a small fee, and without even touching you, he can put it right so that you will be more in balance with yourself. Money passes in one direction, and hands are waved airily in the other, and the transaction is complete. This technique of 'therapeutic touch' is claimed to do things from helping children make sense of the world to helping to bring some dead back to life.

Therapeutic touch has been debunked in a superb paper in JAMA [6]. There are three good things about this paper. One is the background explanation of the 'theory' behind the practice. Another is the systematic review of the literature which shows that 'at most only 1 of the 83 {studies} may have demonstrated independent confirmation of any positive study'. The third is a terrific randomised study by a 9-year-old girl showing that the practitioners cannot substantiate their claims.

In the RCT, 21 practitioners were challenged to 'sense the aura' from the girl's hand. They sat with hands extended through a screen with palms up. The girl tossed a coin to determine which hand was going to be tested, and then put her hand 5–10 cm above one of the practitioner's.

By chance practitioners should have guessed 50% correctly. They averaged 47% (Figure 6.1.2). To do better than chance they had to be right at least 8 of 10 times. Only one ever achieved this, then fell back to chance on re-test. All practitioners were confident or very confident that they could pass the test with flying colours.

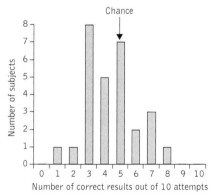

Figure 6.1.2 Number of experienced practitioners of therapeutic touch correctly sensing an aura.

Table 6.1.3 The Oxford Pain Validity Scale (OPVS)

Item		Score (circle one number per item)	Comments
1. Blinding	Was the trial convincingly double-blind?	6	That is, states double-blind and how this was achieved, e.g. double-dummy, identical appearance, etc.
	Was the trial convincingly single-blind or unconvincingly double-blind?	3	That is, states single-blind and how this was achieved, e.g. observer-blind, patient-blind, etc.
	Was the trial either not blind or the blinding is unclear?	0	
2. Size of trial groups	Was the group start size ≥40?	3	Not all groups in the trial will necessarily be relevant to the review question. Rate this item using the smallest group that is relevant to the review question.
	Was the group start size 30–39?	2	
	Was the group start size 20–29?	1	
	Was the group start size 10–19?	0	
3. Outcomes	Look at pre hoc list of most desirable outcomes relevant to the review question:		NB: If the trial has not reported the results of any measures relevant to the review question (even if it described them in methods) it should be excluded from the review.
	Did the paper include results for at least one pre hoc desirable outcome, and use the outcome appropriately?	2	
	There were no results for any of the pre hoc desirable outcomes, or, a pre hoc desirable outcome was used inappropriately.	0	

Table 6.1.3 continued

Item		Score (circle one number per item)	Comments
4. Demonstration of internal sensitivity	Look at the baseline levels for the outcomes relevant to the review question:		One way to demonstrate internal sensitivity is by having an additional active control group in the trial which demonstrates a significant difference from placebo (i.e. the trial design is able to detect a difference).
	For all treatment groups, baseline levels were sufficient for the trialist to be able to measure a change following the intervention (e.g. enough baseline pain to detect a difference between baseline and post-treatment levels). Alternatively, did the trial demonstrate internal sensitivity?	1	For example, by having an extra group treated with an analgesic known to be statistically different from placebo, and by demonstrating this difference. Alternatively, internal sensitivity can be demonstrated with a dose response.
	For all treatment groups, baseline levels were insufficient for the trialist to be able to measure a change following the intervention, or baseline levels could not be assessed, or internal sensitivity was not demonstrated.	0	
5. Data analysis	(i) *Definition of outcomes* Did the paper define the relevant outcomes clearly, including where relevant, exactly what 'improved', 'successful treatment', etc. represented?	1	There must be at least one outcome measure defined clearly to score 1. This item refers to any outcome measure relevant to the review question, not just pre hoc desirables.
	The paper failed to define the outcomes clearly.	0	
	(ii) Data presentation: Location and dispersion Did the paper present either mean data with standard deviations, or dichotomous outcomes, or	1	

median with range, or sufficient data to enable
extraction of any of these?

The paper presented none of the above 0

(iii) *Statistical Testing*

Did the trialist chose an appropriate statistical 1
test, with correction for multiple tests where relevant?

Inappropriate statistical tests were chosen 0
and/or multiple testing was carried out, but with
no correction, or, no statistics were carried out.

(iv) *Handling of Dropouts*

The dropout rate was either ⩾10%, or was 1
>10% and includes an intention-to-treat
analysis in which dropouts were included
appropriately.

The dropout rate was >10% and dropouts were 0
not included in the analysis, or, it is not
possible to calculate a dropout rate from data
presented in the paper.

Total score

Corrections for multiple testing must be put in place when
a series of tests or measures have been carried out
on the same patient group.

The Oxford Pain Validity Scale (OPVS) should only be used on trials which are:
* Randomised.
* have a start group size ⩾10 for all groups relevant to the review question.

Author conclusion: Trial positive/Trial negative
Reviewer conclusion: Trial positive/Trial negative

Fuzzy thinking avoidance

In making evidence-based decisions we have to be more, not less, sceptical. If there is no proof that an intervention works, then the norm should be that it is not used. Claims that it does no harm should be treated with healthy scepticism. Adverse effects of treatments that do much good are treated with proper seriousness – oral contraceptives and rare thrombosis is one example. If we do not know that something works, the chances of knowing that it does *not* do harm are small.

Where an unconventional approach can be shown to work, then we have to treat those claims with appropriate seriousness. Healthy scepticism should not include a closed mind.

A practical guide for individual trials

For the most part, systematic reviews will not be available for many (most) CAT interventions. What is needed is some sort of practical guide to evaluate a trial, looking at its design, size, outcomes, analysis and validity. Fortunately, there is one at hand, the Oxford Pain Validity Scale (Table 6.1.3) [7]. Though designed to be used with trials in painful conditions, it can easily be modified for other clinical circumstances.

Any trial can be run through a set of questions, and scored on each, with a total of between 0 and 16 points. Studies with scores below 8 are likely to have major problems, and should probably not be believed. Those with scores above 8 are better, but may still have problems. A common finding is that clinical trials claim an important effect when there are no statistical differences, or misinterpret statistics, or even get them plain wrong. It is a particular problem for CAT studies, which makes it important to look at any trial carefully [7]. Reviewer's conclusions are often more important than those of the original author, who is likely to be an enthusiast.

References

1. Ernst, E. and Pittler, M. (1998). The effectiveness of acupuncture in treating acute dental pain: a systematic review, *British Dental Journal* 184: 443–7.
2. Smith, L. and Oldman, A. (1999). Acupuncture and dental pain, *British Dental Journal* 186: 158–9.
3. Ezzo, J. *et al.* (2000). Is acupuncture effective for the treatment of chronic pain? A systematic review, *Pain* 86: 217–25.
4. Vickers, A. *et al.* (1998). Do certain countries produce only positive results? A systematic review of controlled trials, *Controlled Clinical Trials* 19: 159–66.
5. McQuay, H. J. *et al.* (1982). Some patients don't need analgesics after surgery, *Journal of the Royal Society of Medicine* 75: 705–8.
6. Rosa, L. *et al.* (1998). A close look at therapeutic touch, *JAMA* 279: 1005–10.
7. Smith, L. A. *et al.* (2000). Teasing apart quality and validity in systematic reviews: an example from acupuncture trials in chronic neck and back pain, *Pain* 86: 119–32.

6.2 **Supplements and herbal remedies**

Taking food supplements like vitamins or fish oil is now common, as is the use of herbal remedies. Many different types are freely available from pharmacies and health food shops, a big change in the last decade. For some of these there is efficacy, and folate supplementation up to about 400 μg daily is proven to yield benefit in reducing the incidence of cancer and heart disease. What this section seeks to do is examine the evidence for benefits for painful conditions. It will never be comprehensive, because new unsubstantiated treatments seem to emerge weekly. Buyers should beware.

Glucosamine and arthritis

Clinical bottom line. The evidence we have is that glucosamine is effective for some people with arthritis. The size of the benefit, on average, is moderate, and it may take several weeks for benefits to be apparent.

In December 1997 *Bandolier* undertook what was probably the first systematic attempt to review the efficacy of glucosamine in arthritis. There were, and still are, a number of difficulties, the most obvious being the nature and stability of the glucosamine used. In the intervening five years there are claims that glucosamine preparations are now more stable and more consistent, but there is no evidence for this. There is no international pharmaceutical standard for glucosamine (or at least none that we know of). Glucosamine is usually in the form of the sulphate, but this formulation will contain other salts and some water of crystallisation, the actual amount of glucosamine may vary from preparation to preparation, stability may be a problem, and glucosamine may be in combination with chondroitin.

Doses used also vary, as do the number of times a day oral tablets are taken. Usual oral doses are about 1–1.5 g a day. Though oral administration is most common, it has also been given by injection into a joint, and by intramuscular or intravenous injection. There is no substantial evidence that this makes any difference. In the United States, research funded by the National Institutes of Health is directed towards making a standard and stable preparation, and testing it in a large randomised trial.

Problems remain, though, and one of those is what outcome is most useful to patients. We also now have some Cochrane reviews, and other bigger randomised trials. The balance of evidence is that glucosamine probably benefits some people with early arthritic changes, and may protect against further joint degeneration.

Bandolier review

Eight randomised trials involving oral or intramuscular glucosamine were found. Articles on intra-articular injection, or where the material used was not clearly defined as glucosamine were excluded, as were non-randomised case series. The trials used oral and/or intramuscular glucosamine in patients with arthritis over periods of up to 8 weeks. Most had well-described methods and six had quality scores of 3 or more on a five-point scale. Oral doses of glucosamine sulphate were 1.5 g a day, and intramuscular doses were 400 mg twice or three times a week. Outcomes used were pain, or Lequesne index, or global evaluation.

Five trials compared glucosamine with placebo. All showed statistical superiority of glucosamine. Four of these had dichotomous outcomes for calculating NNTs, which ranged from 1.7 to 6.3 in individual trials. Overall the NNT was 5.0 (3.5–8.9). This means that out of every five patients with arthritis who are treated with glucosamine, one would have short-term benefits in reduced pain and tenderness who would not have had if they had been given a placebo. Three trials compared glucosamine with NSAID (phenylbutazone or ibuprofen). There was no difference between ibuprofen (1.2 g/day) and oral glucosamine (1.5 g/day).

Few adverse effects or study withdrawals were reported for glucosamine. They tended to occur less frequently with glucosamine than with NSAID. A large open study of 1208 arthritis patients taking oral glucosamine 1.5 g/day for 13–99 days had 28 patients who stopped taking glucosamine because of adverse effects. Those adverse effects reported in more than 1% of patients were epigastric pain/tenderness, heartburn, diarrhoea and nausea.

McAlindon review

This review [1] sought randomised trials of glucosamine and chondroitin in the treatment of osteoarthritis. In the analysis it pooled outcomes reported as the primary outcomes by authors of the original papers, and pooled pre-defined outcomes at four weeks, arguing that outcomes before that time may be spurious in osteoarthritis. It also pooled oral and intramuscular or intra-articular administration.

Using effect size, it found moderate to large efficacy for glucosamine (effect size 0.4) and chondroitin (effect size 1.0) with the outcomes used by authors of the original papers. Using their own hierarchy of outcomes at four weeks, effect sizes were modest (glucosamine 0.3, chondroitin 0.4). Large trials had smaller effect sizes than small trials.

Towheed review

This Cochrane review [2] was notable because the authors found a number of unpublished studies. In all they identified 16 randomised double-blind studies, with 992 patients randomised to glucosamine and 1037 randomised to placebo or NSAID. The mean age of patients was 61 years. Twelve of the trials could be included in the review. All had quality scores of 3 or greater out of 5, indicating that substantial bias was unlikely.

A number of analyses of efficacy were undertaken, depending on outcome or comparator. The broad conclusion was that glucosamine had a clinically significant benefit compared with placebo based on standardised mean differences. In the review this was 1.4, and standardised mean differences (or effect sizes) of 0.8 or greater are defined as large.

The review also looked at adverse events. It found only 14 patients treated with glucosamine withdrew from treatment because of suspected toxicity, with only 61 reporting any adverse effects. Mean trial duration was only six weeks, so long-term safety might still be an issue. Otherwise they concluded that glucosamine was safe and effective in treating osteoarthritis.

Long-term RCT

A three-year study comparing glucosamine with placebo was reported in 2001 [3]. Patients aged over 50 years and with primary knee osteoarthritis were randomised to 1500 mg oral glucosamine sulphate once daily or placebo. The mean age was 66 years, and the mean duration of their osteoarthritis was 8 years.

The primary outcome was the mean joint space width of the medial compartment of the tibiofemoral joint, with X-rays taken with patients standing, and using a validated measuring system using digitised images. Pain, functioning, stiffness and consumption of analgesics were also measured, and measurements were taken at baseline, and one and three years. Two hundred and twelve patients were randomised, and 71/106 on placebo completed three years and 68/106 with glucosamine.

The average joint space width was about 5.4 mm at baseline. With placebo there was a mean narrowing of 0.3 mm over three years. With glucosamine there was no narrowing. After 3 years, 32/106 patients (30%) on placebo had a significant joint space narrowing of more than 0.5 mm, compared with 15/106 patients (15%) with glucosamine. The relative risk of significant joint space narrowing with glucosamine was 0.5 (0.3–0.9), and the number of patients needed to be treated for 3 years to prevent one patient having significant joint space narrowing compared with placebo was 6.6 (3.8–25).

With placebo there was no overall change in pain or functioning. With glucosamine there was a significant improvement of 20–25%. Stiffness was not affected, and the consumption of analgesics or NSAIDs was not different. Patients used rescue medicines on average once every 6 days.

Adverse events were reported by 95% of patients over the three years. Most were transient and mild, not clearly related to treatment, and there were no differences between glucosamine and placebo. Adverse event withdrawals occurred in 21/106 patients on glucosamine and 18/106 on placebo (relative risk 1.2; 0.7–2.1).

Is glucosamine effective?

The evidence we have from clinical trials is limited, but reasonable. Many people are using glucosamine for their arthritis, and so far there seem to be no reports of rare but serious adverse effects.

Chondroitin sulphate for osteoarthritis

Clinical bottom line. Chondroitin sulphate given orally was found to be effective in reducing pain, improving function, and reducing NSAID and analgesic consumption in seven randomised double-blind trials involving 702 patients with osteoarthritis of hip or knee over three months or more.

Chondroitin sulphate describes complex molecules found in cartilage, though it is not a standardised material. Like glucosamine, this has been considered as a possible modifier of symptoms in osteoarthritis, though mechanisms are not understood, nor doses well worked out, nor pharmaceutical standards available.

A review [4] searched several electronic databases for randomised, double-blind studies of chondroitin sulphate in osteoarthritis of hip or knee. Outcomes of interest were: Lequesne index, patient or physician global evaluation, pain, or walking time, or NSAID or analgesic drug use. Baseline characteristics had to show that patient characteristics were homogeneous.

Information on 16 studies was available, but only seven of these, with 702 patients, were included in the meta-analysis. All were comparisons with placebo, in which additional analgesic drugs could be used. Doses were 800–1200 mg a day.

Pain and Lequesne index fell from baseline over 30–180 days in both groups, but the decreases were always greater for chondroitin sulphate than for placebo. These differences were statistically significant after two to four months, and by six months the level of significance was very high (a chance result had a likelihood of less than 1 in 200).

In all trials patients and/or physicians rated chondroitin sulphate better than placebo. In all trials chondroitin sulphate resulted in a significant reduction in NSAID or analgesic use, and this was much more marked than for placebo. Adverse events were reported more frequently with placebo than with chondroitin sulphate.

Comment

The number of trials and patients are limited, but the results for all outcomes indicate that chondroitin sulphate was superior to placebo. The limitations on what type of chondroitin sulphate, and what dose, limit the general applicability of the review, but it is at least a start in answering the question about whether chondroitin sulphate is any use in osteoarthritis. Like glucosamine, the answer seems to be that it is.

Phytodolor for musculoskeletal pain

Clinical bottom line. Phytodolor provides significant pain and/or symptom relief in arthritic and rheumatic diseases at standard doses of 90–120 drops/day. This was no better than that associated with low doses of diclofenac or indomethacin. More information is required on adverse effects.

Phytodolor is a standardised herbal preparation of Populus tremula, Fraxinus excelsior and Solidago virgaurea (ratio 3 : 1 : 1) used for the treatment of musculoskeletal pain. It may have anti-inflammatory properties, and it is thought to inhibit arachidonic acid metabolism via the cyclooxygenase and lipoxygenase pathways, leading to suppression of inflammation.

A systematic review [5] found 10 trials with 1135 patients. Inclusion criteria were randomised, placebo-controlled, double-blind trials of herbal remedies for musculoskeletal pain; published and unpublished reports.

Reviewers provided a descriptive summary of included trials, including main outcome and main result.

Trials were carried out in a number of conditions – predominantly osteo- and rheumatoid arthritis, rheumatic diseases and epicondylitis. Most trials examined standard doses (3 × 30 or 3 × 40 drops/day) for 2–4 weeks. Reviewers did not supply information to enable assessment of the reliability of data collection methods and pain assessment.

Six trials in 315 patients compared phytodolor with placebo over 3–4 weeks. All trials showed significant benefit of phytodolor compared with placebo on main outcomes (pain, morning stiffness, physical impairment, grip strength and rescue medication use). One of these trials found significant benefit with half strength phytodolor (3 × 15 drops/day) and with double strength (3 × 60 drops/day) for pain on movement, and significant reduction in chronic pain with double strength only.

Four trials of 820 patients reported on double-blind comparisons of phytodolor with an active treatment over two to four weeks. In all four trials there was no significant difference between treatments (diclofenac 3 × 25 mg/day or indomethacin 2 × 50 mg/day) assessed using similar outcomes to placebo trials. One of these trials was at a high dose equivalent to 2 × 100 drops/day. However, none of these trials were designed to demonstrate internal sensitivity, and may be lacking in statistical power.

No adverse effects were reported in any placebo-controlled trial. Four of four active controlled trials reported adverse effects. Two of four trials reported similar rates per group, and two reported higher rates with diclofenac (14.2% versus 7.4% and 'tolerance better with phytodolor'). Reviewers did not describe these effects or whether they resulted in study withdrawal.

Comment

The problems here are several. A major one is the availability of these preparations, and the other is the short duration of the trials. Modern trials of analgesics and anti-inflammatory drugs in arthritis have a one-year duration. The trials we have do not exclude some minor transient benefit that is not sustained.

Feverfew for migraine prophylaxis

Clinical bottom line. Overall, these studies suggest that feverfew may be beneficial for the prevention of migraine attacks. However, the effectiveness has not been established beyond reasonable doubt. More information is needed to determine which dose and formulation should be prescribed, and how effective it is.

Feverfew (Tanacetum parthenemium L) is a popular herbal remedy recommended for the prevention of migraine. The pharmacological properties of feverfew have been extensively investigated but remain unclear. A review [6] sought randomised, double-blind placebo-controlled trials using feverfew for the prevention of migraine. Searching was comprehensive, included asking manufacturers for unpublished studies, and papers were included only if feverfew was used alone.

Five studies were found, one of which was published only as an abstract. Two crossover trials (70 patients total, one an abstract looking at serotonin uptake and platelet activity) showed no effects over 2–4 months. Three other trials, (146 patients, one parallel group, the other two crossover trials) found significant reductions in the attack frequency, pain intensity, and incidence and/or severity of nausea and vomiting.

No meta-analysis was possible because of the disparate outcome measures used in the trials. The level of statistical significance reported in the positive trials was usually high, and often beyond 1 chance in 50. Adverse effects were mild and reversible.

Comment

Such information as is available from high-quality trials favours feverfew over placebo for the prevention of migraine headaches. The effectiveness of feverfew has not been established beyond reasonable doubt. The very high levels of statistical significance found in the positive trials suggest that larger studies looking at standardised feverfew extracts would make sense especially with the low level of adverse effects.

Quinine for nocturnal leg cramps

An updated meta-analysis [7] for quinine for nocturnal leg cramps was interesting because it included unpublished material and provided some empirical evidence of publication bias.

Searching using three computerised databases was up to July 1997. Unpublished data was found through examining an FDA report, enquiries to British and German regulatory authorities, and pharmaceutical companies. For inclusion studies had to be randomised and double blind, and to be in ambulatory patients. Information was abstracted on age and sex of patients, treatment duration, outcome measures, adverse effects and washout periods. The main efficacy outcome was the reduction in nocturnal leg cramps in a 4-week period, severity of cramps, and their duration.

There were four published studies with 73 patients and three unpublished studies with 336 patients. The inclusion criteria meant that patients had to have more than two cramps a week. The dose of quinine was between 200 and 500 mg, and the treatment period was 1–4 weeks (2 weeks or more in six of the seven studies). All studies gave the number of cramps, six described their severity, and only one their duration.

With placebo the number of cramps in a 4-week period (by extrapolation if studies were shorter) was 17 (about four a week) for all studies, 21 in the published studies and 16 in the unpublished studies (Table 6.2.1; Figure 6.2.1). Quinine reduced the number of cramps in a 4-week period by 4, 9 and 3, respectively (Table 6.2.1). There was also evidence that the severity of the cramps was reduced.

Tinnitus was the only adverse effect that occurred with significantly higher frequency when subjects took quinine rather than placebo (8 of 397 patients).

Comment

This is interesting stuff from a number of aspects. First, it confirms that quinine is effective for nocturnal cramps. For someone who has about four cramps a week, quinine can be expected to reduce this to three a week. There was clear publication bias. Unpublished trials had

Table 6.2.1 Results of published and unpublished randomised studies of quinine for nocturnal leg cramps

	Number of		Over a four-week period (95% CI)	
	Trials	Patients	Cramps on placebo	Cramps avoided with quinine
Published	4	73	20.6 (14.9–26.6)	8.8 (4.2–13.5)
Unpublished	3	336	16.3 (14.7–17.9)	2.5 (0.2–5.6)
All	7	409	17.1 (15.4–18.8)	3.6 (2.2–5.1)

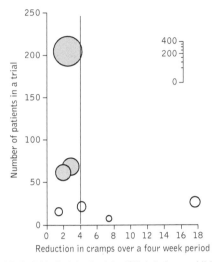

Figure 6.2.1 Individual trials of quinine (filled circles unpublished, open circles published).

a smaller size of effect than published ones. But the published trials were small, and much of the extra effect came from two trials with 27 patients in one and eight in the other. The lesson may not be about publication bias, but the possibility of small trials, however well conducted, giving the wrong answer because of the random play of chance.

Overall comment

There are relatively few supplements and herbal therapies for painful conditions, but that is balanced with some evidence of efficacy. Reports of harmful effects seem to be minor, reversible and uncommon. For people with arthritis, especially mild arthritis, supplements may be preferable, and safer, than taking daily doses of NSAIDs.

References

1. McAlindon, T. E. *et al.* (2000). Glucosamine and chondroitin for treatment of osteoarthritis. A systematic quality assessment and meta-analysis, *JAMA* 283: 1469–73.

2. Towheed, T. E. *et al.* Glucosamine therapy for treating osteoarthritis (Cochrane Review), in: The Cochrane Library, Issue 1, 2001, Update Software, Oxford.

3. Reginster, J. Y. *et al.* (2001). Long-term effects of glucosamine sulphate on osteoarthritis progression: a randomised, placebo-controlled clinical trial, *Lancet* 357: 251–6.

4. Leeb, B. E. *et al*. (2000). A metaanalysis of chondroitin sulfate in the treatment of osteoarthritis, *Journal of Rheumatology* 27: 205–11.

5. Ernst, E. (1999). The efficacy of Phytodolor for the treatment of musculoskeletal pain – a systematic review of randomized clinical trials, *Natural Medicine Journal* 2 : 14–17.

6. Vogler, B. K. *et al*. (1998). Feverfew as a preventive treatment for migraine: a systematic review, *Cephalalgia* 18: 704–8.

7. Man-Son-Hing, M. and Wells, G. (1998). Quinine for nocturnal leg cramps. A meta-analysis including unpublished data, *Journal of General Internal Medicine* 13: 600–6.

6.3 **Acupuncture**

Acupuncture is commonly used as a routine treatment in many parts of eastern Asia, and is becoming more commonly available in western societies. It is often used for chronic painful conditions, and there are standards for using and performing acupuncture. There is more than one type of acupuncture technique, and this age-old method is now becoming technological, with different types of acupuncture needles, and stimulation (heat, electric current), as well as different acupuncture points representing different schools of thought.

Trying to make sense of this evidence will not be easy. The question will often be not how good is the evidence, but whether there is any evidence at all that we can trust. The simple fact is that for any particular combination of needles, stimulation, duration, school, and collection of points, there will be absolutely no evidence at all.

Acupuncture for back pain

Clinical bottom line. Acupuncture is ineffective for back pain.

A systematic review of acupuncture in back pain [1] demonstrates the importance of quality of study design.

Very considerable efforts went into trying to find all the trials. These included MEDLINE, Cochrane Library, and a database specialising in complementary medicine. Authors publishing within the last five years or so were also contacted. Studies were selected on the basis that they were randomised, that dry needles were inserted into the skin, and which was described by the authors as acupuncture. Studies were assessed methodologically both in terms of methodological quality (randomisation, blinding, withdrawals) and on the quality of the acupuncture as judged independently (and blind) by six experienced medical acupuncturists.

Most of the included studies used sham acupuncture as control, though waiting list controls and lidocaine injections were also used. The outcomes were almost always short-term pain relief, as judged by the patient in some instances, and by the practitioner in others. There were few long-term outcomes.

Of the 12 included studies, only four were blinded. Adequacy of acupuncture was judged (on a 0–2 scale, where 2 is best) as 2 in one, 1 in eight and 0 in three. Not all these studies had extractable outcome data. Four blinded studies showed no difference from control (Figure 6.3.1; Table 6.3.1).

Fifty-seven percent of patients improved with acupuncture and 50% with control, a relative benefit of 1.2 (0.9–1.5). The NNT with

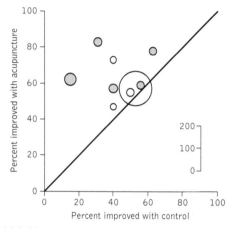

Figure 6.3.1 Blind (white symbols) and open studies (dark symbols) for acupuncture in back pain.

Table 6.3.1 Effects of acupuncture on short-term outcomes in back pain

Type of study	Number of trials	Improved with acupuncture (%)	Improved with control (%)	Relative benefit (95% CI)	NNT (95% CI)
Blind	4	73/127 (57)	61/123 (50)	1.2 (0.9–1.5)	13 (5 to no benefit)
Non-blind	5	78/117 (67)	33/87 (38)	1.8 (1.3–2.4)	3.5 (2.4–6.5)

acupuncture for one patient with back pain to achieve a short-term improvement was 13 (5 to no benefit). Five non-blinded studies did show a difference from control, with 67% improved with acupuncture and 38% with control. Here the relative benefit was significant at 1.8 (1.3–2.4) and the NNT was 3.5 (2.4–6.5).

Comment

Acupuncture trials are often difficult to assess. There are issues of whether the acupuncture has been done correctly, about the appropriateness of control interventions, whether trials can be truly blinded, and about the relevance of outcomes. Ernst and White examined these in their review, and made thoughtful comments on all of them.

Perhaps the biggest problem is that these trials, as a group, have avoided the hard question of longer-term outcomes. Even if acupuncture provides short-term relief, its place in management of back pain remains unknown.

The question is whether this review provides evidence of lack of effect, or lack of evidence of effect. The inability of the four highest quality blinded trials to show a statistically significant short-term improvement must be worrying for those providing acupuncture services, and for the health services or individuals who purchase acupuncture. A sceptical view seems to be most appropriate until trials of high quality prove that to be wrong.

Acupuncture for neck and back pain

Clinical bottom line. There is no convincing evidence demonstrating that acupuncture is more effective than placebo for the relief of back or neck pain. The higher quality (double blind) studies were all negative. The trials with positive outcomes were all of low quality (not blind) with serious methodological flaws.

This review found 13 randomised controlled trials [2] with 251 patients in active groups and 241 in sham control groups. Control groups included sham acupuncture, sham TENS, no treatment or waiting list controls. The main outcomes were pain intensity, pain relief or global measures of treatment efficacy.

Inclusion criteria were randomised controlled trials comparing acupuncture, with or without electrical stimulation, or laser acupuncture with an inactive control group; acute or chronic back or neck pain; group size of at least 10 patients and pain outcomes.

Trials were generally of low quality with a number of methodological flaws including lack of blinding, small group sizes, poorly defined or inappropriate outcome measures, lack of internal sensitivity and poor data analysis. The duration of acupuncture treatments varied from single to multiple sessions, and type of acupuncture included traditional Chinese acupuncture and manual or electrical stimulation of trigger or non-traditional points.

Based on a vote counting exercise, five trials concluded that acupuncture was effective and eight did not. A sensitivity analysis between the trial result (positive or negative) and OPVS score showed a significant relationship between validity of the trial and the reviewer's conclusions ($p = 0.023$). Trials with lower validity scores were more likely to show a benefit of acupuncture whereas trials with higher scores were more likely to show no benefit of acupuncture over placebo.

Three of the 13 trials reported on adverse effects. In one trial two patients had pain at the acupuncture site and one acupuncture patient had a fever. In one trial one patient withdrew who received TENS and the other trial report stated that none of the patients experienced any adverse effects.

Comment

This review demonstrates that a number of original papers come to the opposite conclusion from their data. On top of that it shows again that trials of greater validity are more likely to have negative outcomes.

Acupuncture for fibromyalgia

Clinical bottom line. There is no evidence for efficacy of acupuncture in fibromyalgia.

Because fibromyalgia is a difficult painful condition with no easy treatment options, acupuncture is often used. One reason is that 'patients want it'. One wonders whether patients are fully informed. So what is the evidence that acupuncture is effective? A review tells that there is little or no evidence of benefit, but that it might make things worse [3].

A complementary medicine group in Baltimore with a deserved reputation for good work did the review. In particular, searching was exemplary, using not only electronic database searching, but special registries, their own registry of complementary medicine in pain and letters to nearly 100 specialised institutions or individuals.

There were three randomised trials, three prospective cohort studies, and one retrospective cohort study. The randomised trials involved 135 patients. Two of them were of low methodological quality. All the cohort studies were deemed to be of low quality.

That left a single randomised trial that compared electro-acupuncture with sham electro-acupuncture over three weeks in 70 patients, with no long-term outcomes. Acupuncture was reported to be better than sham acupuncture for several outcomes, but there were differences in sex split and duration of disease at baseline, so that it looked as if there had been a randomisation failure.

Comment

This is an example of an exemplary review, but an exemplary review of nothing. There is no evidence that acupuncture works for fibromyalgia.

Acupuncture for osteoarthritis

Clinical bottom line. There is no evidence that acupuncture is more effective than sham/placebo acupuncture for the relief of joint pain due to osteoarthritis. Most of the existing trials have serious methodological flaws. The two most methodologically rigorous trials showed no difference between the effect of acupuncture and sham acupuncture for pain relief. The trials comparing acupuncture to active treatment controls were of insufficient methodological rigour to determine efficacy.

Acupuncture is amongst the most frequently used complementary therapies for osteoarthritis (OA). About half of all consultations with British acupuncturists are for OA conditions. A review of 13 trials with 437 patients [4] included controlled trials, patients with symptomatic OA of any joint, traditional Chinese and non-traditional acupuncture and an adequate control group (not defined further).

The author conducted a comprehensive search including the databases MEDLINE and CISCOM (a database specialising in complementary medicine) and references of retrieved reports and also sent requests to experts in the field. The reviewer provided a descriptive summary of included trials as pooling of data was impossible due to their disparate nature.

Most trials used formula acupuncture (needling of a predefined set of points according to conventional diagnosis) as opposed to Chinese acupuncture (needling of individualised sets of points according to traditional Chinese diagnosis). The majority of the trials were of a poor quality with severe methodological flaws (Table 6.3.2). These included lack of randomisation, blinding and statistical testing, small group sizes, and diagnostic criteria for OA and outcome measures were not well defined.

Only two trials were both randomised and double-blind providing the most valid data. Both trials compared formula acupuncture to sham acupuncture, one trial gave acupuncture once a week for 8 weeks and the other gave acupuncture three times a week for 3 weeks. For each trial there was no difference between treatment groups for pain and tenderness outcomes.

Although these are the highest quality trials in this review, they still have methodological flaws. Both trials were small with only

Table 6.3.2 Trials of acupuncture for osteoarthritis, including different study designs

Number of trials	Type of study	Control groups	Trial conclusion
3	CCT (not R, not B)	piroxicam (1)	positive
		physiotherapy (2)	1 positive, 1 negative
		no treatment (1)	positive
4	RCT (not blind)	sham TENS (1)	positive
		sham acupuncture (2)	1 positive, 1 no difference
		TENS (1)	no difference
4	RCT (SB)	sham TENS (1)	no difference
		no treatment (1)	positive
		sham acupuncture (1)	no difference
2	RCT (DB)	sham acupuncture (2)	no difference

Abbreviations: CCT = controlled clinical trial; R = randomised; B = blind; SB = single-blind; DB = double-blind; TENS = transcutaneous electrical nerve stimulation.

20 patients in each treatment group. It is not clear from the review when or how the outcomes were measured, whether the results were statistically tested, or what diagnostic criteria for OA was used.

Taking all 13 trials together, six trials recorded greater pain relief in the acupuncture group than in the control group, seven trials showed no difference. The lower the methodological quality of the trial the more likely it was to show a positive effect. Only one of six blinded trials had a positive result, compared with five out of seven that were not blinded.

Comment

Better quality trials give no support for the use of acupuncture for osteoarthritis. High quality, large, and long-term trials that would really test the efficacy of the technique are lacking.

Overall comment

Acupuncture is widely used for treating chronic pain. It is a concern that there is little evidence that it is effective, that better quality study design consistently produces results showing acupuncture to be ineffective, and even these trials have the major problem of being of relatively short duration in conditions, like osteoarthritis, that are long-lasting. The confusion of different types of acupuncture, and different claims about how acupuncture is best delivered, should not cloud the fact that there is no evidence that it works.

Acupuncture is not without harm. Examining acupuncture for life-threatening adverse reactions [5] shows a number of potential problems, not all of which are recognised commonly. Fifty-six articles were identified, examining two main areas.

Infections linked to acupuncture and the improper handling of needles or their reuse without adequate sterilisation included hepatitis B and C, HIV, bacterial endocarditis and staphylococcal septicaemia. These studies included overviews, epidemiological surveys and case reports.

There are apparently over 60 cases of pneumothorax caused by acupuncture reported. Other traumatic events include cardiac tamponade and punctured heart, including at least one actual death.

This refreshing little review points out that the seemingly innocuous, if done improperly or without care, can result in serious harm. The numbers of patients harmed by acupuncture in this literature review is difficult to assess, but runs into the hundreds. Choosing acupuncture because it is deemed harmless may be a poor choice.

References

1. Ernst, E. and White, A. R. (1998). Acupuncture for back pain: A meta-analysis of randomised controlled trials, *Archives of Internal Medicine* 158: 2235–41.

2. Smith, L. A. *et al*. (2000). Teasing apart quality and validity in systematic reviews: an example from acupuncture trials in chronic neck and back pain, *Pain* 86: 119–32.

3. Berman, B. M. *et al*. (1999). Is acupuncture effective in the treatment of fibromyalgia? *Journal of Family Practice* 48: 213–18.

4. Ernst, E. (1997). Acupuncture as a symptomatic treatment of osteoarthritis. A systematic review, *Scandinavian Journal of Rheumatology* 26: 444–7.

5. Ernst, E. and White, A. (1997). Life-threatening adverse reactions after acupuncture? A systematic review, *Pain* 71: 123–6.

Table 6.4.2 Trial quality and outcome in homeopathy

Quality score (out of 5)	Number of trials	Odds ratio
0	2	6.9 (1.5–31.4)
1	15	3.6 (2.1–6.1)
2	32	3.2 (2.3–4.6)
3	19	1.8 (1.4–2.3)
4	11	1.4 (1.0–2.0)
5	10	2.0 (1.4–2.9)

where we are mixing up different interventions, with different clinical situaltions, with different outcomes, and for different durations of treatment, and with different (and perhaps not always adequate) controls. The authors of the letter comment that:

some (but by no means all) methodologically astute and highly convincing homeopaths have published results that look convincing but are, in fact, not credible. Viewed in this way, the reanalysis . . . can be seen as the ultimate epidemiological proof that homeopathic remedies are, in fact, placebos.

Quod erat demonstrandum, perhaps, because quality is but one issue in clinical trials. The other is validity. Trials have to look at sensible and useful outcomes, or be performed in situations that make clinical and scientific sense. There is still a point that even this sensitivity analysis mixes up all kinds of different trials in all kinds of different clinical situations. Pooling them makes no logical sense. Even Linde and his co-authors [2] admit that many of the more recent high quality studies are quite negative.

Homeopathy for osteoarthritis

Clinical bottom line. There were only four randomised trials, of short duration, in which there was no convincing evidence that homeopathy was particularly beneficial for osteoarthritis.

The systematic review [5] found four randomised controlled trials with 406 patients in active and placebo groups with various outcomes.

The four randomised studies were of short duration (2–5 weeks), and each used a different homeopathic remedy. Outcomes were different in each trial, though involved mainly pain on movement, or at rest, or joint tenderness.

- One study showed no difference between intra-articular homeopathy and intra-articular hyaluronic acid.
- One showed no difference between a sublingual homeopathic remedy and paracetamol.
- One showed no difference between a homeopathic remedy and placebo, though fenoprofen was superior to both.

- One showed no difference between a topical homeopathic remedy and topical piroxicam gel on one outcome, but did on another.

Comment

The main problem with these studies is that they were short. Major randomised trials comparing conventional therapy against placebo in studies where pain is severe because of a 'flare' in arthritis have shown that use of placebo is associated with reduction in pain. This can be due to patients using escape medicines (over-the-counter analgesics and NSAIDs), and because pain may be falling without treatment. The ability of the studies to detect a true difference for continued treatment is low or non-existent. Individually or together these studies show that there is no convincing evidence that homeopathy is of any value for osteoarthritis.

Homeopathic prophylaxis for migraine

Clinical bottom line. A systematic review of methodologically strong trials suggests that homeopathy is ineffective for migraine. This is supported by a subsequent randomised trial of very high quality.

The searching strategy in this review [6] was extensive, and used not only electronic searching of several databases, but hand searching of specialist journals and use of specialist databases. Four randomised, double-blind, placebo-controlled studies comparing homeopathic remedies with placebo were found.

The three studies with the strongest methods showed no difference between homeopathy and placebo. One methodologically weak study did show a difference, and some de-blinding was reported to have been possible.

Comment

It is known that trials of poor reporting quality (as in the one positive study) can produce exaggerated treatment effects. What we have is this – that there is no evidence that homeopathy has any benefit for preventing migraine or headaches.

Overall comment

That just about sums up the evidence for homeopathy and pain. There's not much. What there is generally poor. The better the quality of a trial, the more likely it is to be negative.

References

1. Linde, K. *et al.* (1997). Are the clinical effects of homeopathy placebo effects? A meta-analysis of placebo-controlled trials, *Lancet* 350: 834–43.

2. Linde, K. *et al.* (1997). Impact of study quality on outcome in placebo controlled trials of homeopathy, *Journal of Clinical Epidemiology* 52: 631–6.

3. Ernst, E. and Pittler, M. H. (2000). Re-analysis of previous meta-analysis of clinical trials of homeopathy, *Journal of Clinical Epidemiology* 53: 1188.

4. Jadad, A. R. (1996). Assessing the quality of reports of randomized clinical trials: is blinding necessary? *Controlled Clinical Trials* 17: 1–12.

5. Long, L. and Ernst, E. (2000). Homeopathic remedies for the treatment of osteoarthritis: a systematic review, *British Homeopathic Journal* 90: 37–43.

6. Ernst, E. (1999). Homeopathic prophylaxis of headaches and migraine? A systematic review, *Journal of Pain and Symptom Management* 18: 353–7.

6.5 **Other complementary or alternative therapies for pain**

It is close to impossible to categorise all complementary therapies for pain under a single heading, after herbal, acupuncture and homeopathy have been dealt with. This section will therefore examine a number of systematic reviews of different therapies in different conditions.

Physiotherapy exercises for back pain

Clinical bottom line. Trials are of insufficient quality to draw a clear conclusion. It is not clear whether physiotherapy is better than other conservative treatments, or whether it is better than no treatment. It is not possible to establish which types of exercises are the most effective.

Physiotherapy is widely used for back complaints, usually exercise therapy given alone or in combination with other treatments (e.g. massage, heat, traction, ultrasound or short wave diathermy).

A systematic review [1] found 16 trials in which control groups were active/no intervention/placebo and the main outcomes pain and mobility.

Of the 16 trials included, most were of poor methodological quality, and trials were generally not adequately designed to assess the intervention – small group sizes, high rates of loss-to-follow-up, lacking internal sensitivity, poor statistical analysis. Type of exercise, control interventions and length of intervention varied between trials. Ten trials had negative conclusions and six had positive conclusions. Reviewers noted that there was a general trend for higher quality trials to have positive results. Blinding status was unclear, but 10 of 16 appeared to be evaluator-blind.

Inactive/placebo comparisons. Four trials compared exercise therapy with no therapy or placebo therapy. One of four trials showed a benefit of exercise therapy for pain and activity at four and 12 weeks, but this did not persist to three months. The remaining trials showed no benefit for acute pain, sciatic symptoms and chronic low back pain.

Active comparisons. Seven trials compared exercise therapy with other conservative treatments. Two of seven trials showed significant benefit compared with hot packs and rest and with mini back school (i.e. one session). The second study showed benefit was still present at one year. Five of seven trials showed no benefit when compared with manual therapy, home care instructions, non-steroidal anti-inflammatory drugs, manipulation, manipulation and mobilisation or short wave diathermy.

Different exercise therapies compared. Eight trials compared different types of exercise therapy – mainly isometric flexion exercises compared with extension exercises. Four of eight trials showed no difference (although all were flawed). Four showed some benefit – one favouring three months of intensive dynamic back extensor exercises over a less intensive treatment plus massage and heat, one favoured extension over flexion exercises, and two favoured flexion exercises over mobilisation plus other exercises and, in one trial, massage and heat.

Comment

This review was completed before much of the knowledge about sources of bias in trial design was established. It should be viewed with caution, and probably updated.

Balneotherapy for arthritis

Clinical bottom line. No high quality evidence exists to show whether taking baths helps people with arthritis. The studies were methodologically flawed and of insufficient power. No meaningful information on efficacy was reported.

Balneotherapy (spa therapy) is the act of bathing in thermal or mineral waters at temperatures of about 34°C. The hydrostatic force of the water is thought to bring about pain relief, which may result from taking stress off the affected joint, relaxation or other factors. It is most commonly prescribed for patients with psoriatic or rheumatoid arthritis.

The review [2] sought clinical trials in patients with arthritis; assessed balneotherapy; used at least one WHO or ILAR endpoint for rheumatoid arthritis (e.g. pain). Study quality was assessed and reports were divided by methodological design. A descriptive analysis was conducted.

Rheumatoid arthritis. Four randomised trials assessed balneotherapy in 147 patients over three months. One study was double blind, the others were single blind. Three showed improvement in outcomes (e.g. duration of morning stiffness, 15 min walk time, hand grip strength); one single blind study drew no conclusion. None compared differences between treatment groups. There were three non-randomised, unblinded studies (135 patients) with one-year follow-up in one study and no follow-up in three. All were positive.

Other forms of arthritis. Three randomised trials assessed 91 patients over six or 18 weeks. Two studies were single (observer) blind, the others were not blind. All reported improvement with hydrotherapy with or without exercises. Three non-randomised, unblinded studies assessed 240 patients; all were positive.

Comment

The reviewers stated that although most studies reported improvement with balneotherapy, the number of patients improved in each trial was not mentioned. No useful information about efficacy was reported in these trials. Whether 19 studies excluded because they did not meet inclusion criteria for language could provide any useful information is unknown. The studies lacked power (all but one had fewer than 25 patients per treatment group) and the lack of adequate blinding meant that bias was likely. The quality scores for these trials were poor; the randomised trials only scored about half of the maximum score in the system used. Improvement was not defined so it is unknown whether that reported constituted clinically relevant improvement.

Exercise therapy for osteoarthritis of the hip or knee

Clinical bottom line. There is limited evidence that exercise provides modest reductions in pain and disability in patients with mild or moderate osteoarthritis of the hip or knee. The majority of trials were small, of low validity and had insufficient power.

The systematic review [3] included randomised controlled trials which assessed exercise therapy in patients with osteoarthritis of the hip or knee and with the outcomes of pain, self-reported disability, observed disability, or patient's global assessment of treatment effect. The validity of the trials and their power to detect a difference between treatments were assessed. Effect sizes, with 95% confidence intervals, were calculated.

Eleven studies were included. Only one study assessed osteoarthritis of the hip. Two trials were described as being of adequate validity and sufficient power and are discussed here. These assessed the effect of aerobic or resistance exercises in patients with mild-to-moderate osteoarthritis of the hip or knee over 12 weeks. There were between 100 and 146 patients per treatment group.

Pain. In one study aerobic exercise was more effective than resistance exercise; the effect sizes were 0.31 (0.28–0.34) and 0.47 (0.44–0.5) respectively. The second trial assessed a combination of strengthening and range-of-motion exercises and functional training; the effect size for pain was higher, 0.58 (0.54–0.62).

Disability. Modest improvements were reported in the two high quality studies. The effect sizes were highest for patients randomised to aerobic exercise for both self-reported disability, 0.41 (0.38–0.44), and for observed disability in walking, 0.89 (0.85–0.93).

Comment

The reviewers stated that different outcome measurement tools were used in the trials, most were small and no information about the long-term, beneficial or adverse effects, of exercise were provided. The reviewers concluded that there is some evidence for small to modest beneficial effects of exercise in the treatment of osteoarthritis of the hip or knee. These conclusions are based mainly on the results of the two trials of adequate validity and power. The studies of lower validity and inadequate power showed variable results and reported on few of the outcomes of interest.

Fasting and vegetarian diet in rheumatoid arthritis

Clinical bottom line. Few trials likely to be bias free (randomised, blind), and valid (longer duration) exist. The results are mixed, but a cautious interpretation may be that there is no evidence of lack of effect, while what evidence we have suggests some benefit.

Clinical observation has been that diet may improve the symptoms of rheumatoid arthritis. The biology underlying any dietary influences is not exact. Some food additives are taken by patients with rheumatoid arthritis. It has also become traditional in some centres for patients to fast, followed by a vegan or vegetarian diet with add-back of foods not associated with symptom worsening. This may be accompanied by holistic approaches involving physiotherapy, exercise, and psychotherapy. A systematic review has examined the evidence-base for fasting and vegetarian diet.

The review included trials with follow-up information for at least three months, and full journal publication.

There were 31 reports. Only one was randomised. A further randomised report with just under three months duration was also included. The other reports were observational studies, or controlled studies. Most were very small, with few having more than 30 patients in total, or 30 patients per group. The main findings in each study are reported, including clinical and biochemical or immunological findings.

Pooling of clinical finding data was done for two randomised and two non-randomised studies separately and together, showing an overall effect size of about 0.8. This is quite a large effect.

Comment

No-one would want any approach to treatment not to work in a difficult and protracted disease like rheumatoid arthritis. This review does a good job in drawing the published work together, and commenting on it sensibly, so we can see the whole picture. That picture may not be pretty, but has a few good points. There is preliminary evidence (no more than that) that fasting and a vegetarian diet may improve biochemistry and symptoms.

Low level laser therapy for osteoarthritis

Clinical bottom line. Based on little data there is no evidence that low-level laser therapy (LLLT) is more effective than placebo in reducing osteoarthritis pain. There were few trials of disparate design and quality and overall they produced negative results for most outcome measures.

Low level laser therapy uses a light source that is thought to generate photochemical reactions in the cells and is used as a non-invasive treatment for OA.

The systematic review [5] had the following inclusion criteria: randomised controlled trials (RCTs) or controlled clinical trials (CCTs); clinical and/or radiological confirmation of the diagnosis of OA; adults; all types of LLLT; placebo and active controls; pain or functional outcomes. Reviewers calculated a standard mean difference, or an odds ratio for sub-sets of trials based on methodological quality of trials, duration and dose of treatment and site of OA involvement.

Four of the included trials were RCTs, one was a non-randomised controlled trial and is not commented on further here. Of the four RCTs, only one was cited as being double-blind, the blinding status of the other three was unclear but they were probably patient blind. All compared laser therapy with placebo. Trials varied in the number of laser treatments given, type of laser and wavelength used and outcome measures. Treatment sessions varied from twice daily for 10 days to 2–3 a week for three to four weeks.

Two of three trials found no significant difference between laser and placebo for the primary outcome of pain, overall there was no significant difference with standard mean difference of −0.23 (95% CI: −1.0 to 0.57). For two trials that measured patient assessed global disease activity there was no difference between laser and placebo, odds ratio 0.96 (0.44–2.1). There were no significant differences between laser and placebo for functional status, swelling, muscle strength or joint tenderness.

No adverse effects were reported and no evidence of harm was found.

Comment

Not enough evidence for routine use would be the obvious conclusion.

Low level laser therapy for rheumatoid arthritis

Clinical bottom line. There is some evidence that a minimum of four weeks of LLLT is more effective than placebo in reducing rheumatoid arthritis pain and stiffness. However, this conclusion should be interpreted with caution due to limited data.

Low level laser therapy LLLT uses a light source that is thought to generate photochemical reactions in the cells and has been used as a non-invasive treatment for rheumatoid arthritis for about 10 years.

The systematic review [6] had the following inclusion criteria: randomised controlled trials; adults, clinical or radiological confirmation of rheumatoid arthritis diagnosis; all types LLLT; placebo or standard treatment control, pain or other outcome measures recommended for rheumatoid arthritis trials. Reviewers calculated a standard mean difference, or an odds ratio for sub-sets of trials based on methodological quality of trials, duration and dose of treatment and site of rheumatoid arthritis involvement.

Five double-blind RCTs were included in the analysis. Quality scores ranged from one to five, the median score was three. All compared laser therapy with placebo. Trials varied in the number of laser treatments given, type of laser and wavelength used and outcome measures. Treatment sessions were two to three per week for three to four weeks for all trials except one, which treated patients for 10 weeks, three times a week. Pain was reduced from baseline in LLLT group but not in placebo group by 14–36% in three trials. Standardised mean differences of pooled results found a statistically significant improvement in pain with LLLT, standardised mean difference −0.53 (95% confidence interval: −0.85 to −0.22). Statistically significant improvements were also found for morning stiffness and tip to palm flexibility. All other outcomes were negative.

No adverse effects were reported and no evidence of harm was found.

Comment

Not enough evidence for routine use would be the obvious conclusion.

Physiotherapy for soft tissue shoulder disorders

Clinical bottom line. Evidence suggests that ultrasound is not useful in alleviating the symptoms associated with soft tissue shoulder disorder. There is insufficient reliable information to assess the efficacy of other physiotherapy interventions, including different electrical therapies, cold therapy, thermotherapy and different exercise and manipulation therapies. However, based on information from poor quality trials, there is currently no evidence to support these interventions. More information from high quality trials is needed.

Pain is the primary symptom associated with shoulder disorders affecting the soft tissue. Cumulative annual incidence of shoulder disorders varies from seven to 25 per 1000 general practitioner consultations. Half of the episodes will resolve within 6 months, but many will persist beyond a year. Treatment includes advice, analgesics, nonsteroidal anti-inflammatory drugs, steroid injection and physiotherapy.

In the systematic review [7] inclusion criteria were randomised, controlled trials of physiotherapy interventions for soft tissue shoulder disorders; physiotherapy interventions include ultrasound, transcutaneous electrical nerve stimulation (TENS), electrotherapy, pulsed electromagnetic fields, magnetic treatment, cold therapy, thermotherapy, exercises, manipulation and mobilisation; outcomes included success rate, pain, mobility or functional status; full journal publication. Reviewers assessed trials for validity and extracted information on outcomes of interest on an intention-to-treat basis. The main outcomes were success rate, pain, mobility or functional status.

Included trials were of mixed quality, with only half satisfying at least 50% of the validity checks. Included patients ranged from those who met specific narrow diagnostic criteria, to general soft tissue shoulder disorders. Most trials were too small to test reliably for differences between groups. Reviewers did not provide information on the blinding status of trials, making it difficult to judge whether reports of significant benefit were likely to be biased.

Ultrasound. Six trials examined ultrasound. Most of these trials have been considered in a separate review of ultrasound for musculoskeletal disorders, which concluded that the evidence suggests that ultrasound is not effective compared with placebo and active treatments.

Electrical therapies. Based on two small trials, TENS was no more effective than ultrasound at six weeks, or than constant voltage electrotherapy at three weeks. Of two trials looking at pulsed electromagnetic field therapy, both reported benefit compared with placebo. However, in one case reviewers were able to extract intention-to-treat data, which showed no benefit. One small trial looked at magnetic treatment plus heat and exercise, and reported no benefit compared with heat and exercise alone.

Cold therapy. One trial showed no benefit of ice packs compared with ultrasound or steroid injection. One small trial showed no benefit of ice packs plus medication and pendular exercises compared with mobilisation, facilitation exercises, steroid injection, all given with medication and pendular exercises, and no benefit compared with medication and pendular exercises alone.

Thermotherapy. Two small trials compared different types of thermotherapy with steroid injection, analgesics and/or muscle relaxants, and found no benefit.

Exercise therapy. One trial showed exercise therapy was as effective as surgery in patients with a stage II impingement syndrome at six months, and was more effective than placebo laser therapy. Three small trials showed no benefit of exercises alongside a range of other treatments compared with the treatments given alone.

Comment
Another example where a commonly-used method is unsupported by evidence.

Relaxation for acute and chronic pain
Clinical bottom line. There is no convincing evidence that relaxation therapy is at all helpful.

Relaxation techniques have been used to produce freedom from anxiety and skeletal muscle tension, and there have been suggestions that relaxation techniques can be useful for relief of acute and chronic pain. Two excellent systematic reviews [8, 9] indicate that, at best, this is not proven.

Both reviews used extensive searching techniques to establish that all published material had been found. Inclusion criteria were full journal publication, relaxation being used alone and not as part of a multimodal therapy, randomised studies, pain outcomes and numbers of treated patients no fewer than 10 per group.

Acute pain. There were seven studies with 362 patients, predominantly after surgery. Controls were generally non-treatment, waiting list controls, or use of music tapes. Three studies (61 patients received relaxation) showed significantly less pain with relaxation, while four (128 patients received relaxation) did not.

Chronic pain. Nine studies with 414 patients studied relaxation in chronic pain, seven in non-malignant pain and two in cancer pain. Controls were again of various types, including waiting lists or studies compared different relaxation techniques.

Three studies showed some efficacy for relaxation at early assessments, but none was effective beyond four months of treatment. In several instances control interventions (splints, hydro-galvanic baths or bio-feedback) produced lower pain scores than relaxation.

Comment

Evidence for the pain-relieving effects of relaxation is underwhelming. In acute pain, for instance, it was interesting to note that the studies with larger numbers tended to be negative while those with smaller numbers tended to be positive. Vote-counting of positive and negative studies has to be tempered by the weight of evidence, and here the weight of 3:4 against relaxation being effective on vote counting becomes 1:2 by using patients on active treatments. When we add the knowledge that there are instances of smaller trials tending to over-estimate treatment efficacy, the weight may become as high as 1:3 against or even more.

This is also an area where goalposts are easily moved: new method, technical expertise and so on. The fact is that although 16 randomised trials were found and evaluated, most were small, and few found any beneficial effect beyond that which might be obtained from taking a couple of aspirin.

Relaxation may still make people feel better. It was Earl St Vincent who said of Napoleon's invasion force 'I do not say they cannot come, I only say they cannot come by sea'. Perhaps of relaxation we can say that we do not deny that it may have a benefit, we merely say it does not relieve pain.

Cervical spine manipulation and mobilisation for neck pain and headache

Clinical bottom line. Based on poor quality trials and diverse treatments studied, it is difficult to clearly assess benefits of manipulation and mobilisation. There does not appear to be any consistent benefit of manipulation for chronic neck pain when given alone or in conjunction with other treatments. There is a lack of evidence for manipulation for acute neck pain and for mobilisation for acute and chronic neck pain. There is a lack of evidence for manipulation and mobilisation for tension headache and migraine. In all cases, where benefit was seen, it was sporadic and of short duration, and therefore of questionable clinical relevance.

A number of different therapists carry out spinal manipulation and mobilisation for pain relief, including osteopaths, chiropractors and physiotherapists. In general, manipulation involves a high velocity thrust to a joint beyond its restricted range of movement, and mobilisation uses low velocity passive movements within or at the limit of the joint range.

The systematic review [10] included blinded and unblind studies of manipulation and mobilisation for cervical spine pain (e.g. neck pain, headache, whiplash, face pain, cervical angina); trials of complications of cervical spine manual therapy; acute (less than 3 weeks), subacute (3–13 weeks) and chronic (greater than 13 weeks) pain; any language.

Reviewers pooled information from randomised controlled trials where appropriate, and provided a descriptive summary of included studies. Pooled data were used to calculate effect size using a random effects model. This was assessed for clinical relevance by estimating what the pooled effect size represented on a 100 mm visual analogue scale. Trials involving manipulation and mobilisation were classified as manipulation trials. Only randomised controlled trials are considered in this summary. It was difficult to assess from the review the nature of blinding in trials.

Quality of included randomised controlled trials varied, but was generally low. Trial methodologies, included patients and control groups varied greatly. Interventions varied from one session to 3 months of up to twice weekly sessions. No statement was made about the appropriateness of statistical testing, which is of particular importance in these trials where many outcomes are measured over long periods of time – risk of false positives is therefore high. No statement was made about the levels of baseline pain or the power of these trials to detect a change – risk of false negatives is therefore high. Only five of the 14 trials made any attempt to blind patients/evaluators.

Neck pain: acute. No trials looked at manipulation.

Three trials were considered. One trial of 30 patients showed no statistical difference between mobilisation plus collar, transcutaneous electrical nerve stimulation plus collar and collar alone at 1, 3 and 12 weeks (cervical mobility and pain). However, all patients were allowed to consume analgesics. Two trials of quite intensive Maitland mobilisation for acute flexion–extension sprains showed better pain relief and range of movement compared with control. All patients consumed analgesics as needed. The first of these trials (61 patients) showed benefit at four and eight weeks, and also showed a similar benefit with patients receiving a neck collar and advice (control group, rest and analgesics). The second (170 patients) showed benefit at 4 and 8 weeks compared with collar.

Neck pain: subacute and chronic. Five trials looked at manipulation. Data were pooled for 3 week pain outcomes for 155 of these patients. Effect size showed no benefit (0.42, 95% confidence interval −0.005 to 0.85), and the improvement seen represented approximately 10 mm on a 100 mm visual analogue scale. Of the included trials, the highest quality trial (100 patients) showed no benefit on a number of outcomes immediately after treatment, and a second, very small (9 patients), low quality trial showed benefit. Both compared a single treatment session of manipulation with mobilisation. Looking at longer-term benefit, one trial with some blinding in 39 patients showed no benefit after a single session of manual therapy plus diazepam compared with diazepam alone. One trial of 52 patients showed no benefit of one to three sessions of manipulation plus azapropazone versus azapropazone only. The fifth trial in 64 patients compared up to three months of manipulation with exercise/massage over a 12-month period. There was a very modest benefit based on a measure of functional status 12 weeks only, and no differences in pain.

One trial of mobilisation in 63 patients was identified. Significant benefit of mobilisation plus salicylate was seen at one week post-treatment compared with salicylate plus massage and electrical stimulation and traction and compared with salicylate only. At 3 weeks only, there was greater cervical mobility.

Muscle tension headache. Three trials looked at manipulation in chronic headache sufferers. One trial of 126 patients compared twice weekly manipulation plus heat and light massage with daily amitriptyline, both given for 6 weeks (analgesics allowed as required). No differences were seen between groups immediately after treatment; four weeks later treatment benefits were more likely to persist with manipulation compared with amitriptyline. One trial of 19 patients compared two sessions of manipulation with cold packs for posttraumatic headache and found significantly better pain relief at 2 weeks with manipulation, but not at 5 weeks. The third trial in 22 patients compared one session of manipulation with palpation and with supine rest. Benefit was seen at 5 min. No long-term assessments were made.

Migraine. One trial in 85 patients looked at two months of twice-weekly manipulation compared with mobilisation. At 2 months, manipulation given by chiropractors showed significantly less pain, greater reduction in frequency compared with mobilisation. However, physiotherapy manipulation was not better than mobilisation, and neither type of manipulation reduced mean frequency of attacks, mean duration of attacks or mean disability.

Adverse effects. Reviewers specifically included reports containing information on complications of manipulation and mobilisation. This information did not come from randomised controlled trials, and risk cannot therefore be quantified. Based on 118 case reports, reviewers noted that most complications from manipulation involve vertebrobasilar accidents, including brain stem or cerebellar infarction, obstruction of the posterior inferior cerebellar artery, occlusion of basilar artery, spinal cord compression, vertebral fracture, tracheal rupture, diaphragm paralysis, internal carotid hematoma and cardiac arrest. Of these 118 cases, 21 patients died, and 52 survived with serious neurological deficit, paralysis or permanent functional impairment. Work of others estimates risk at 1 in 40,000 manipulations for mild complications and 1 in 4000,000 to over 1 million for serious complications.

Comment
A remarkable lack of evidence for interventions carried out so commonly, together with some risk of serious complications.

Ultrasound therapy for musculoskeletal disorders

Clinical bottom line. Ultrasound is not effective for reducing pain or functional disability associated with lateral epicondylitis (tennis elbow), soft-tissue shoulder disorders or ankle distortions. Based on three trials, ultrasound showed some benefit for general improvement of symptoms. The NNT for ultrasound for 'at least satisfactory general improvement of symptoms' compared with placebo at 4 to 8 weeks was 6.0 (95% confidence interval 3.2–40). There was no convincing evidence for ultrasound for degenerative rheumatic disorders, heel pain, myofascial trigger points, supraspinatus tendinitis or lateral epicondylitis. However, more trials of higher quality are required to confirm this. Ultrasound in combination with exercise therapy did not offer any further benefit.

Therapeutic ultrasound is often used in the treatment of musculoskeletal disorders. In Canada 94% of physical therapists use ultrasound. Ultrasound is assumed to have thermal and mechanical effects on the target tissue resulting in an increased local metabolism, circulation, extensibility of connective tissue and tissue regeneration.

The systematic review [11] included randomised controlled trials of ultrasound for pain and/or restriction of range of motion associated with musculoskeletal disorders; ultrasound alone or as an adjuvant to exercise therapy; placebo (sham ultrasound) or active comparisons; any language.

Reviewers provided a descriptive summary of trials taking quality into account. Evidence for ultrasound was assessed according to quality and quantity of data from trials. Data were pooled where trials represented clinical homogeneity with respect to diagnosis, intervention and outcome measures. Only high quality trials were considered for data pooling. For general improvement outcomes (dichotomous information on numbers with symptom improvement), differences in success rates between study groups were calculated with 95% confidence intervals, together with the NNT point estimate. For non-dichotomous information, differences between groups in change from baseline or differences in post-treatment scores were calculated. Effect sizes were calculated as the difference between the mean (change) scores in the compared groups divided by their pooled standard deviation. In this summary we have calculated the relative benefit with 95% confidence interval for the pooled data as a measure of statistical significance, together with the NNT with 95% confidence intervals. We have not reported on individual effect sizes from trials as individual trials are either too small or of insufficient quality to provide useful clinical information.

Included trials were of mixed quality and blinding status, and were generally of small size. Eighteen trials included a placebo control. Number of treatment sessions was not stated.

Lateral epicondylitis (tennis elbow). Data were pooled from three high quality, placebo-controlled trials in 185 patients looking at outcomes over 4–8 weeks. Two of three reported no difference, but the pooled relative benefit showed some benefit of ultrasound compared with placebo for general improvement in symptoms, 1.4 (95% confidence interval 1.04–2.0). The NNT for ultrasound for 'at least satisfactory general improvement of symptoms' compared with placebo at 4–8 weeks was 6.0 (95% confidence interval 3.2–40). The remaining three trials were of poor quality, and reported a significant benefit compared with no treatment (one trial), and inconsistent results compared with other therapies (four comparisons). Evidence suggests that ultrasound may be of benefit for treating tennis elbow.

Soft-tissue shoulder disorders. None of the seven trials showed any benefit of ultrasound over control. This included five placebo comparisons, three no-treatment comparisons, and three active comparisons. Evidence suggests that there is no benefit of ultrasound for soft-tissue shoulder disorders.

Degenerative rheumatic disorders. Ten trials were identified. These trials were mainly active comparisons, and findings were mixed. However, trials were of insufficient size to measure this adequately, and quality of trials was poor. There is therefore a lack of evidence for ultrasound in this area.

Ankle distortions. Three of three high quality controlled trials showed no benefit of ultrasound over placebo, suggesting that ultrasound is ineffective.

Temporomandibular joint pain or myofascial pain. Four low quality trials reported no benefit in most cases. There is therefore a lack of evidence for ultrasound in this area.

Other diagnoses. Seven trials considered patients with a variety of musculoskeletal disorders (heel pain, myofascial trigger points, supraspinatus tendinitis or lateral epicondylitis). Description of results was unclear, but there was no convincing evidence for ultrasound in these disorders.

Ultrasound in combination with exercise therapy. Of the included trials, 13 considered ultrasound in combination with exercise therapy. The four high quality trials all reported no benefit of ultrasound plus exercise compared with exercise alone, suggesting no additional benefit of ultrasound.

Comment
There was no convincing evidence that ultrasound was of much use, and where a soft outcome of at least satisfactory general improvement was used, confidence intervals around a calculated NNT were very wide.

Overall comment
What all these reviews have in common is that the trials are a mixed bag of quality and validity. Most are poor, in both regards. Where they are more adequate, generally, but not always, there is not much in the way of clinical effect, and nowhere were large and impressive clinical effects seen. For chronic pain where other therapies have had limited efficacy in individual patients, it is understandable that those patients seek some alternate therapy. Professional carers should not encourage them to believe that miraculous results are likely.

References
1. Koes, B. W. *et al.* (1991). Physiotherapy exercises and back pain: a blinded review, *BMJ* 302: 1572–6.
2. Verhagen, A. P. *et al.* (1997). Taking baths: The efficacy of balneotherapy in patients with arthritis. A systematic review, *Journal of Rheumatology* 24: 1964–71.
3. Van Baar, M. E. *et al.* (1999). Effectiveness of exercise therapy in patients with osteoarthritis of the hip or knee, *Arthritis and Rheumatism* 42: 1361–9.
4. Müller, H. *et al.* (2001). Fasting followed by vegetarian diet in patients with rheumatoid arthritis: a systematic review, *Scandinavian Journal of Rheumatology* 30: 1–10.
5. Brosseau, L. *et al.* (2000). Low level laser therapy (classes I, II and III) for the treatment of osteoarthritis (Cochrane Review), in: The Cochrane Library, Issue 2, 2000, Update Software, Oxford.
6. Brosseau, L. *et al.* (2000). Low level laser therapy (classes I, II and III) in the treatment of rheumatoid arthritis (Cochrane review), in: The Cochrane Library, Issue 2, 2000, Update Software, Oxford.

7. van der Heijden, G. J. M. G. *et al.* (1997). Physiotherapy for patients with soft tissue shoulder disorders: a systematic review of randomised clinical trials, *BMJ* 315: 25–30.
8. Seers, K. and Carroll, D. (1998). Relaxation techniques for acute pain management: a systematic review, *Journal of Advanced Nursing* 27: 466–75.
9. Carroll, D. and Seers, K. (1998). Relaxation techniques for chronic pain: a systematic review, *Journal of Advanced Nursing* 27: 476–87.
10. Hurwitz, E. L. *et al.* (1996). Manipulation and mobilization of the cervical spine: a systematic review of the literature, *Spine* 21: 1746–60.
11. van der Windt, D. A. W. M. *et al.* (1999). Ultrasound therapy for musculoskeletal disorders: a systematic review, *Pain* 81: 257–71.

Section 7
Cancer and palliative care

7.1 **Cancer and palliative care**

Writing about the evidence for the different treatments used to relieve pain due to cancer presents several difficulties.

1. Trials in this group of trials are notoriously difficult to conduct, because of multiple symptoms, many co-interventions, and the fact that these are often sick people.

2. Following from (1), for many treatments we do not have evidence of sufficient quality of or sufficient quantity (from trials in cancer pain alone) to allow definitive conclusions to be drawn.

3. Following from (2) we need then to draw on the evidence from pain in other contexts, acute (including postoperative) and chronic non-cancer pain, in order to provide high quality evidence.

Much of what we do, and do successfully, in symptom control in advanced cancer is derived from hard-won experience, not from randomised trials. It works no less well because of this, and the wisdom others can deliver high quality care. The best single source of this wisdom, we believe, is the book on symptom control in far advanced cancer by Twycross and Lack [1].

Wisdom is dynamic, changing as more evidence becomes available. This wisdom is behind the development of the WHO ladder for cancer pain relief (Figure 7.1.1).

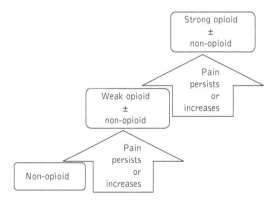

Figure 7.1.1 WHO ladder for cancer pain.

Morphine

For advanced cancer, pain control relies on morphine (though not necessarily alone). There is no systematic review of morphine clinical trials that we know of, and precious few trials. Therefore, in this introduction, two systematic reviews on morphine clinical pharmacology are offered. The first is a systematic review of factors affecting the ratios of morphine and its major metabolites. The second is a systematic review of the maximum plasma concentration of morphine (and the time at which the maximum occurs). The final section reviews the trials of oral morphine in the cancer pain setting. In the conclusion we set out the areas where we think there is a clear research agenda, and the lessons we have learned about the design and conduct of future trials in cancer pain management.

Morphine is an old established and very effective drug. In some ways it is simple to use and there are good guidelines about how to use it effectively in particular situations. Its mechanism of action is complicated by the fact that it has an active metabolite, morphine-6-glucuronide (M6G), and that there is suspicion (on no good evidence) that the other metabolite morphine-3-glucuronide (M3G) can act as an antagonist at high concentrations. Clearly there is a need to understand those circumstances where the relationship between morphine and its metabolites is deranged, and that could affect the effect obtained from a given dose.

Morphine and its major metabolites

Clinical bottom line. The effects of age, renal impairment, route of administration and method of analysis were examined for their effects on the ratio in plasma between morphine and its major metabolites, M3G and M6G. Neonates produced less glucuronide than children or adults. Metabolite ratios were higher in renal impairment. Routes of administration that avoided first pass metabolism (intravenous, transdermal, rectal, intramuscular) resulted in lower metabolite production than oral, buccal or sublingual. Metabolite production was similar for single or multiple dosing.

Systematic review

Faura, C. C. *et al.* (1998). Systematic review of factors affecting the ratios of morphine and its major metabolites, *Pain* 74: 43–53.

The review sought reports of plasma concentrations of morphine and its metabolites in human subjects, using a number of electronic databases. The date of the last search was March 1997. Neonates were defined as children within one month of birth, children as defined by the original authors. Molar ratios of morphine to M3G, morphine to M6G and M3G to M6G were calculated. The mean results were weighted by the size of the study.

Findings

There were 57 studies with 1232 patients in 91 clinical groups.

Effect of age

Neonates had low ratios of morphine glucuronides to morphine. This was higher in children, and higher again in adults. Figure 7.1.2 shows the relationship for M6G and morphine.

Effect of renal impairment

With impaired renal function the ratios of morphine glucuronides to morphine increased significantly, whether the morphine was given by oral or intravenous route of administration (Figure 7.1.3).

Single or multiple doses

For oral administration there was no difference in ratios between single and multiple dosing.

Method of analysis

Similar results were obtained for chromatographic and immunological methods of analysis.

Ratio of M3G to M6G

This ratio remained constant in all subgroups analysed (Figure 7.1.4). This suggests that morphine glucuronidation is predominantly under the control of a single enzyme system.

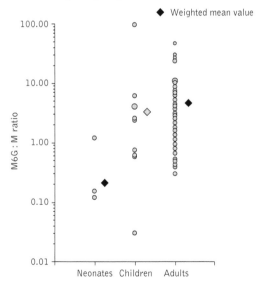

Figure 7.1.2 M6G to morphine ratios in neonates, children and adults.

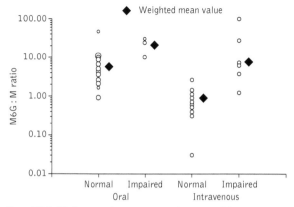

Figure 7.1.3 M6G to morphine ratios according to renal function.

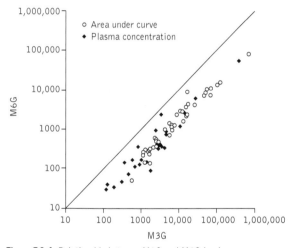

Figure 7.1.4 Relationship between M6G and M3G in plasma.

Comment

These results are useful in understanding some of the background to using morphine in clinical situations. Active metabolites will be higher in patients with impaired renal function, and lower in children and especially neonates.

Peak plasma concentrations after oral morphine

Clinical bottom line. The type of formulation profoundly affects the plasma concentration of morphine after oral administration. Peak morphine concentrations are about 6 nmol/L/mg after immediate release morphine, 3 nmol/L/mg for controlled release morphine and 0.5 nmol/L/mg for once-daily morphine. The time to peak concentration was 1, 2.7 and 8.5 h respectively.

There are many reports of plasma morphine concentrations after oral administration. Almost none are randomised trials, and the studies are complicated by different formulations, different types of patients (healthy volunteers and patients) and different measurement methods. The result has been something of a minefield for interpretation. A systematic review brings some light to the darkness.

Systematic review

Collins, S. L. *et al.* (1998). Peak plasma concentrations after oral morphine: a systematic review, *Journal of Pain and Symptom Management* 16: 388–402.

The review sought studies investigating the plasma concentrations after oral morphine in adult human subjects, and included searching according to 39 brand names in at least four electronic databases. The date of the last search was July 1997. Reports had to have enough pharmacokinetic information to reliably estimate a maximum plasma concentration and the time to maximum concentration. Extracted was information on the maximum plasma concentration and the time to maximum plasma concentration, together with the dose of morphine, together with the formulation. These were divided into immediate release (four to six times a day), controlled release (twice a day), and once daily formulations. For maximum concentration, values were corrected by dividing the concentration by the dose administered (in mg).

Findings

There were 129 reports in total, of which 69 met inclusion criteria, and with information on 2146 subjects (454 patients and 1692 healthy volunteers). Healthy volunteers and patient data were similar, but that from healthy volunteers was less variable, perhaps reflecting the, sometimes inadequate, descriptions of patient condition. There was considerable variability between studies, though method of assay was not an issue, and there was no difference in the range of results between single and multiple dosing.

Peak morphine concentration

The maximum concentration, corrected for dose, was higher for immediate release (5.8 nmol/L/mg) than for controlled release (3.2 nmol/L/mg) and once-daily morphine (0.5 nmol/L/mg) (Figure 7.1.5).

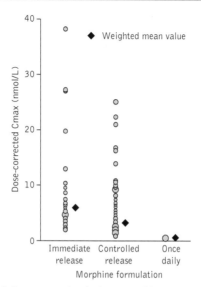

Figure 7.1.5 Dose-corrected peak plasma morphine concentration with different formulations.

Time to peak concentration

The time to maximum was 1.1 h for immediate release, 2.7 h for controlled release, and 8.5 h for once-daily morphine (Figure 7.1.6).

Comment

This is a useful study because it confirms the different release properties of formulations often used for pain treatment in cancer. It also serves to demystify much of the confusion around morphine measurements – for instance, demonstrating that measurement methods make little difference to the results. There was a comment on the wayward standards of reporting, with authors failing to state what they were measuring, and the phrase morphine concentration hides much confusion that itself contributes to the variability.

Trials of oral morphine

Randomised trials of morphine in cancer pain were sought, using various different search strategies to identify the eligible reports in MED-LINE (1966–1996), EMBASE (1980–1996), the Cochrane Library (1997, issue 2) and the Oxford Pain Relief Database (1950–1994). The last electronic search was conducted in December 1996. The words 'morphine', 'diamorphine', 'heroin' were used to identify relevant reports, using a combination of free text words and MeSH terms, and without restriction to language. Additional reports were identified

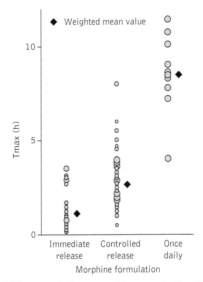

Figure 7.1.6 Time to peak plasma morphine concentration with different formulations.

from reference lists of retrieved reports, review articles, and specialist textbooks. Inclusion criteria were full journal publication of randomised controlled trials which included treatment groups of oral morphine, cancer pain, blinded design, adult patients, and pain assessments. Review articles, letters or abstracts were not included.

Reports were screened to eliminate those without pain outcomes, those which were definitely not randomised, or were abstracts or reviews. Each report which could possibly be described as a randomised controlled trial was read independently by each of the authors and scored using a three item, 1–5 score, quality scale. The maximum score of an included study was 5 and the minimum score was 1.

Trials comparing normal release with controlled release formulations

Eleven trials met inclusion criteria. Although often of low power, these by and large support the contention that controlled release morphine can substitute for normal release morphine while maintaining analgesia and posing no extra adverse effect burden. Two further trials showed that different ways of giving the same total dose of a controlled release formulation, one high dose tablet versus several smaller dose tablets, produced the same outcome.

Such trials are necessary for registration of novel formulations, but otherwise add surprisingly little to our bank of knowledge. We had hoped to reap good information about adverse effects from these trials, which were the majority of the oral morphine cancer trials, but the information simply was not there, and the duration of study was often disappointingly brief. One might hope that investigators doing similar trials in the future will take note of the deficiencies. The reality is that few people are in a position to do quality investigations in cancer pain, and that if those scarce resources are fully occupied with registration trials then it will be a long time before we will have adequate answers to the more fundamental questions.

Comparisons of different normal release formulations

Three trials showed that there was no clinical advantage of the Brompton mixture over morphine solution alone and that morphine hydrochloride solution and tablets produced similar outcomes.

Oral versus other routes ± other drugs

A number of disparate and interesting trials come under this heading. The trials by Beaver *et al.* and by Kalso and Vainio focused on equipotent dose across route, and provide short duration answers for morphine, oxycodone and oxymorphone. The problem that clinicians face is the applicability of such three day answers to patients on chronic dosing. The gulf between the acute 6 : 1 ratio quoted for oral to parenteral morphine and the 2 or 3 : 1 which clinicians have found valid in chronic use is wide, and emphasises the difficulty faced in future studies. Study duration must be adequate to represent chronic dosing.

The comparisons of oral morphine with morphine by other routes are also largely unsatisfactory. Because they are small trials, or because of design inadequacies, they do not permit definitive answers for the various cells in Figure 7.1.7.

Comparisons	Outcome	
	Efficacy	Adverse effects at equi-analgesic dosing
Same route, different drug		
Same drug, different route		
Subcutaneous		
Epidural		
Intrathecal		
Rectal		
etc.		

Figure 7.1.7 Trying to define the important questions.

The future

The research agenda is simple. If we require answers to the different questions posed in Figure 7.1.7 then some organisation is required. The lessons learned from this set of trials are that trials have to be of adequate size and design if they are to produce useful answers. The additional problem, stressed repeatedly in this report, is that trials in cancer pain patients are particularly difficult. Unless and until the nettle is grasped and adequate multi-centre trials are done our practice will remain based on custom and practice.

Reference

1. Twycross, R. G. and Lack, S. A. (1983). *Symptom control in far advanced cancer*, Pitman Books Ltd, London, ISBN 0-272-7917-0.

7.2 **Non-steroidal anti-inflammatory drugs for cancer pain**

Clinical bottom line. Non-steroidal anti-inflammatory drugs (NSAIDs) are effective in relieving cancer pain. Single doses of an NSAID are effective at 6 h, and multiple doses of NSAID are effective at ten to 14 days. This review did not attempt to compare the efficacy of different NSAIDs. For single doses, NSAIDs appear to be as effective as intramuscular morphine 5–10 mg, weak opioids or opioid combinations and the same NSAID given at higher doses. For multiple doses, there was no difference between NSAIDs and weak opioids or opioid combinations. No other comparisons were possible. Upper gastrointestinal upset, dizziness and drowsiness were the most common adverse effects for single and multiple dose trials. In multiple dose trials, NSAIDs were associated with fewer adverse effects than intramuscular morphine 5–10 mg.

NSAIDs are widely used in the treatment of cancer-related pain. World Health Organisation guidelines recommend NSAIDs as the sole treatment of mild to moderate cancer pain, and in combination with opioids for moderate to severe pain.

Systematic review

Eisenberg, E., Berkey, C. S., Carr, D. B., Mosteller, F. and Chalmers, T. C. (1994). Efficacy and safety of nonsteroidal antiinflammatory drugs for cancer pain: a meta-analysis, *Journal of Clinical Oncology* 12: 2756–65.

Date review completed: 1992

Number of trials included: 25

Number of patients: 1545

Control group: Placebo and other active

Main outcomes: Pain intensity, pain relief, adverse effects

Inclusion criteria were randomised, double blind, controlled trials of NSAIDs with or without combination opioid for cancer pain; full journal publication; English language.

Reviewers extracted data on dosing regimens, adverse effects and pain. Pain data were patient ratings of pain intensity or pain relief scores using visual analogue or other quantitative scales. From this, peak pain intensity or pain relief difference was calculated and summed pain intensity difference (SPID) or total pain relief (TOTPAR). These were converted to percentages (percent of maximum). Means were weighted by sample size.

Comparison groups were placebo, different dose of NSAID including recommended versus supramaximal dose, weak opioid/weak opioid combination and morphine. Weak opioid was defined as those doses/drugs appropriate for treating mild to moderate pain.

Findings

Most trials reported on various types of cancer pain or did not specify type of cancer.

Single dose trials: 6 h outcome

Placebo versus NSAID comparisons: there were between eleven and 14 placebo comparisons for each measure, looking at up to six different NSAIDs. Doses were not stated. NSAIDs were superior to placebo at six hours on each of the four pain measures (percentage values of TOTPAR or SPID and of peak pain relief or peak pain intensity difference) ($p < 0.05$). Percentages for these measures ranged from 31% to 60% for NSAIDs compared with 15–36% for placebo).

Weak opioid/weak opioid combination versus NSAID comparisons: there were eight to nine comparisons for two measures (peak pain intensity and SPID) looking at a range of drugs/doses. There were no statistical differences between groups on either measure.

Intramuscular morphine 5–10 mg versus NSAID comparisons: there were four to five comparisons for two measures (SPID and TOTPAR). There were no statistical differences between groups on either measure.

Other comparisons: no significant differences were found comparing aspirin with other NSAIDs or comparing different doses of the same NSAID, including recommended dose with supramaximal dose.

Multiple dose trials: 10–14 day outcomes

Only weak opioid/weak opioid combination versus NSAID comparison was possible. There were two comparisons: one of ketorolac 10 mg versus acetaminophen 600 + codeine 60 mg and one of ketorolac 10 mg versus pentazocine 50 mg. Neither showed a significant difference on peak pain relief or TOTPAR.

Adverse effects

Common adverse effects for single and multiple dose trials included upper gastrointestinal upset, dizziness and drowsiness. For single dose trials, when all adverse effects were pooled, there were no significant differences between NSAIDs and placebo or NSAIDs and intramuscular morphine 5–10 mg. However, there were significantly more adverse effects with weak opioid or opioid combinations than with NSAIDs (20 versus 14 episodes per 100 patients).

With multiple dose trials it was only possible to compare NSAIDs with weak opioids/opioid combinations. There were no significant differences when all adverse effects were pooled.

7.3 **Radiotherapy for painful bone metastases**

Clinical bottom line. Radiotherapy can provide effective analgesia for painful bone metastases. Over 40% of patients can expect at least 50% pain relief, and just under 30% can expect complete pain relief at one month. There appears to be little difference in efficacy between the fractionation schedules and between different doses using the same schedule.

Radiotherapy is commonly used to provide pain relief for localised painful bone metastases. It is, however, difficult to provide accurate estimates of the proportion of patients achieving relief, and the extent and duration of relief owing to the variations within the condition and in the primary cancer itself. Contemporaneous interventions and supplementary analgesics further complicate the picture.

Systematic review

McQuay, H. J., Carroll, D., Moore, R. A. (1997). Radiotherapy for painful bone metastases: a systematic review, *Clinical Oncology* 9: 150–4.

Date review completed: March 1996

Number of trials included: 13

Number of patients: 1373 for total pain relief/1486 for 50% pain relief (1 month outcomes)

Controls: For one month relief = assumed naturally resolving total pain relief rate of 1/100

Main outcomes: NNT at one month (complete and at least 50% pain relief) and at any time during the trial. Onset and duration of pain relief.

Inclusion criteria were full journal publication; randomised controlled trial of radiotherapy in the palliative treatment of painful bony metastases; radiotherapy schedule; radiotherapy versus isotope injection; isotope injection versus placebo; pain outcomes. The nature of the trial designs and illness variations prohibited classic pooling of data, so the review generated best possible quantitative estimates.

Findings

Main findings are in Table 7.3.1. The NNTs for various pain relief outcomes are as follows.

Complete pain relief one month after radiotherapy. Twenty-seven per cent of patients achieved total pain relief. The NNT was 3.9 (3.5–4.4).

Table 7.3.1 NNTs for various pain relief outcomes with radiotherapy

Outcome	Data set	Number of patients benefited/total	NNT (95% CI)
Complete pain relief one month after radiotherapy	5 trials (all schedules)	368/1373	3.9 (3.5–4.4)
50% pain relief one month after radiotherapy	5 trials (all schedules)	437/1486	3.6 (3.2–3.9)
50% pain relief at any time after radiotherapy	23 treatment groups (all schedules)	628/1486	Not given

50% pain relief one month after radiotherapy. Twenty-nine percent of patients achieved 50% pain relief. The NNT was 3.6 (3.2–3.9).

50% pain relief at any time after radiotherapy. Forty-two percent of patients achieved 50% pain relief (all schedules), with little difference between the fractionation schedules. Pain relief was similar for the various fractionation schedules adopted, and for single and multiple fraction schedules.

Speed of onset of relief and duration. Based on the largest trial, median duration of complete relief was 12 weeks (759 patients). It took four weeks for half of the patients achieving complete relief to do so.

Radioisotopes and radiotherapy for generalised disease. Based on three trials (192 patients) radioisotopes alone produced a similar degree of relief with a similar onset and duration to that provided by radiotherapy. There were significantly fewer new pain sites in the strontium groups compared with controls. Hemibody irradiation and radioisotopes have the potential to reduce the number of new sites of bone pain, but radioisotopes do have increased haematological toxicity. Radiotherapy plus strontium produced better quality of life scores than radiotherapy plus placebo.

Adverse events

Reviewers state that reporting was poor. There were no obvious differences between the various schedules with nausea and vomiting, diarrhoea or pathological fractures.

7.4 **Strontium 89 therapy for painful bony metastases**

Clinical bottom line. Strontium 89 is useful in prostatic and breast cancer. Although it may not necessarily reduce pain from existing bony metastases, it appears to decrease the number of new sites developing. Strontium 89 appears to have similar clinical response rates to other radiopharmaceuticals with selective bone localisation.

Most secondary bone lesions arise from primary carcinoma of the prostate, breast or lung, and external beam radiation therapy palliates 70% of lesions. However, this is not always adequate treatment for patients with multiple lesions and end-stage disease. In such cases pain relief is an important aspect of treatment. Radiopharmaceutical therapy can be given as an adjunct to external beam radiation for managing pain caused by skeletal metastases. Several radiopharmaceuticals, including strontium chloride 89 exist with selective bone localisation and the ability to irradiate bony metastases from within by short-range radiation.

Systematic review

Robinson, R. G., Preston, D. F., Schiefelbein, M. and Baxter, K. G. (1995).
Strontium 89 therapy for the palliation of pain due to osseous metastases, *JAMA* 274: 420–4.

Date review completed: December 1994

Number of trials included: Approximately 8 (2 randomised controlled trials)

Number of patients: Approximately 1000

Control group: None, non-radioactive strontium, external beam therapy

Main outcomes: Pain (analgesic requirement), clinical response rate (e.g. changes in mobility, sleep, daily activities, etc.), new painful sites

Inclusion criteria were trials of intravenous strontium chloride 89 for painful osteoblastic bony metastases; outcomes included analgesic requirement, group size at least 10; three month follow-up; treatment of one injection of strontium 89; haemotoxicity data reported; English language reports.

Data on baseline and periodic pain and on baseline and periodic hemotoxicity were extracted from original reports. These data were not pooled. Response rates were defined (although not clearly) as some improvement on a relevant measure and as complete pain relief.

Findings

Included trials were mainly of patients with prostate or breast cancer. Doses of strontium 89 ranged from 0.6 MBq/kg (16 μCi/kg) to 400 MBq/kg (10.8 mCI). Only two were randomised controlled trials.

Randomised controlled trials

One trial compared strontium 89 with external beam therapy in 305 patients with painful prostatic metastatic cancer. Patients were assessed for suitability for local or hemibody radiation, and were then randomised to receive either radiotherapy or 200 MBq (5.4 mCi) of strontium 89. Pain relief at three months was similar (no significant differences in analgesic intake), but development of painful new sites occurred in significantly fewer patients receiving strontium 89 compared with local and hemibody radiation (both p values < 0.05). Significantly fewer strontium 89 patients needed radiotherapy to painful sites of pain compared with patients receiving local radiotherapy ($p < 0.01$), but not hemibody radiotherapy.

Toxicity: There was a significantly higher incidence of adverse gastrointestinal tract effects among both groups of radiotherapy treated patients (local radiation 27%; hemibody radiation 43%) compared with strontium 89 (10%).

A second trial compared strontium 89 plus conventional radiotherapy with radiotherapy alone in 126 patients with hormone-refractory metastatic prostatic cancer (dose not stated). All patients received local field irradiation, and were then randomised to placebo or strontium 89. Overall symptom relief and survival were similar in the two groups. However strontium 89 was associated with significantly fewer new pain sites (59% versus 34%), less analgesic intake, less time to radiotherapy, fewer serum tumour markers compared with placebo, thus demonstrating a slowing of the disease process.

Toxicity: This was more common in the strontium 89 group compared with placebo, with significantly higher white blood cell toxicity and platelet toxicity.

Trials without a control

These can be summarised as producing response rates (i.e. any change in sleep pattern, analgesic intake, work history, daily activities or mobility – as measured in trials), which varied between 50% and 90% at approximately 3–6 months. Hematologic toxicity is summarised as mild and reversible. This is similar to response rates for other radiopharmaceuticals used for cancer pain palliation. Samarium 153 ethylenediaminetetramethylenephosphonic acid (EDTMP Sm 153) has a response rate of 65–80% over 3.8 months, and rhenium 186 hydroxyethylenediphosphonic acid (HEDP Re 186) has a response rate of 50–80% over 5 weeks. Both have hematologic toxicity described as mild and reversible.

7.5 Intracerebroventricular opioid therapy compared with epidural and subarachnoid opioids for intractable cancer pain

Clinical bottom line. Intracerebroventricular (ICV) opioid therapy appears to be at least as effective as epidural or subarachnoid opioid therapy in patients with intractable cancer pain. Adverse effects and catheter/system related problems do not clearly favour one route. These should be carefully weighed when making a decision about method of delivery, but more rigorous data are needed in order to assess whether ICV is an appropriate first-line neuraxial treatment.

Central or neuraxial opioid treatments have been used for the small number of cancer patients who do not respond to systemic treatment. Epidural, subarachnoid and ICV catheters can all be used for chronic treatment, although the additional devices such as pumps and reservoirs which have been designed to prolong catheter life also increase cost and require a surgical procedure.

Systematic review

Ballantyne, J. C., Carr, D. B. Berkey, C. S., Chalmers, T. C. and Mosteller, F.
(1996). Comparative efficacy of epidural, subarachnoid, and intracerebroventricular opioids in patients with pain due to cancer, *Regional Anesthesia* 21: 542–56.

Date review completed: February 1991

Number of trials included: 83

Number of patients: Intracerebroventricular 268, epidural 909, subarachnoid therapy 410

Main outcomes: Pain relief, adverse effects, catheter and system complications

Inclusion criteria were trials of intracerebroventricular (ICV), epidural or subarachnoid administration of opioids for cancer pain; extractable data.

Reviewers did not find any controlled trials, and therefore carried out a meta-analysis to analyse the accumulated incidence data on efficacy and side effects/complications for uncontrolled trials. Reviewers note the limitations of this approach, namely that patient groups may not be comparable (e.g. patients receiving ICV treatment may be those who have failed spinal opioid treatment), and that the data will be more biased than that of properly randomised controlled trials.

Pain data were extracted and categorised as either excellent or good, or unsatisfactory. Adverse effects were categorised as either transient or protracted. When this was unclear, adverse effects were regarded as protracted. Catheter/system complications were categorised as major infection, minor infection, other (pump failure, reservoir malfunction, leakage, blockage and misplacement). Adverse effects and complications data were compared using the difference in the percent rates with standard error of the difference. These were used to indicate likely statistical differences – that is, a difference more than two standard errors was regarded as a probable significant difference between two groups.

Findings

Thirteen trials of ICV (268 patients), 29 of epidural (909 patients) and 21 of subarachnoid therapy (410 patients) were found. ICV trials were of ICV plus implanted reservoir. Epidural and subarachnoid trials were of catheter alone, catheter with reservoir or catheter with pump. Included trials did not measure pain relief using standardised measures.

Reviewers compared numbers of patients receiving excellent pain relief across routes, in seven ICV, 13 epidural and nine subarachnoid trials. There were no differences between numbers of patients reporting excellent pain relief for ICV versus epidural (75% versus 72%) and ICV versus subarachnoid (75% versus 58%).

Reviewers compared numbers of patients receiving unsatisfactory pain relief across routes, in seven ICV, 23 epidural and 14 subarachnoid trials. There was a significant difference between numbers of patients reporting unsatisfactory pain relief for the ICV versus epidural comparison (4% versus 10% $p = 0.045$), but not the ICV versus subarachnoid comparison (4% versus 6%).

Adverse effects

ICV versus subarachnoid delivery: ICV was associated with less persistent nausea, persistent and transient urinary retention, persistent and transient pruritus compared with subarachnoid delivery. These were regarded as probable statistical differences. There were no differences for transient nausea or respiratory depression.

ICV versus epidural delivery: ICV was associated with less persistent nausea, persistent urinary retention, persistent and transient pruritus compared with epidural delivery. Epidural was associated with less transient nausea and less respiratory depression than ICV. These were regarded as probable statistical differences. There were no differences for transient urinary retention.

Adverse events

Most commonly reported other effects for ICV were sedation (4% and 9% of patients reporting protracted and transient sedation) and confusion (5% and 16%). These symptoms were rare for other routes. Constipation was reported less frequently with ICV (3%) compared with a statement that it occurred in the majority of patients using other routes.

Catheter/system complications: ICV is probably associated with more major infections compared with other pump routes, but probably fewer complications involving removal compared with epidural with or without reservoir.

7.6 **Neurolytic coeliac plexus block (NCPB) for cancer pain**

Clinical bottom line. Based on data from uncontrolled trials, neurolytic coeliac plexus block is an effective method for relieving pain associated with pancreatic and non-pancreatic intra-abdominal malignancies, with approximately 90% of patients achieving at least partial pain relief short term (two weeks) and long term (three months and beyond). There appears to be no added benefit from NCPB with any form of radiological guidance. Common transient adverse effects were local pain, diarrhoea and hypotension. More severe adverse effects included neurological and non-neurological adverse effects, both of which occurred in 1% of patients.

Between 2% and 5% of patients with advanced cancer receiving hospice care have nerve blocks as part of cancer pain management. Neurolytic blocks, that is, those which destroy the nerve, are only used in patients with short life expectancies or where other simpler techniques have failed. In this situation neurolytic coeliac plexus block (NCPB) is used to treat pain associated with upper abdominal cancer.

Systematic review

Eisenberg, E., Carr, D. B. and Chalmers, C. T. (1995). Neurolytic coeliac plexus block for treatment of cancer pain: a meta-analysis., *Anesthesia and Analgesia* 80: 290–5.

Date review completed: Mid 1993

Number of trials included: 24 (2 randomised controlled trials)

Number of patients: 1145

Control group: Predominantly uncontrolled trials

Main outcomes: Pain relief

Inclusion criteria were randomised and non-randomised trials of NCPB for cancer pain; controlled and uncontrolled trials; full journal publication; English language.

Reviewers analysed the results of randomised controlled trials separately from those of other studies. Pain and other data were extracted. Pain data were categorised as either complete pain relief, partial pain relief and minimal/no relief. Results were categorised as acute (up to two weeks) or long-term (two or more weeks). Where pooling was possible, calculating weighted means using a random effects model assessed the estimate of the success rate of the intervention.

Findings

Of the included trials specifying cancer type, 707/1117 patients had pancreatic cancer, and 410/1117 had non-pancreatic intra-abdominal malignancies. Duration of patient pain was approximately 2–7 months, and where reported (four trials) was classified as severe.

Randomised controlled trials

Two trials were included. One compared three different types of NCPB technique and the second compared NCPB with oral analgesic. Unfortunately reviewers did not fully report the findings of these trials. In one trial 10/10 patients reported at least partial pain relief at 2 weeks and 7/10 at three to 10 weeks (control information not given). In the second trial 70–80% of patients reported at least partial pain relief at two weeks, and 60–75% at three months and beyond (control information not given).

Uncontrolled trials

Short-term analgesic efficacy: Eighteen trials in 989 patients were included. 89% of these had at least partial relief. Of the patients experiencing at least partial relief, 59% experienced complete relief by two weeks.

Long-term efficacy: Ninety percent of 273 patients experienced at least partial relief at three months or beyond.

Six trials with 53 patients reported pain at time of death. 73–92% of patients had at least partial relief.

There were no apparent differences in pain relief in pancreatic compared with non-pancreatic cancer.

Procedure methods

Most patients underwent radiologically guided NCPB (including computed tomography, radiography and less commonly fluoroscopy or ultrasound). Overall, the success rates (at least partial pain relief) varied from 86% to 95%.

NCPB with no radiological guidance was reported for 238 patients from uncontrolled trials. There was a mean success rate of 95% (92–98%).

One randomised, controlled trial reported a 90% success rate with radiographic guidance. A further 271 patients from uncontrolled trials had a mean success rate of 91% (87–94%).

Computed tomography was reported for 271 patients from uncontrolled trials. There was a mean success rate of 88% (83–97%).

One randomised trial reported a 70–80% success rate with fluoroscopy. A further 36 patients from an uncontrolled trial had a mean success rate of 86%.

Adverse effects

There were three commonly reported transient adverse effects: local pain was reported in 96% of patients (two trials), diarrhoea in 44% of patients (five trials), and hypotension in 38% of patients (10 trials).

More severe effects were reported in 13 trials. Neurological complications such as lower extremity weakness and paresthesia, epidural anaesthesia and lumbar puncture were reported in 1% of patients. Significant non-neurological adverse effects, including pneumothorax, shoulder, chest and pleuritic pain, hiccuping and haematuria occurred in a further 1% of patients.

It was not possible to establish whether different procedures were associated with particular adverse effects.

7.7 **Nilutamide plus orchidectomy for metastatic prostatic cancer**

Clinical bottom line. Nilutamide is associated with pain relief in patients who have undergone orchidectomy for prostatic cancer. Although nilutamide has an NNT of 7.5 (5–15) for any pain relief at six months compared with placebo, it remains to be established whether this is of clinical relevance.

The most effective treatment for prostatic cancer with metastases is thought to be removal of the testicular and adrenal androgens. Orchidectomy and luteinizing hormone releasing hormone agonists (LHRH agonists) or oestrogens suppress testicular androgens. Anti-androgens such as nilutamide, flutamide or cyproterone acetate are used to suppress the effects of adrenal androgens. Nilutamide (Anandron) is an oral non-steroidal anti-androgen, and like other anti-androgens is associated with a number of adverse effects.

Systematic review

Bertagna, C., De Gery, A., Hucher, M., Francois, J. P. and Zanirato, J. (1994). Efficacy of the combination of nilutamide plus orchidectomy in patients with metastatic prostatic cancer. A meta-analysis of seven randomized double-blind trials (1056 patients), *British Journal of Urology* 73: 396–402.

Date review completed: Most recent included trial, 1986

Number of trials included: 6

Number of patients: 1056

For pain: 839 (439 orchidectomy plus nilutamide/400 orchidectomy plus placebo)

Control group: Placebo anti-androgen

Main outcomes: Pain, biochemical measures, disease regression, survival

Inclusion criteria were randomised double-blind placebo-controlled trials of orchidectomy plus nilutamide for stage D prostate cancer; no previous hormone treatment; hormone treatment started not later than three months after orchidectomy; short- and long-term outcomes.

Data were extracted from original trials. Short-term outcomes were defined as symptoms at 6 months. Patients were categorised as improved, unchanged or deteriorated compared with baseline. For tumour markers, this was defined as a 25% change. Long-term outcomes were summed progression outcomes (of 6-month measures) and the summed survival outcome (of 12-month measures). For pain, reviewers presented 6-month data, with patients either percent improved, unchanged or deteriorated in comparison with baseline measures (pain measure not stated). Definition of improved was not given so it is assumed this was any change, however small.

Reviewers pooled dichotomous data and calculated odds ratios with 95% confidence intervals. We used the same data to calculate relative benefit and NNT with 95% confidence intervals.

Findings

Six trials on 839 patients were included in the analysis. Five trials had a dosing regime of 300 mg/day of nilutamide, and one trial gave nilutamide 300 mg/day for one month and then 150 mg/day from then on. Length of follow-up varied within and across trials. The largest trial had a follow-up period ranging from 1 to 3.5 years. The other trials had follow-up periods ranging from approximately 2–4, 5 or 6 years.

Four of six trials had significant relative benefits, suggesting significant pain relief with nilutamide compared with placebo. This included the lower dose trial. The overall relative benefit was significant, 1.4 (1.2–1.7), and nilutamide had a NNT of 7.5 (5–15) for any pain relief over 6 months compared with placebo.

Data on other outcomes are clearly presented in the paper. However, there is a more recent review (listed below) which, although it has no pain outcomes, has more up-to-date survival and regression data.

Adverse effects

Reviewers did not report on adverse effects.

Further references

The following review is more recent, but does not report on pain outcomes:
Caubet, J. F. *et al.* (1997). Maximum androgen blockade in advanced prostate cancer: a meta-analysis of published randomized controlled trials using nonsteroidal antiandrogens, *Urology* 49: 71–78.

The following review reports on use of flutamide, but with no pain outcomes:
Bennett, C. L. *et al.* (1999). Maximum androgen-blockade with medical or surgical castration in advanced prostate cancer: a meta-analysis of nine published randomized controlled trials and 4128 patients using flutamide, *Prostate Cancer and Prostatic Diseases* 2: 4–8.

7.8 **Complementary therapy at the end of life**

Clinical bottom line. There is no solid evidence that complementary and alternative therapies have any value for treating pain, dyspnoea or nausea and vomiting at the end of life.

Systematic review

Pan, C. X. *et al.* (2000). Complementary and alternative medicine in the management of pain, dyspnea, and nausea and vomiting near the end of life: a systematic review, *Journal of Pain and Symptom Management* 20: 374–87.

Six electronic databases were searched for papers about pain, dyspnoea, and nausea and vomiting at the end of life. The intention was to find papers that clearly studied interventions for these conditions, rather than surveys. The authors found 21 studies, 11 of which were randomised trials, two non-randomised controlled studies, and eight case series. Most of the studies investigated highly individual treatments in highly individual situations, so the likelihood of data pooling was low.

Findings

Pain

Fourteen studies addressed pain. Six different therapies were studied:

- TENS was evaluated in one RCT with 15 patients, one non-randomised controlled study with 60, and two case-series with 38.

- Acupuncture was evaluated in one RCT with 239 patients and two case series with 275 patients. There was no difference between real and sham acupuncture in the RCT.

- Massage was evaluated in one RCT with 28 patients and one case series with 9, and with additional aromatherapy in one case series with 103 patients.

- Psychological therapies were evaluated in one RCT with 94 patients. This showed highly significant improvements for oral mucositis pain ($p < 0.01$) compared with usual treatment.

- Music therapy was evaluated in one RCT with nine patients.

- Hypnosis was evaluated in one RCT with 58 patients.

Dyspnoea

- Acupuncture was evaluated in one RCT with 24 patients and one case series with 20.

- Acupressure was evaluated in one RCT with 31 patients.
- Breathing retraining was evaluated in one RCT with 20 patients.
- Psychoanalysis was evaluated in one RCT with 65 patients.
- Coping and counseling was evaluated in one RCT with 20 patients.

Nausea/vomiting
- Acupressure was evaluated in one non-randomised controlled study with nine patients.

Comment
Most of these studies could show some benefit of treatment with some outcome. The problems, though, are manifest. First, most were far too small to tell anything, even if their conduct was immaculate. Secondly, their conduct was not immaculate. Few were blinded, and most had what would normally be considered major structural flaws. There really is no solid evidence that complementary and alternative therapies have any value for treating pain, dyspnoea or nausea and vomiting at the end of life.

7.9 **Palliative care delivery systems**

Clinical bottom line. We are far from identifying high-quality, effective, and appropriate palliative care services.

Systematic review

Critchley, P., Jadad, A. R., Taniguchi, A., Woods, A., Stevens, R., Reyno, L. and Whelan, T. J. (1999). Are some palliative care delivery systems more effective and efficient than others? A systematic review of comparative studies, *Journal of Palliative Care* 15: 40–47.

Date review completed: October 1998

Number of papers included: 41

Number of patients: 4135

The studies compared hospices with beds, hospices with home care or traditional oncology wards. Searches were to March 1997: MEDLINE (from 1966); HealthStar (from 1975), CINAHL (from 1982), CancerLit (from 1982); The Cochrane Library, issue 2 of 1997 plus manual search of the reference lists of eligible studies identified and reference lists of textbooks on palliative care. Data were extracted using a predefined instrument. A descriptive analysis was conducted.

Articles were included if they:

1. were published as a full report in a peer-reviewed journal, in any language;
2. were comparative studies of any methodological design; reported results from patients of any age described as palliative, or as having end-stage or terminal conditions;
3. included comparisons of two or more ways of providing care for the above group of patients;
4. included data on outcomes related to the patients, their family members, health care providers, or health care system.

Findings

Forty-one studies were included: they were published between 1978 and 1996. Thirty-three were found in electronic databases and eight were found in reference lists. Eighteen were published in 1988 and later. All were published in English. 11 were RCTs; 30 were non-randomised comparative studies. Only four of the 41 studies provided information on all of the clinically relevant elements selected a priori: type of care provided, type of health care providers, setting, and outcomes. It was clear that most efforts have focused on adults with cancer and little has been done to increase understanding of palliative care in paediatric or non-cancer populations. In addition, research has focused on individual rather than system issues.

- Hospice groups used fewer interventional therapies and diagnostic tests compared with conventional care.
- Patients served by hospices without beds spent more time at home, were more likely to die at home and care was cheaper than for patients in other groups.
- Home care services did not reduce the length of any hospital stay if a patient needed to be admitted.
- Pain relief and symptom control was marginally better in hospices with beds.

Comment

The authors recognise that health services research in a palliative care population brings particular practical and ethical challenges, however they argue that it should be possible to use appropriate methodology to evaluate the needs of the palliative care population.

Section 8
Management issues

8.1 **Easy targets are not always the right ones**

Once more a government committee has taken a side-swipe at combination analgesics – this time their machinations appear in the British National Formulary (BNF). It says [1]:

> the most expensive range of less suitable drugs are those that work on the central nervous system, such as some of the painkillers. The BNF says combinations of aspirin or paracetamol with opioids, such as codeine, are a bad idea.

> Those that contain a full dose of opioid . . . also have the full range of opioid side effects, from drowsiness, nausea and vomiting and constipation to the risk of long-term dependence. Yet Solpadol cost the country £8,270,000 and Tylex £10,237,000.

These arguments seem to recur regularly in the developed world and rarely meet opposition from those involved in treating pain.

Effectiveness and convenience

The first argument is that the combinations are no more effective than their components. Even in single doses this is incorrect. Figure 8.1.1 shows a league table of relative efficacy of oral analgesics used in single doses for postoperative pain (section 2.2).

Adding codeine to paracetamol 600 mg provides analgesia equivalent to a bigger (1 g) dose of paracetamol, and paracetamol 1 g with

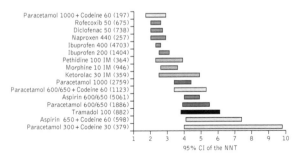

Figure 8.1.1 Number-needed-to-treat (NNT) for oral postoperative analgesics to achieve at least 50% relief of severe or moderate pain compared with placebo.

codeine 60 mg is the best performer. As yet we do not have the similar analysis for multiple dosing, but extensive clinical experience over many years attests that this will show an even greater effect for patients with chronic pain. We also know that other combinations also do particularly well, like paracetamol and tramadol [2].

We know that the combinations work on different mechanisms to relieve pain. Yes, we could give the components separately, which would delight the purists who dislike combinations of drugs with different kinetics. But the convenience of just one medication to take is worthwhile, especially for elderly patients on many other drugs. We prescribe sustained release morphine formulations (at huge cost) because it is perceived as more convenient.

Adverse effects

The BNF quote then moves on to adverse effects. Of course these combinations have opioid adverse effects, but we need a touch of common sense. Many elderly patients really should not be prescribed NSAIDs because of their high risk of gastrointestinal haemorrhage (section 5.6). Women over 65 years are at several times the risk of major gastrointestinal complications, and these are precisely the patients who present with pain problems. Female sex, increasing age, high doses, co-morbid conditions and progression to more harmful from less harmful NSAIDs are all factors making NSAIDs a poor choice for many patients.

Despite the new coxibs having fewer gastrointestinal problems, cyclooxygenase-2 inhibition still carries risks for those with impaired renal and cardiac function. These are the same elderly women with co-morbid conditions who have high risks for gastrointestinal problems.

Combination analgesics are a real and necessary alternative to NSAIDs for this expanding group. The risks with NSAIDs always seem to be downplayed in these discussions. The estimate from a systematic review is that the risk of dying from gastrointestinal problems after at least two months on an NSAID or aspirin is of the order of 1 in 1200 [3]. This is a finite risk, to be compared with the 1 in 17,000 risk of dying in a road traffic accident in the UK in any one year. It may be useful to contrast this risk with the risk of dying on therapeutic doses of combinations of paracetamol with opioid, which is negligible.

Removing drugs from the formulary, or damning them with faint praise, would be professionally legitimate if

1. there was no evidence of efficacy,

2. there were adverse effect concerns.

In the case of these combinations we would argue that there is evidence of efficacy and that concerns about adverse effects which do not take account of the problems with the alternatives are naïve. The only remaining motive would be financial. Again removal of the combinations might make short-term savings, but prescription costs of the alternatives would far outweigh any short term saving. We know that 1 in 2800 NSAID prescriptions in the elderly will lead to an episode of ulcer bleeding [4]. We also know that the overall cost of NSAID-related gastrointestinal adverse effects to the NHS is a conservative £250 million a year [5].

The considerable costs of dealing with these complications would then need to be subtracted from the 'savings' produced by removal of the combinations. A great deal more money would be saved if ibuprofen was prescribed instead of diclofenac. Ibuprofen is three times safer, eight times cheaper and there is no evidence that diclofenac is any more effective than ibuprofen [6]. Joined up thinking rather than budget-led constraints would make this clear.

The three-pot system

A terrible irony of this denigration of the paracetamol combinations is that it comes at a time when the evidence summarised above is being implemented to improve clinical care in both acute and chronic pain. This has led to advocacy of a three-pot system: paracetamol, paracetamol and opioid combination and NSAID.

Two schemes are in use, one for those who can take NSAIDs, one for those who cannot. Both minimise exposure to opioid and to NSAID. The schemes are shown in Figures 8.1.2 and 8.1.3. These draw on leaflets in use in Chesterfield UK. Before and after comparisons of implementation of the three-pot system are under way.

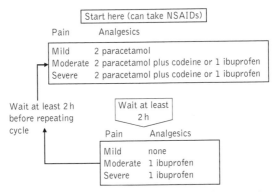

Figure 8.1.2 A simple scheme (three-pot) for acute and chronic pain relief using paracetamol/opioid combination drugs for patients who can take NSAIDs.

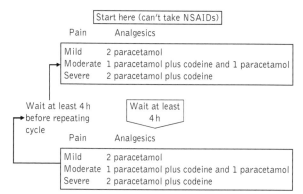

Figure 8.1.3 A simple scheme (three-pot) for acute and chronic pain relief using paracetamol/opioid combination drugs for patients who cannot take NSAIDs.

The three-pot system is based on best evidence, and uses cheapest available analgesics. It will work for most patients, incorporates the spirit of the WHO analgesic ladder and will minimise the number of patients who need to progress to stronger analgesics such as morphine. The proposals to attack combinations of simple analgesics with opioids are ill-informed and misguided.

Present and future problems

The three-pot system has the benefit of maximising effectiveness while minimising harm and minimising cost. It could be adjusted to use coxibs instead of NSAIDs and it could use different combinations of paracetamol and opioid (tramadol instead of codeine, perhaps?). Clearly it needs to be examined in a pragmatic trial. Who will pay? There is no mileage there for pharmaceutical companies, and government is indifferent, while charities chase genetic silver bullets. Yet simple, pragmatic solutions are what is required for people whose quality of life is diminishes by constant, everyday pain.

References

1. Boseley, S. (1998). £100 m bill for wrong NHS drugs, *Guardian* October 27 1998.
2. Edwards, J. E. *et al.* (2002). Combination analgesic efficacy: Individual patient data meta-analysis of single dose oral tramadol plus acetaminophen in acute postoperative pain, *Journal of Pain and Symptom Management* 23: 121–30.

3. Tramèr, M. R. *et al.* (2000). Quantitative estimation of rare adverse effects which follow a biological progression – a new model applied to chronic NSAID use, *Pain* 85: 169–82.

4. Hawkey, C. J. *et al.* (1997). Prescribing of nonsteroidal anti-inflammatory drugs in general practice: determinants and consequences, *Alimentary Pharmacology and Therapeutics* 11: 293–8.

5. Moore, R. A. and Phillips, C. J. (1997). Cost of NSAID adverse effects to the NHS, *Journal of Medical Economics* 2: 45–55.

6. Collins, S. L. *et al.* (1998). Oral ibuprofen and diclofenac in postoperative pain: a quantitative systematic review, *European Journal of Pain* 2: 285–91.

8.2 **Better prescribing of NSAIDs**

Providing information to doctors about better prescribing, also called academic detailing, has been shown to be a good thing. A Cochrane review [1] of 18 randomised or quasi-randomised trials found positive effects on practice in all trials, but only one measured a patient outcome. A new study from Adelaide [2] demonstrates an apparent remarkable decrease in admissions for perforations, ulcers and gastrointestinal bleeding following detailing about appropriate use of NSAIDs.

Study

The study was conducted in a particular area of metropolitan Adelaide with a population of 154,000. Two surgery visits were made in 1992. These visits focussed on better use of prescribed NSAIDs. The visits were preceded by a review of the literature, with a written summary of useful information prepared, and externally reviewed by experts and opinion leaders. Printed materials providing a source of 'balanced, unbiased information' were then left at each doctor visit. The programme highlighted the extensive use of NSAIDs and large number of adverse reactions, specifically in high use and high-risk groups.

Just under 90% of the 210 doctors practising in the area (80% of whom were GPs) received the service conducted by pharmacists with teaching hospital clinical experience. A neighbouring comparison area of 72,000 people did not have the intervention.

Outcomes measured for NSAID use were defined daily doses of NSAIDs prescribed per person per day, and units of NSAIDs delivered to pharmacies from manufacturers and wholesale suppliers. Hospital admissions for persons with ICD codes indicating ulceration or bleeding events in the upper GI tract with or without bleeding were obtained in the intervention or comparison area.

Findings

NSAID prescribing in the intervention area fell (Table 8.2.1). Two to 4 years after the visits prescribing in the intervention area was 9% lower in the intervention area compared to the control area. Two years after the intervention supplies of NSAIDs to pharmacies were 25% lower.

Over the period 1986–98 hospital admission rates for upper GI tract ulceration or bleed in the comparison area was unchanged at about

Table 8.2.1 Outcomes of NSAID prescribing – use of NSAIDS and hospital admissions for perforation and ulcers

Outcome	Period	Intervention area	Comparison area
NSAID prescribed	94–96 compared with 91	−16%	−7%
NSAID delivered to pharmacies	94 compared with 91	−23%	+5%
Hospital admissions for perforation or ulceration	1992	20/100,000	14/100,000
Hospital admissions for perforation or ulceration	1998	6/100,000	14/100,000

14 per 100,000 people. In the intervention area rates were rising before the intervention to a peak of about 20 per 100,000 before the intervention. Thereafter rates began to fall, and by 1998 were about 6 per 100,000, a fall of 70% from the peak.

Comment

There is much to say about this. The study could be criticised in a number of ways, but studies of every day interventions are remarkably hard to do. The results are remarkable because we are given patient outcomes, starkly unchanged in the comparison area but with big changes in the intervention area. The size and duration of the effect astonish.

But wait. If one thing shines out from this study it is the way in which the intervention was made. Evidence was gathered, it was weighed, it was honed by experts and opinion leaders, and it was 'balanced, unbiased information'. The doctors who received it were treated as the responsible people they were, and not like mushrooms.

Perhaps this is the secret. If so, this is a clear lead for how PCGs, of about the same average size as the intervention area in this study, could make a difference.

References

1. O'Brien, T. *et al.* (1999). Educational outreach visits: effects on professional practices and health care outcomes (Cochrane Review) in: The Cochrane Library 1999 issue 4. Update Software, Oxford.
2. May, F. W. *et al.* (1999). Outcomes of an educational-outreach service for community medical practitioners: non-steroidal anti-inflammatory drugs, *Medical Journal of Australia* 170: 471–4.

8.3 **Quality improvement by audit: Pain relief after day surgery**

Examples of how delivery of healthcare can be done effectively – often called 'doing the right thing right' – are rare. Given the academic slant of many of our medical journals, these must seem pretty mundane, and it must be hard to catch an editor's eye.

Pain relief after day surgery

In an 8-week period in 1993, 150 adults having surgery in a day surgery unit in Cardiff (general surgery, gynaecology, ophthalmic or ENT) were audited using a postal questionnaire for pain at home after their operation. At 24 and 72 h they rated their pain as mild, moderate or severe, and recorded analgesic drugs used over three days. The hospital had an analgesic prescribing policy covering about half these patients.

The results of the audit showed that of the 111 usable questionnaires returned, 29 patients (26%) reported severe pain at least one time, and 12 patients (11%) contacted their GP or were readmitted to hospital because of poor pain control. For some operations (hernia repair, for instance), almost all the patients had severe pain and over a third sought GP advice or were re-admitted.

Action taken

Briefly, the prescribing policy was revised to include 'missing' procedures. Procedures were ordered into those where mild pain was expected (e.g. cataracts), moderate pain was expected (e.g. varicose veins), or severe pain was expected (e.g. hernia repair). Prescribing policy was adjusted to take account of the expected pain level:

- *mild pain*: Paracetamol 1000 mg four times a day;
- *moderate pain*: Co-codamol 1 or 2 tablets four times a day;
- *severe pain*: Co-codamol 1 or 2 tablets four times a day plus naproxen 500 mg twice a day

(with, of course, appropriate adjustments for certain patients with ulcers or asthma).

In addition a system of 'rubber-stamping' prescription forms was devised so that appropriate prescriptions were given for appropriate operation types.

Results of this action

An audit of 200 patients over a 10-week period in 1994 showed that the prescribing policy was followed in 89% of cases. There were 130 returned questionnaires. They showed that the number of patients reporting severe pain at 24 or 72 h at home had been reduced almost to zero (about 10% reporting severe pain in but four of 12 operation types). No patient had cause to contact their GP for provision of postoperative pain relief.

Comment

Simple really, when put like this. Some thought, some organisation, and a will to do things better, and everyone benefits.

Reference

1. Haynes, T. K., Evans, D. E. and Roberts, D. (1995). Pain relief after day surgery: quality improvement by audit, *The Journal of One-Day Surgery*, Summer: 12–15.

8.4 **Improving oral postoperative analgesia**

Promoting an evidence-based approach at Stoke Mandeville Hospital, Aylesbury.

Why was the initiative launched?

Successive initiatives in the 1990s at Stoke Mandeville Hospital had made progress in using new analgesic techniques like epidural, spinal, patient and nurse controlled analgesia. But management of subsequent 'step-down' prescribing of oral analgesics was not keeping pace. Patients' postoperative care was not the best because of the inadequacy of the oral component. Prescribing at this stage was unstructured, with a wide range of oral analgesics in routine use, without any evidence base. Expenditure on oral analgesia was rising rapidly.

There was a growing feeling that something needed to be done. An opportunity for action came following the publication in 1997 of a review of the effectiveness of prescribing for pain relief which offered the basis for implementing an evidence-based approach [1].

What was done?

A team of people (Trevor Jenkins, Principal Pharmacist and Elaine Taylor, Nurse Specialist, supported by Dr John Sale, Consultant Anaesthetist) took the initiative in the early months of 1998 to find ways to tackle the situation. Their initial analysis suggested three issues needed attention:

+ It was not clear who had responsibility for the education of prescribers, nurses or pharmacists.

+ New junior doctors were asking nurses 'which oral analgesic is usually prescribed' rather than thinking about what was best for patients.

+ There were blurred inter-professional relationships at ward level between prescribers, nurses and pharmacists.

Creating a framework for action

The review provided a basis for recommendations for effective oral postoperative analgesics and a framework for care. Findings from local audit studies illustrated the diversity of local prescribing practice: 13 different medicines were prescribed to 45 patients.

The framework was designed to be evidence-based (on analgesic efficacy), to focus choice on appropriate medicine, route, and mode of delivery and be simple and safe to use. It aimed at enhancing multi-professional working. The recommended medicines included diclofenac and paracetamol with or without codeine. Diclofenac 50 mg was recommended to minimise the number of changes required, and because of the range of preparations available.

To promote discussions the team arranged for their analysis and recommendations to be discussed with medical staff at a meeting in Autumn 1998 as part of the Trust's clinical audit programme. The session encouraged debate about diversity, about personal preferences, about the research evidence, and about responsibilities and training. After rigorous discussion, all anaesthetic and surgical consultants endorsed the framework: junior doctors welcomed the evidence-based approach. The meeting allowed progress to be made in planning how the changes would be implemented from 1st January 1999.

Training

A training initiative took the message to clinical staff: they did not believe that it would be practical to reach all those involved through educational lectures. The nurse specialist arranged visits to each ward to explain the new approach to nursing staff. Care was taken to ensure that these visits were convenient and that all nurses on the wards were involved. These ward-based workshops covered the new approach and how to advise medical staff on best choice and prescribing when asked, 'what does this hospital usually prescribe for pain relief?' The Principal Pharmacist arranged similar sessions for clinical pharmacists in the hospital. Again care was taken with timing and location to ensure that all pharmacists were involved.

A fact sheet was prepared to link the evidence-base to the recommendations and provide a flow chart for managing prescribing. Posters of the framework, with a prescribing example, were put up on surgical wards to remind staff about the new approach. A clinical guideline (available on Bandolier Internet site) was issued to all professions involved with postoperative care of patients. The team also involved patients in their work, by creating information leaflets for patients undergoing day surgery and adolescent in-patients.

Did it make a difference?

Two indicators show that the quality of prescribing has increased significantly at no extra cost, that is,

- increased use of recommended oral analgesics, especially paracetamol;
- the apparent cost per surgical in-patient finished consultant episode (FCE) remained broadly the same or even fell.

Anecdotally, nurses say that patients' postoperative pain is better controlled and patients' co-operation has improved. Pain control is being pre-empted and dealt with more effectively without any wait for alternative analgesia. The initiative has had the added benefit of promoting the roles of the Acute Pain Nurse Service and Pharmacists within the hospital. It has encouraged clinical staff to seek advice to improve patients' pain control.

The training initiatives have been particularly successful. Nurses now feel empowered and more confident when they have an evidence base on which to advise junior doctors. The flow chart has bred new confidence in all staff when advising patients, relatives and colleagues on effective pain control. The 6-monthly arrival of new junior medical staff provides a regular opportunity to reinforce the messages about the local approach. Within induction programmes the Acute Pain Service explain the use of the flowchart.

This work is a good example of collaboration between specialities working for the benefit of the patient:

- patients are receiving the most effective analgesics;
- step-down from PCA and epidural is efficient and effective;
- nurses and midwives have a simple, safe tool to manage postoperative pain;
- junior doctors learn evidence-based practice.

Reference

1. McQuay, H. J. *et al.* (1997). Treating acute pain in hospital, *BMJ* 314: 1531–35.

8.5 **Do-it-yourself pain control**

Introducing self-medication for mothers after Caesarean section at Warwick Hospital.

Why was the initiative launched?

The successful implementation of an acute pain service prompted questions about how pain control was managed for women after Caesarean section. Methods used there had evolved over time. Midwives and doctors thought it could be improved, but for different reasons, while no-one knew what mothers thought because they had not been asked.

What was done?

Two parallel paths of action were set in hand in 1996. One was a baseline audit to establish the nature of pain control being provided to mothers. The other was a review of the evidence about effective analgesic prescribing.

The audit involved case note review and interviews with 30 mothers in late 1996. Although mothers generally expressed satisfaction when asked, the audit suggested that pain control was not always satisfactory. Pain limited function, stopping some mothers from feeding and bathing their babies. Pain was not being routinely assessed.

The audit prompted the formulation of a local protocol for the management of post-Caesarean pain. From the review of evidence, an oral regime was adopted based on the Oxford league table and Chesterfield system of individual patient titration. This three-step approach relied on the appropriate use of paracetamol, NSAIDs and oral morphine. Key features of the protocol were the introduction of formal pain assessments, the use of pre-printed prescription labels to apply to drug charts and the introduction of self-medication by mothers.

The self-medication aspect of the protocol became practical after the Trust was persuaded to change its policy for Oramorph. Previously the Trust had treated all concentrations of Oramorph as controlled drugs even though there was no legal requirement to treat low concentrations (10 mg/5 ml) in this way. Information obtained from the Department of Health, the Royal Pharmaceutical Society and the United Kingdom Central Council for Nursing and Midwifery (UKCC) helped to convince the Trust that deregulating Oramorph would be acceptable.

A local education programme was introduced by professionals from the Acute Pain Service by individual face-to-face sessions (doctor to doctor, nurse to nurse) rather than through seminars. This ensured that the process had minimal impact on clinical commitments. The tutorials were designed to reflect the likely concerns and anxieties of professionals. For example, midwives were being asked to move away from the traditional approach to the control of drugs to one placing responsibility on mothers. They would no longer be responsible for signing out drugs and needed to be assured of the legitimacy of the new approach.

The introduction of self-medication was supported by a patient information leaflet. Reflecting the three-step approach, the leaflet explained how mothers should handle mild, moderate and severe pain and how to seek advice if needed. These leaflets have a sell-by date ensuring they are kept up to date and are maximally helpful to mothers.

Is it working?

The new protocol was introduced in early 1997. The Acute Pain Service has monitored its implementation and ensured that any problems are tackled. The new approach has proved to be popular with mothers and is improving the management of pain. A re-audit in 31 mothers showed that:

- Maternal function was much improved. Only seven mothers were not caring for their babies with just one giving pain as the reason (the other six were in a special care baby unit). In the baseline survey, the numbers were 13 and 10 respectively.

- The incidence of severe pain at rest and on movement was down by about 30%.

- Mothers were more satisfied with their pain control. Over 40% (13) rating pain control as excellent compared with about 20% (7) in the baseline (Figure 8.5.1).

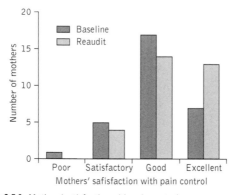

Figure 8.5.1 Mothers' satisfaction with pain control.

The audit findings were encouraging in demonstrating progress, but it also helped to identify aspects of the care where further improvement could be achieved. For example, it identified that most pain was occurring as the regional anaesthetic wore off, before the self-administered analgesics were commenced. The first dose should be administered early enough to take effect before the spinal anaesthetic has worn off. The protocol has been revised to reflect this approach.

The length of stay of mothers was not recorded in the baseline audit but subsequent examination of hospital records revealed an encouraging reduction of one day between the baseline and re-audit. Based on the hospital's average number of Caesarean sections (438 a year), the average reduction of one postoperative day suggests a saving of about £95,000 per annum or 438 bed days. It could be argued that these savings are a direct consequence of the new protocol because there have been no other policy or operational changes in the care of mothers after Caesarean section.

Section 9
Appendices

9.1 **Glossary**

Absolute risk reduction (ARR). See treatment effects

Case–control study. A study which involves identifying patients who have the outcome of interest (cases) and control patients without the same outcome, and looking back to see if they had the exposure of interest.

Case series. A report on a series of patients with an outcome of interest. No control group is involved.

Clinical practice guideline. A systematically developed statement designed to assist clinician and patient decisions about appropriate health care for specific clinical circumstances.

Cohort study. Involves identification of two groups (cohorts) of patients one which received the exposure of interest, and one which did not, and following these cohorts forward for the outcome of interest.

Confidence interval (CI). Quantifies the uncertainty in measurement. It is usually reported as 95% CI, which is the range of values within which we can be 95% sure that the true value for the whole population lies. For example, for an NNT of 10 with a 95% CI of 5–15, we would have 95% confidence that the true NNT value was between 5 and 15.

Control event rate (CER). See treatment effects.

Cost-benefit analysis. Assesses whether the cost of an intervention is worth the benefit by measuring both in the same units; monetary units are usually used.

Cost-effectiveness analysis. Measures the net cost of providing a service as well as the outcomes obtained. Outcomes are reported in a single unit of measurement.

Cost-minimisation analysis. If health effects are known to be equal, only costs are analysed and the least costly alternative is chosen.

Cost-utility analysis. Converts effects into personal preferences (or utilities) and describes how much it costs for some additional quality gain (e.g. cost per additional quality-adjusted life-year, or QALY).

Crossover study design. The administration of two or more experimental therapies one after the other in a specified or random order to the same group of patients.

Cross-sectional study. The observation of a defined population at a signal point in time or time interval. Exposure and outcome are determined simultaneously.

Decision analysis (or clinical decision analysis). The application of explicit, quantitative methods that quantify prognoses, treatment effects, and patient values in order to analyse a decision under conditions of uncertainty.

Ecological survey. A survey based on aggregated data for some population as it exists at some point or points in time: to investigate the relationship of an exposure to a known or presumed risk factor for a specified outcome.

Event rate. The proportion of patients in a group in whom the event is observed. Thus, if out of 100 patients, the event is observed in 27, the event rate is 0.27. Control event rate (CER) and experimental event rate (EER) are used to refer to this in control and experimental groups of patients respectively. The patient expected event rate (PEER) refers to the rate of events we would expect in a patient who received no treatment or conventional treatment. See treatment effects.

Evidence-based health care. Extends the application of the principles of evidence-based medicine (see below) to all professions associated with health care, including purchasing and management.

Evidence-based medicine. The conscientious, explicit and judicious use of current best evidence in making decisions about the care of individual patients. The practice of evidence-based medicine means integrating individual clinical expertise with the best available external clinical evidence from systematic research.

Experimental event rate (EER). See treatment effects.

Incidence. The proportion of new cases of the target disorder in the population at risk during a specified time interval.

Inception cohort. A group of patients who are assembled near the onset of the target disorder.

Intention-to-treat analysis. A method of analysis for randomised trials in which all patients randomly assigned to one of the treatments are analysed together, regardless of whether or not they completed or received that treatment.

Likelihood ratio (LR). The likelihood that a given test result would be expected in a patient with the target disorder compared with the likelihood that the same result would be expected in a patient without the target disorder.

Meta-analysis. A systematic review that uses quantitative methods to summarise the results.

N-of-1 trials. In such trials, the patient undergoes pairs of treatment periods organised so that one period involves the use of experimental treatment and the other involves the use of an alternate or placebo therapy. The patient and physician are blinded, if possible, and outcomes are monitored. Treatment periods are replicated until the clinician and patient are convinced that the treatments are definitely different or definitely not different.

Negative predictive value. Proportion of people with a negative test who are free of the target disorder. See also likelihood ratio.

Number needed to treat (NNT). The inverse of the absolute risk reduction and the number of patients that need to be treated to prevent one bad outcome. See treatment effects.

Odds. A ratio of the number of people incurring an event to the number of people who have non-events.

Odds ratio (OR). The ratio of the odds of having the target disorder in the experimental group relative to the odds in favour of having the target disorder in the control group (in cohort studies or systematic reviews) or the odds in favour of being exposed in subjects with the target disorder divided by the odds in favour of being exposed in control subjects (without the target disorder).

Patient expected event rate (PEER). See treatment effects.

Overview. See systematic review.

Positive predictive value. Proportion of people with a positive test who have the target disorder. See also likelihood ratio.

Post-test odds. The odds that the patient has the target disorder after the test is carried out (pre-test odds $\times$ likelihood ratio).

Post-test probability. The proportion of patients with that particular test result who have the target disorder (post-test odds/[1 + post-test odds]).

Pre-test odds. The odds that the patient has the target disorder before the test is carried out (pre-test probability/[1 − pre-test probability]).

Pre-test probability/prevalence. The proportion of people with the target disorder in the population at risk at a specific time (point prevalence) or time interval (period prevalence). See also likelihood ratio.

Randomisation (or random allocation). Method analogous to tossing a coin to assign patients to treatment groups (the experimental treatment is assigned if the coin lands 'heads' and a conventional, 'control' or 'placebo' treatment is given if the coin lands 'tails').

Randomised controlled clinical trial (RCT). A group of patients is randomised into an experimental group and a control group. These groups are followed up for the variables/outcomes of interest.

Relative risk reduction (RRR). See treatment effects.

Risk ratio (RR). The ratio of risk in the treated group (EER) *t* risk in the control group (CER) – used in randomised trials and cohort studies: RR = ERR/CER.

Sensitivity. Proportion of people with the target disorder who have a positive test. It is used to assist in assessing and selecting a diagnostic test/sign/symptom. See also likelihood ratio.

SnNout. When a sign/test/symptom has a high Sensitivity: a Negative result rules out the diagnosis. For example, the sensitivity of a history of ankle swelling for diagnosing ascites is 93%; therefore if a person does not have a history of ankle swelling, it is highly unlikely that the person has ascites.

Specificity. Proportion of people without the target disorder who have a negative test. It is used to assist in assessing and selecting a diagnostic test/sign/symptom. See also likelihood ratio.

SpPin. When a sign/test/symptom has a high Specificity; a Positive result rules in the diagnosis. For example , the specificity of a fluid wave for diagnosing ascites is 92%; therefore if a person does have a fluid wave, it rules in the diagnosis of ascites.

Systematic review. A summary of the medical literature that uses explicit methods to perform a thorough literature search and critical appraisal of individual studies and that uses appropriate statistical techniques to combine these valid studies.

Treatment effects

Control event rate (CER). The rate of events occurring with control (for example, the number (percent, proportion) of patients with adequate pain relief with placebo).

Experimental event rate (EER). The rate of events occurring with treatment (for example, the number (percent, proportion) of patients with adequate pain relief with an analgesic).

Relative risk reduction (RRR). The proportional reduction in rates of bad outcomes between experimental and control participants in a trial, calculated as |EER − CER|/CER, and accompanied by a 95% CI.

Absolute risk reduction (ARR). The absolute arithmetic difference in rates of bad outcomes between experimental and control participants in a trial, calculated as |EER − CER|, and accompanied by a 95% CI.

Number needed to treat (NNT). The number of patients who need to be treated to achieve one additional favourable outcome, calculated as 1/ARR and accompanied by a 95% C1. If, for instance, 75% of patients have adequate analgesia with treatment (EER) and 25% with control (CER), the NNT is $1/(0.75 − 0.25) = 1/0.5 = 2$. The NNT has to specify treatment, control, outcome and duration (of treatment and effects).

Number needed to harm (NNH). The number of patients who, if they received the experimental treatment, would lead to one additional patient being harmed, compared with patients who received the control treatment, calculated as 1/ARR and accompanied by a 95% CI.

9.2 **Using the Oxman and Guyatt scoring system for reviews**

The purpose is to evaluate the scientific quality (i.e. adherence to scientific principles) of research overviews (review articles) published in the medical literature. It is not intended to measure literary quality, importance, relevance, originality, or other attributes of overviews.

The index (Table 9.2.1) is for assessing overviews of primary (original) research on pragmatic questions regarding causation, diagnosis, prognosis, therapy, or prevention. A research overview is a survey of research. The same principles that apply to epidemiological surveys apply to overviews; a question must be clearly specified, a target population identified and accessed, appropriate information obtained from that population in an unbiased fashion, and conclusions derived, sometimes with the help of formal statistical analysis, as is done in 'meta-analyses'. The fundamental difference between overviews and epidemiological surveys is the unit of analysis, not scientific issues that the questions in this index address.

Since most published overviews do not include a methods section it is difficult to answer some of the questions in the index. Base your answers, as much as possible, on information provided in the overview. If the methods that were used are reported incompletely relative to a specific item, score that item as 'partially'. Similarly, if there is no information provided regarding what was done relative to a particular question, score it as 'can't tell', unless there is information in the overview to suggest either that the criterion was or was not met.

For Question 8, if no attempt has been made to combine findings, and no statement is made regarding the inappropriateness of combining findings, check 'no'. If a summary (general) estimate is given anywhere in the abstract, the discussion, or the summary section of the paper, and it is not reported how that estimate was derived, mark 'no' even if there is a statement regarding the limitations of combining the findings of the studies reviewed. If in doubt mark 'can't tell'.

For an overview to be scored as 'yes' on Question 9, data (not just citations) must be reported that support the main conclusions regarding the primary question(s) that the overview addresses.

The score for Question 10, the overall scientific quality, should be based on your answers to the first nine questions. The following guidelines can be used to assist with deriving a summary score: If the

Table 9.1.1 Scoring system

The Oxman & Guyatt index of scientific quality			
1	Were the search methods used to find evidence on the primary question(s) stated?	No	Partially	Yes
2	Was the search for evidence reasonably comprehensive?	No	Can't tell	Yes
3	Were the criteria used for deciding which studies to include in the overview reported?	No	Partially	Yes
4	Was bias in the selection of studies avoided?	No	Can't tell	Yes
5	Were the criteria used for assessing the validity of the included studies reported?	No	Partially	Yes
6	Was the validity of all the studies referred to in the text assessed using appropriate criteria?	No	Can't tell	Yes
7	Were the methods used to combine the findings of the relevant studies (to reach a conclusion) reported?	No	Partially	Yes
8	Were the findings of the relevant studies combined appropriately relative to the primary question of the overview?	No	Can't tell	Yes
9	Were the conclusions made by the author(s) supported by the data and/or analysis reported in the overview?	No	Partially	Yes
10	How would you rate the scientific quality of this overview?			

		Flaws				
Extensive		**Major**		**Minor**		**Minimal**
1	2	3	4	5	6	7

'can't tell' option is used one or more times on the preceding questions, a review is likely to have minor flaws at best and it is difficult to rule out major flaws (i.e. a score of 4 or lower). If the 'no' option is used on Questions 2, 4, 6 or 8, the review is likely to have major flaws (i.e. a score of 3 or less, depending on the number and degree of the flaws).

9.3 **Bandolier's 10 tips for healthy living**

This is a quick summary of ten lifestyle tips to help avoid seeing a doctor about heart disease or cancer, based on good quality information. For more details, see the healthy living pages off the Bandolier home page at www.ebandolier.com.

1. Eat whole grain foods (bread, or rice, or pasta) on four occasions a week. This will reduce the chance of having almost any cancer by 40%. Given that cancer gets about 1 in 3 of us in a lifetime, that's big advice.

2. Don't smoke. If you do smoke, stop. Nicotine patches, gum or inhaler won't help much, and acupuncture won't help at all. Try to reduce your smoking, as there is a profound dose-response (the more you smoke, the more likely you are to have cancer, or heart or respiratory disease). So cut down to below five cigarettes a day and leave long portions of the day without a cigarette.

3. Eat at least five portions of vegetables and fruit a day, and especially tomatoes (including ketchup), red grapes and the like, as well as salad all year. This protects against a whole variety of different nasty things:
   - it reduces the risk of stroke dramatically;
   - it reduces the risk of diabetes considerably;
   - it will reduce the risk of heart disease and cancer.

4. Use Benecol or other stanol-containing spreads instead of butter or margarine. It really does reduce cholesterol, and reducing cholesterol will reduce the risk of heart attack and stroke even in those whose cholesterol is not particularly high.

5. Drink alcohol regularly. The type of alcohol probably doesn't matter too much, but the equivalent of a couple of glasses of wine a day or a couple of beers is a good thing. The odd day without alcohol won't hurt either. Think of it as medicine.

6. Eat fish. Eating fish once a week won't stop you having a heart attack in itself, but it reduces the likelihood of you dying from it by half.

7. Take a multivitamin tablet every day, but be sure that it is one with at least 200 mg of folate. The evidence is that this can substantially reduce chances of heart disease in some individuals, and it has been shown to reduce colon cancer by over 85%. It may

also reduce the likelihood of developing dementia. Folate is essential in any woman contemplating pregnancy because it will reduce the chance of some birth defects.

8. If you are pregnant or have high blood pressure, coffee is best minimised. For the rest of us drinking four cups of coffee a day is likely to reduce our chances of getting colon cancer and Parkinson's disease.

9. Get breathless more often. You don't have to go to a gym or be an Olympic marathon runner. Simply walking a mile a day, or taking reasonable exercise three times a week (enough to make you sweat or glow) will substantially reduce the risk of heart disease. If you walk, don't dawdle. Make it a brisk pace. One of the benefits of regular exercise is that it strengthens bones and keeps them strong. Breaking a hip when elderly is a very serious thing.

10. Check your height and weight on a chart to see if you are overweight for your height. Your body mass index is the weight in kilograms divided by the height in metres squared: for preference it should be below 25. If you are overweight, lose it. This has many benefits. There is no good evidence on simple ways to lose weight that work. Crash diets don't work. Take it one step at a time, do the things that are possible now, and combine some calorie limitation with increased exercise. The good news is that in a few years time we may have some appetite suppressants to make it easier.

9.4 **Cochrane Collaboration and pain**

The Cochrane Collaboration is an international, non-profit organisation that aims to help people make well-informed decisions about health-care by preparing and maintaining 'systematic reviews' of the effects of treatments. A Cochrane systematic review is an up-to-date summary of reliable evidence of the benefits and risks of a particular treatment. Cochrane reviews are published in the Cochrane Library which is available through the Internet or quarterly on CD-ROMs. For more information see: www.cochrane.org.

There is no doubt that the Cochrane Collaboration is one of the truly great innovations of the last decade or so. That many people from all over the world can work collaboratively to produce good evidence is wonderful, and it is a credit to those people who strived to make it happen, despite great difficulties. The product, the Cochrane Library, has about 1300 reviews. Even better, it is the single best source of controlled clinical trials, with over 250,000 of them, many found through hand-searching the literature.

Bandolier's admiration is not unqualified, though. Too many reviews make too much of too little information, some reviews pay too little attention to quality issues, and some are just plain wrong. But it is getting better, and bigger. We should use it more.

In pain, there are several review groups doing important work. The most obvious point of contact is PaPaS. The Cochrane Pain, Palliative Care and Supportive Care Group (PaPaS) focuses on reviews for the prevention and treatment of pain; the treatment of symptoms at the end of life; and supporting patients, carers and their families through the disease process. The Editorial office for the PaPaS group is at the Pain Research Unit at the Churchill Hospital in Oxford, UK. They work with researchers and health care professionals worldwide. Their Internet site is www.jr2.ox.ac.uk/cochrane/, and contact details are:

Frances Fairman – Review Group Co-ordinator, or Yvonne Roy – Review Group Administrator at the address below:
Pain, Palliative and Supportive Care Group
Pain Research Unit
Churchill Hospital
Oxford
UK OX3 7LJ
Tel.: +44 1865 225762
Fax: +44 1865 225400
E-mail: frances.fairman@pru.ox.ac.uk
yvonne.roy@pru.ox.ac.uk

Useful Cochrane reviews

The following is a list of titles of Cochrane reviews that might be of interest because they relate to pain.

- Acupuncture for idiopathic headache
- Acupuncture for lateral elbow pain
- Acupuncture for low back pain
- Advice to stay active as a single treatment for low back pain and sciatica
- Alpha2 adrenergic agonists for the management of opioid withdrawal
- Analgesia and non-aspirin, non-steroidal anti-inflammatory drugs for osteoarthritis of the hip
- Anaesthesia for hip fracture surgery in adults
- Anticonvulsant drugs for acute and chronic pain
- Antimalarials for treating rheumatoid arthritis
- Auranofin versus placebo in rheumatoid arthritis
- Azathioprine for treating rheumatoid arthritis
- Back schools for non-specific low back pain
- Balneotherapy for rheumatoid arthritis and osteoarthritis
- Bed rest for acute low back pain and sciatica
- Behavioural treatment for chronic low back pain
- Bisphosphonates for the relief of pain secondary to bone metastases
- Combined oral contraceptive pill (OCP) as treatment for primary dysmenorrhoea
- Conservative treatment for whiplash
- Cyclophosphamide for treating rheumatoid arthritis
- Cyclosporine for treating rheumatoid arthritis
- Danazol for pelvic pain associated with endometriosis
- Deep transverse friction massage for treating tendinitis
- Dietary interventions for recurrent abdominal pain (RAP) in childhood
- Dynamic exercise therapy for rheumatoid arthritis
- Electrical stimulation for preventing and treating post-stroke shoulder pain
- Electrical stimulation for the treatment of rheumatoid arthritis
- Electromagnetic fields for the treatment of osteoarthritis
- Eletriptan for acute migraine
- Epidural blood patching for preventing and treating post-dural puncture headache

- Epidural local anaesthetics versus opioid-based analgesic regimens on postoperative . . .
- Epidural versus non-epidural analgesia for pain relief in labour
- Exercise therapy for low back pain
- Feverfew for preventing migraine
- Glucosamine therapy for treating osteoarthritis
- Gonadotrophin-releasing hormone analogues for pain associated with endometriosis
- Herbal and dietary therapies for primary and secondary dysmenorrhoea
- Herbal therapy for treating osteoarthritis
- Herbal therapy for treating rheumatoid arthritis
- Hydromorphone for acute and chronic pain
- Injectable gold for rheumatoid arthritis
- Injection therapy for subacute and chronic benign low back pain
- Interventions for preventing and treating pelvic and back pain in pregnancy
- Interventions for shoulder pain
- Interventions for treating chronic pelvic pain in women
- Interventions for treating plantar heel pain
- Laparoscopic surgery for pelvic pain associated with endometriosis
- Lidocaine-prilocaine cream for analgesia during circumcision in newborn boys
- Low level laser therapy (Classes I, II and III) for treating Osteoarthritis
- Low level laser therapy (Classes I, II and III) for treating rheumatoid arthritis
- Lumbar supports for prevention and treatment of low back pain
- Massage for low back pain
- Methotrexate for treating juvenile idiopathic arthritis
- Methotrexate for treating rheumatoid arthritis
- Moderate-term, low-dose corticosteroids for rheumatoid arthritis
- Modern combined oral contraceptives for pain associated with endometriosis
- Multidisciplinary Bio-Psycho-Social Rehabilitation for Chronic Low Back Pain
- Multidisciplinary biopsychosocial rehabilitation for subacute low back pain among working age
- Multidisciplinary rehabilitation for fibromyalgia and musculoskeletal pain in working age adults

- Non-aspirin, non-steroidal anti-inflammatory drugs for treating osteoarthritis of the knee
- Non-steroidal anti-inflammatory drugs (NSAIDs) for treating lateral elbow pain in adults
- Non-steroidal anti-inflammatory drugs for low back pain
- Orthotic devices for treating patellofemoral pain syndrome
- Penicillamine for treating rheumatoid arthritis
- Patient education for adults with rheumatoid arthritis
- Perioperative local anaesthesia for reducing pain following tonsillectomy
- Pharmacological interventions for recurrent abdominal pain (RAP) in childhood
- Posture and fluids for preventing post-dural puncture headache
- Prevention of NSAID-induced gastroduodenal ulcers
- Progestagens and anti-progestagens for pain associated with endometriosis
- Prophylactic intravenous preloading for regional analgesia in labour
- Prophylactic use of oxytocin in the third stage of labour
- Psychological therapies for sickle cell disease and pain
- Radiotherapy for the palliation of painful bone metastases
- Rizatriptan for acute migraine
- Rofecoxib for the treatment of rheumatoid arthritis
- Shock wave therapy for lateral elbow pain
- Single dose dextropropoxyphene, alone and with paracetamol (acetaminophen), for postoperative pain
- Single dose dihydrocodeine for acute postoperative pain
- Single dose oral aspirin for acute pain
- Single dose oral ibuprofen and diclofenac for postoperative pain
- Single dose oxycodone and oxycodone plus paracetamol (acetominophen) for acute postoperative pain
- Single dose paracetamol (acetaminophen), with and without codeine, for postoperative pain
- Single dose piroxicam for acute postoperative pain
- Single-dose dipyrone for acute postoperative pain
- Sucrose for analgesia in newborn infants undergoing painful procedures
- Surgery for lateral elbow pain
- Surgical interruption of pelvic nerve pathways for primary and secondary dysmenorrhoea

- Sulfasalazine for treating rheumatoid arthritis
- Therapeutic ultrasound for postpartum perineal pain and dyspareunia
- Therapeutic ultrasound for treating patellofemoral pain syndrome
- Therapeutic ultrasound for osteoarthritis of the knee
- Thermotherapy for treating rheumatoid arthritis
- Topical agents or dressings for pain in venous leg ulcers
- Transcutaneous electrical nerve stimulation and acupuncture for primary dysmenorrhoea
- Transcutaneous electrical nerve stimulation for knee osteoarthritis
- Transcutaneous electrical nerve stimulation (TENS) for chronic low back pain
- Transcutaneous electrical nerve stimulation (TENS) for chronic pain
- Types of intra-muscular opioids for maternal pain relief in labour

9.5 **Evidence based organisations, websites and resources**

National electronic Library of Health

www.nelh.nhs.uk/

NeLH is a first port of call for many of us. It's getting better all the time, and many of us are using it a lot. There's some good stuff there, but some of it is unfortunately limited to NHS professionals.

University of York, NHS Centre for Reviews and Dissemination
www.york.ac.uk/inst/crd/welcome.htm

The NHS Centre for Reviews and Dissemination (CRD) was established in January 1994 to provide the NHS with important information on the effectiveness of treatments and the delivery and organisation of health care. The CRD, a research unit within the University, carries out systematic reviews on selected topics, has a database of good quality reviews, a dissemination service and an information service, and seeks to promote research-based practice in the NHS. The CRD has a database of systematic reviews available on the Cochrane Library (see below).

University of Sheffield, School of Health and Related Research (ScHARR)
www.shef.ac.uk/~scharr

ScHARR carries out applied and methodological health services research, consultancy and teaching programmes for health services staff. It works closely with the Department of Health and NHS health authorities and trusts.

Aggressive Research Intelligence Facility (ARIF)
www.hsrc.org.uk/links/arif/arifhome.htm

ARIF is a specialist unit based at the University of Birmingham. Its role is to help health care workers access and interpret research evidence, particularly systematic reviews of research, in response to particular problems they are experiencing. It is the research and development department of the NHS Executive, West Midlands.

National Centre for Clinical Excellence (NICE)
www.nice.org.uk/nice-web

NICE – The National Institute for Clinical Excellence – was set up as a Special Health Authority for England and Wales on 1 April 1999. It is part of the National Health Service (NHS), and its role is to provide patients, health professionals and the public with authoritative, robust and reliable guidance on current 'best practice'. The guidance covers both individual health technologies (including medicines, medical devices, diagnostic techniques, and procedures) and the clinical management of specific conditions.

NHS R&D Health Technology Assessment Programme
http://www.ncchta.org/main.htm
This is now becoming a really useful site, and the amount of research grows. The most useful feature is that almost all reports are available free in downloadable PDF formats.

Scottish Intercollegiate Guidelines Network
www.sign.ac.uk/
The Scots do some things better. The SIGN guidelines are often terrific, and link evidence with the real world.

PubMED, National Library of Medicine
www.ncbi.nlm.nih.gov/entrez/query.fcgi
Entrez is a search and retrieval system that integrates information from databases at the NCBI. These databases include MEDLINE, which can be accessed through PubMed. The advantages of searching PubMed are that records not yet indexed fully for MEDLINE appear in their pre-MEDLINE state, and articles can often be downloaded directly in electronic form.

BioMed Central
www.biomedcentral.com
An electronic journal with free access to users. It is an independent publishing house with immediate access to peer-reviewed articles covering over 50 fields of biomedical research.

Cochrane Collaboration:
www.cochrane.org
A worldwide collaboration of researchers and practitioners which prepares, maintains and promotes systematic reviews of healthcare interventions. These can be found on the Cochrane Library. The Cochrane Collaboration has many specialist sub-groups which cover different disease areas.

Cochrane Library:
www.update-software.com
The Cochrane Library is an electronic publication designed to supply high quality evidence to inform people providing and receiving care, and those responsible for research, teaching, funding and administration at all levels. It is published quarterly on CD-ROM and the Internet, and is distributed on a subscription basis.

NHS R&D Centre for Evidence-Based Medicine (CEBM)
http://cebm.jr2.ox.ac.uk

The CEBM has been established in Oxford as the first of several centres around the country whose broad aim is to promote evidence-based health care and provide support and resources to anyone who wants to make use of them. The centre runs regular training courses and workshops.

Bandolier
www.ebandolier.com
Bandolier is a print and Internet journal about health care, using evidence-based medicine techniques to provide advice about particular treatments or diseases for healthcare professionals and consumers.

Critical Appraisal Skills Programme (CASP)
www.public-health.org.uk/casp

CASP's aim is to help health service decision makers, and those who seek to influence decision makers, to develop skills in the critical appraisal of evidence about effectiveness, in order to promote the delivery of evidence-based health care. The Critical Appraisal Skills Programme is part of the Public Health Resource Unit, working at the Institute of Health Sciences in Oxford, to help bring the principles and practice of evidence-based practice to as wide an audience as possible.

Agency for Health Care policy and Research (USA)
www.ahcpr.gov
The Agency for Healthcare Research and Quality (AHRQ) is a US government agency that provides evidence-based information on health care outcomes; quality; and cost, use and access.

InterTASC (Technology Assessment Services Collaboration)
www.soton.ac.uk/~interdec
InterTASC is a collaboration of organisations which have been established to provide commissioners in health authorities and primary care groups and NHS Trusts with research knowledge about the effectiveness and cost-effectiveness of acute service interventions. Formerly known as InterDEC.

Other EBM sites worth a look

The Health Information Research Unit (HIRU) at McMaster University
http://hiru.mcmaster.ca

The Unit for Evidence-Based Practice and Policy, UCL
http://www.ucl.ac.uk/primcare-popsci/uebpp/ uebpp.htm#How

International Network of Agencies for Health Technology Assessment
http://www.inahta.org

Centre for Research Support
http://www.ceres.uwcm.ac.uk/

Effective health care bulletins (University of York)
http://www.york.ac.uk/inst/crd/ehcb.htm

Scottish Health Purchasing Information Centre
Details at: http://www.nhsconfed.net/shpic/index.htm

Many useful EBM sites listed at

http://www.wsufftrust.org.uk/Library/InternetLinks/
EvidenceBasedHealth.htm
This site includes links to specialist EBM sites such as nursing, dentistry and child health.

Healthcare Information Resources

North Glasgow University NHS Hospital Trust
www.northglashealthinfo.org.uk
A comprehensive information resource, including a new library and comprehensive database.

Date Due

NOV 2 9 2019			

Printed in the U   **BRODART, CO.**   Cat. No. 23-233   Printed in U.S.A.
May 16, 2014

589522.001